MIASMATIC PRESCRIBING

ITS PHILOSOPHY, DIAGNOSTIC CLASSIFICATIONS, CLINICAL TIPS, MIASMATIC REPERTORY MIASMATIC WEIGHTAGE OF MEDICINES AND CASE ILLUSTRATIONS

SECOND EXTENDED EDITION

by

DR SUBRATA KUMAR BANERJEA
GOLD MEDALIST
BHMS (HONOURS IN NINE SUBJECTS OF CALCUTTA UNIVERSITY)
FELLOW: AKADEMIE HOMOOPATHISCHER DEUTSCHER ZENTRALVEREIN (GERMANY)
DIRECTOR: BENGAL ALLEN MEDICAL INSTITUTE
PRINCIPAL: ALLEN COLLEGE OF HOMOEOPATHY, ESSEX. ENGLAND

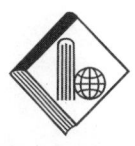

B. Jain Publishers (P) Ltd.
USA—EUROPE—INDIA

MIASMATIC PRESCRIBING

First Edition: 2001
Second Extended Edition: 2006
Second extended Indian Edition: 2010
8th Impression: 2019

All rights reserved. No part of this book may be reproduced, stored in a retrieval system or transmitted, in any form or by any means, mechanical, photocopying, recording or otherwise, without any prior written permission of the publisher.

© with the author

Published by Kuldeep Jain for
B. JAIN PUBLISHERS (P) LTD.
B. Jain House, D-157, Sector-63, NOIDA-201307, U.P. (INDIA)
Tel.: +91-120-4933333 • *Email:* info@bjain.com
Website: **www.bjain.com**

Printed in India by
J.J. Offset Printers

ISBN: 978-81-319-0943-0

DEDICATION

Dedicated to commemorate 'Our Love', the Love of 'Two Similias'!

PREFACE

I was born and brought up in a homoeopathic family and in an environment of homoeopathic philosophy and am proud to say that homoeopathy is in my blood. I am a fourth generation homoeopath, my great-grandfather Dr Kalipada Banerjee was born in a town near Kolkata (India) in 1844 and was a practising homoeopathy for 38 years. His son, my grandfather, Dr Kishori Mohan Banerjee, was born in 1886 and followed in his father's footsteps qualifying as a homoeopath in Kolkata, which by this time had acquired a reputation as the 'Mecca of homoeopathy'. My grandfather however, had a great desire to broaden his knowledge and travelled to America where he learned the art of miasmatic prescribing directly from the great Dr John Henry Allen. After returning to his native country, Dr Kishori Mohan Banerjee founded The Bengal Allen Homoeopathic Medical College and Hospital in 1924 naming it after his much loved and respected tutor, Dr Allen. Sadly, he died at a young age of 55 but his legacy lived on through his son, my uncle, Dr Naba Kumar Banerjee, by whose inspiration my own love for homoeopathy was discovered and nurtured. Although my father Dr R.K. Banerjee is a pathologist, he has always rendered support in my study of this great art and science of homoeopathy, as has my aunt, Dr Kamala Banerjee, whose love and affection was key to many of my earlier academic laurels. My family have always held true to Hahnemannian-Kentian principles and since my grandfather's time incorporated miasmatic diagnosis into their plans of treatment. It is this approach, which I believe, was intrinsic to their success as homoeopathic physicians and I offer you this book not only in their memories but also for the future of homoeopathy.

The inclusion of miasm in a homoeopathic prescription is becoming more and more important in this modern world of suppression. Hahnemann with his infinite wisdom recognised some two hundred years ago the prominence of one-sided diseases with a scarcity of proper characteristic symptoms and the increasing usage of modern drugs has intensified this to a degree that such cases are becoming increasingly common today. There can only be one approach if a complete cure is sought and this is to systematically remove each layer of suppression and miasmatic dyscrasia before proceeding to nip the underlying cause of disease in the bud. This book is designed for homoeopathic practitioners and students alike and for this reason I am assuming a degree of knowledge as befits both. However, I feel it is worthwhile at the outset to define the homoeopathic context of the word miasm as an invisible, inimical, dynamic principle, an inherited weakness, a stigma or vacuum in the constitution and to share with you the analogy of the peeling away of petals from the lotus flower, a representation of the removal of each different layer of suppression or disease and their corresponding dyscrasia which I use in my lectures to demonstrate the curative art of miasmatic prescribing.

With proper application, miasmatic prescribing can uproot the underlying cause of disease and nip the bud of increased susceptibility to future diseases, so it is not only curative but also preventative, something for which our patients will surely thank us in the long run. There are no shortcuts to complete and permanent cure and it is up to us and our patients to play our parts in striving towards successful treatment in as many cases as possible. It is by the incorporation of miasmatic prescribing into our treatments that this can become possible.

There are six main sections to this book as detailed below:

Part I — Philosophy and Utility of Miasm: Here I have taken the opportunity to discuss the philosophical background of miasm and to share my views regarding suppression and the need for miasmatic prescriptions in the modern world. Key words are presented to reflect the miasmatic tendencies.

Part II — Miasmatic Diagnostic Classifications: Starting with the mental symptoms, this is a head to foot schematic classification of the four miasms, including my tips for rapid miasmatic diagnosis.

Part III — Miasmatic Diagnosis of Clinical Classifications: In this section, I have shared all the possible clinical nosological names under their respective miasmatic headings with a view to enable fast diagnosis of the corresponding miasm.

Part IV — Miasmatic Ancestral Tips: All the tips of my four generations of miasmatic prescribers.

Part V — Miasmatic Repertory : This is a totally new concept and once again aimed for your quick miasmatic diagnosis.

Part VI — Miasmatic Weightage of Medicines: A comprehensive guide to the weight, value or gradation of the medicines and listings of the leading anti-miasmatics.

I have worked for six years in completing this book and in last twenty-two years or so, have lectured on miasms all over the world wherever homoeopathy is known. It is always a pleasure to lecture on miasm as I can share my great love and passion for this subject. This venture however would not have possible without the constant support, care and co-operation, love and affection of my partner Janet and I am deeply touched and indebted to her.

I would also like to sincerely acknowledge the help given by Fiona Wray, who has painstakingly edited the contents of the book; would also like to extend my gratitude towards Debasish Mukherjee for his technical support in typing the manuscript and Manas Nayak for his help with the printing.

I welcome any constructive suggestion towards the improvement of future editions. All the information mentioned herein has some verifications and it is with this foreknowledge and my own experience that I have been successfully incorporating miasmatic prescribing into my practices for many years. I entreat you to publish the failure of miasmatic incorporation in prescribing, if any and if ever, to the world!

It is my hope that you will both learn from and enjoy this book; the benefits of prescribing miasmatically will be experienced by both yourselves and your patients.

Subrata Kumar Banerjea
Essex, England.
September 6, 2001
(My birthday)

PREFACE TO SECOND EDITION

By including three new chapters in this second edition, I have expanded upon the concepts in the original to make this book more comprehensive. On review, I decided that to include case illustrations and to expand on the ideas with a clinical, practical approach would be even more useful to the practising homoeopath.

Part VII — Practical approach - Classical Prescribing: In this chapter I have illustrated how to handle the cases that come to us in the current climate of suppression in a practical and useful way without deviating from the classical approach of prescribing. As I have stated throughout the book, time tested scientific miasmatic and classical approach to prescribing is a structured formula for solid reliable prescribing.

Part VIII — Case Illustrations: I have included a few cases to demonstrate how incorporation of miasm helped to reach the similimum when there were apparent close remedy possibilities. This method has proved to colleagues, my students and me over the years that this enhances the depth of the prescription and the certainty of good improvement in the case.

Part IX — Look and Diagnose; Personality assessment through Miasm: This is a chapter, which I have found interesting. The development of these ideas has revealed to me another aspect of miasmatic diagnosis and subsequent prescription. I was always encouraged by my teachers and my uncle to observe the attitude, posture, and behaviour of people and to refine those observational skills into the practice. I have applied those same principles of observing, for remedy selection, into observation of the dominant miasm and found it to be hugely beneficial.

I would like to sincerely acknowledge the constant support and love of my wife, Janet, which I treasure, say thank you to my student Kathryn who has typed some of the manuscripts and to Debasish Mukherjee for his technical support in typing the body of the manuscript, thanks also to Manas Nayak for his help with the printing.

I welcome any constructive suggestion towards the improvement of future editions and feedback on your success using the methods outlined here. All the information given in this book has been verified and it is with this knowledge and my own experience that I have been, successfully, incorporating miasmatic prescribing into my practice for many years.

It is my hope that you will both learn from and enjoy this book and that the benefits of prescribing miasmatically will be experienced by both yourself and your patients.

Subrata Kumar Banerjea
September 6, 2006

ALLEN COLLEGE OF HOMOEOPATHY,
"Sapiens"
382 Baddow Road,
Great Baddow, Chelmsford CM2 9RA.
Essex, England.
Tel & Fax : 44 (0) 1245 505859
E.Mail: allencollege@btinternet.com
Web Site: www.homoeopathy-course.com

MIASM:
DR BANERJEA'S DEFINITION

I define miasm as 'an invisible, inimical, dynamic principle which permeates into the system of a living creature, creating a groove or stigma in the constitution which can only be eradicated by a suitable anti-miasmatic treatment. If effective anti-miasmatic treatment does not take place then the miasm will persist throughout the life of the person and will be transmitted to the next generation'.

MIASM: DR BANERJEA'S TEN PRINCIPLES

I. Miasm is a dynamic energy which cannot be seen.

II. Every living creature on earth, bacteria, virus etc., has its own miasm.

III. Miasm is hostile to the life preserving energy (inimical to the vital force) of any living creature.

IV. It is dynamic, as it affects the dynamic plane and thereby dynamically deranges the life preserving energy of any living creature.

V. The basic pre-condition of a miasmatic infection is susceptibility.

VI. When a person or any living creature is susceptible (characterised by hypo-immunity = psora) the inimical, invisible dynamic principle of miasm gets the chance to permeate into the body (as the immunity is low and thereby the person is susceptible to receive such infection), this is known as miasmatic infection.

VII. After entering in the body, it tends to join the fundamental miasms already existing in the body.

VIII. Then it takes the upper hand; as the miasmatic force from outside plus the miasmatic force already dormant in the body conjoin together and dynamically affect the vital force (life preserving energy) thereby dynamic derangement of the vital force occurs.

IX. So, the miasmatic force dynamically deranges the vital force and that results in disease. There is always a battle going on inside the body between the vital force and the miasmatic force; in health the vital force wins and in disease, the miasmatic force wins.

X. The miasmatic force creates a stigma or vacuum in the constitution, which can only be eradicated by suitable anti-miasmatic medicine, otherwise it is transmitted to the next generation. Miasmatic dissection and incorporation of the same in each case will help (a) to open up a case, where there is a scarcity of symptoms due to various physical, emotional or iatrogenic suppressions, by the centrifugal action of deep acting anti-miasmatic medicines. Also, of importance is the value of selecting an anti-miasmatic medicine which covers the nature and character of the individual in absence of any recognisable totality. Thus, the anti-miasmatic medicine covers the essence of the person and opens up the case; (b) to be more confident in prescribing by including the surface miasm in the consideration of the totality, as miasm, the dyscrasia of the person, constitutes a major part of the totality; (c) to evaluate the necessity of change of the plan of treatment or change of the remedy; as few symptoms have disappeared after the first remedy, yet the miasmatic totality indicates the preponderance of the same miasm in the surface which was originally covered by the initial remedy, therefore it foretells that we can stay with the previous remedy; (d) to evaluate the homoeopathic prognosis of the case, as removal of layers of suppression manifest as clarity of symptoms and can be accompanied by a quantum jump in the sense of well being; (e) to fulfil Hahnemann's three injunctions of cure: rapid, gentle and permanent; and (f) anti-miasmatic medicines help to clear up the suppressions (in relation to the past); clear up the presenting symptoms from its root or origin (in relation to the present); and clear up the susceptibility to get infection and thereby strengthens the constitution (in relation to the prophylactic aspect or future).

CONTENTS

PREFACE .... iv-v

MIASM :
DR BANERJEA'S DEFINITON vi

MIASM :
DR. BANERJEA'S TEN PRINCIPLES vii

PART-I :
PHILOSOPHY AND UTILITY 1-39

Introduction 1-5

The Utility and Incorporation
of Miasm in Prescribing. 1-5

Contaminated Picture. 1

Conjoint Picture. 2

Scarcity of Symptoms. 2

Uncovering the Layers 2

Classical Miasmatic Prescribing. 3-4

Why should we Know Miasm? 4-5

The Philosophy of Miasm 6

Miasm – The Contagium Vivum 6

Differentiations of Pseudo-
Psora and Tubercular Miasms 6

Key Words and Criterias : 7-8

Basic Criteria of the Four
Great Miasms 7-8

**MIASM : Infection and
Implementation** 9-10

Miasmatic Infection and
it's Criteria 9

The Source of Miasmatic Infection 9

Susceptibility: The Precondition 9

ix

Transmission of Miasmatic Infection and
Dyscrasia: Though Pathologically Sterile 9

Psora is Infectious 9

Artificial Chronic Disease :
Drug-Miasm 9

Vaccinosis : A Miasmatic Dyscrasia
Of Sycosis 9

Miasmatic Interpretation
in Chronic Prescribing 10

Implementation of Miasms
in Prescribing : Conclusion 10

Terminologies 11-12

Acute Miasm 11

Chronic Miasm 11

Miasmatic State
Dr Banerjea's Definition 11

Diathesis 11

Miasmatic Diseases 11

Comparison of Pseudo-psora with Syco-psora 12

Anti-Miasmatic Medicine 12

**Hahnemannian Classification
of Miasms** 13

The Rationality of Miasm 14-16

Miasm: The Expression 14

Expressions of Miasm by other
Authors 14

The Dynamic Pathology of Hahnemann 14

Modus Operandi 15

Three Criteria of
Miasmatic Disease.. 16

The Scientific Basis of
the Miasm Theory 16

**The Clinical and Practical
Utility of Miasms** 17

The Practical Utility of
the Miasmatic Theory... 17

Reappearance of Suppressions
and the Clinical Utility of
Miasmatic Theory... 17

Psora and its States... 18-19

The Qualifying Condition of Psora 18

Primary, Latent, Secondary
and Tertiary Psora 18

Primary Psora 18

Latent Psora.. 18

Secondary Psora 18

Tertiary Psora 18

Order of Progression in Chronic
Disease (applicable to all four miasms)... 19

Hahnemannian Dynamism 20

Hahnemannian Conception and
Modern Bacteriology. 20

Kill the Bacteria, Cure the
Disease, a Futility... 20

Psoric Miasm and Tubercular Bacilli 20

Layers of Miasmatic States.. 21-24

Layers of Predisposition 21

Development of Symptoms 21

Layers of Predisposing Weakness 22

xi

Unfolding of Miasmatic Layers
and Removal of Suppression 23

Plan of Miasmatic Treatment :
Amendment to the Plan as the
Surface Miasm Changes 24

Dr Banerjea's Approach to a
Plan of Miasmatic Treatment 24

The Nature of Miasm 25-27

Hahnemann's Conclusive Evidence
That Psora is not a predisposition but a Disease 25

The Contagious, Infectious
Principle of the Psoric Miasm 25

The Psoric Miasm was not Related
to Itch-mite Disease only 25

Psora and the Cause of Diseases 25

Extirpation of Psora 25

Cessante Cause, Cessat Effectus 25

Suppression of Primary Psora 26

Reappearance of Primary Psora 26

The Cure of Psora 26

Predilections 26

Skin and Psora; Mucous Membranes
and Sycosis: Predilections 26

Miasm and its Dyscrasias 27

**Dr Banerjea's Ancestral
and Clinical Tips on Miasmatic Prescribing** 28-31

Psora 28

Pseudo-Psora 28

Sycosis 28

Syphilis 29

Tubercular 29

Mixed Miasmatic States 29

Miasmatic Characteristics 30

Miasm and Bacteria 31

Philosophy and Misconceptions 32-39

Hahnemannian Conception:
The origin of psora: The itch eruption and its suppression 32

Misconception: Do not Confuse Scabies (Itch) with the Hahnemannian
Conception of the Psoric Itch Eruption 32

Dr Banerjea's Explanatory Logic and Interpretation 33

Kentian Conception: Psora,
the Spiritual Sickness 33

Hahnemannian and Kentian Conception: Psora, the Foundation
of all Sickness 34

Misconception: Psora, the Common Mother 34

Psora, the Foundation of All Sickness – an Inductive Logic
Dr Banerjea's Explanatory Logic and Interpretation 35

Although Psora Causes Susceptibility to Sickness
it is not only a Dyscrasia but a Disease Process Itself 35

Hahnemann's Self Contradiction: He was free from Psora but prone to Acute Ailments:
Dr Banerjea's Explanatory Logic and Interpretation 35

Psora is not a Predisposition but a Disease itself:
Dr Banerjea's Explanatory Logic and Interpretation 36

The Prior State of Predisposition is Susceptibility:
Dr Banerjea's Explanatory Logic and Interpretation 37

Psora: Generally Manifests Functional disorders
but can also result in structuralchanges 37

Misconception: Psora is only a Functional Disease 38

Largest Sarcomatous Tumour Under Psora in its Tertiary Stage:
Dr Banerjea's Explanatory Logic and Interpretation 38

Psora like other fundamental Miasms, Transmits generation to
Generation: Heriditory Transmission ... 38

Misconception: Spontaneous Hereditary Transmission of Psora ... 39

Dymanic Pathology ... 39

PART-II:
MIASMATIC DIAGNOSTIC CLASSIFICATIONS ... 41-157

Comparison of
Mental Symptoms ... 41-51

Comparison of
Characteristics and Nature ... 52-59

Comparison of
Vertigo Symptoms ... 60-61

Comparison of the
Head and Scalp Symptoms ... 62-69

Comparison of
the Eye Symptoms ... 70-72

Comparison of the
Ear Symptoms ... 73-75

Comparison of
Nasal Symptoms ... 76-79

Comparison of
the Oral Symptoms ... 80-82

Comparison of
the Facial Symptoms ... 83-85

Comparison of the
Respiratory Symptoms ... 86-91

Comparison of the
Cardiac Symptoms ... 92-95

Comparison of the
Stomach Symptoms ... 96-101

Comparison of the
Abdominal Symptoms ... 102-104

Comparison of the
Rectal Symptoms ... 105-109

Comparison of the Urinary Symptoms	110-113
Comparison of the Sexual Symptoms	114-121
Comparison of the Dermatological Symptoms	122-128
Comparison of the Nail Symptoms	129
Comparison of the Extremity Symptoms	130-135
Comparison of Sleep Symptoms	136-137
Comparison of Modality Symptoms	138-139
Comparison of Characteristics: A Synopsis	140-157

PART-III : MIASMATIC DIAGNOSIS OF CLINICAL CLASSIFICATIONS 15-171

Psychiatric Clinicals	159
Ophthalmological Clinicals	160
Clinicals of the Ear	161
Clinicals of the Nose	161
Oral Clinicals	161
Clinicals of the Respiratory System	161
Cardiac Clinicals	162
Gastric Clinicals	163
Abdominal Clinicals	164
Clinicals of the Rectum	165
Urinary Clinicals	165
Sexual Clinicals	166

Dermatological Clinicals 167

Clinicals of the Extremities 168

Classification of
Mixed Miasmatic Clinicals 170

**PART-IV: MIASMATIC
ANCESTRAL TIPS** 173-188

Clinical Tips on Natural Characteristics 173

Clinical Tips on Paediatric Characteristics 176

Clinical Tips on Pimples 176

Clinical Tips on Influenza 176

Clinical Tips on Dementias 177

Clinical Tips on Bronchospasm 178

Clinical Tips on Cancer 180

Ten Symptomatological Enunciations of Cancerous
Manifestations and their Corresponding Miasmatics 180

Prophylactic Aspect of Homoeopathic
Medicine in Cancer 181

Clinicals Tips on Rheumatism 181

Miasmatics of Rheumatic
Manifestations 181

Miasmatics of Rheumatic Modalities 181

Clinical Tips on Eczema 182

Clinical Tips on Aids 183-186

Miasmatic Interpretation of the
Various Symptomatic Manifestations of Aids 183

Clinical Tips on Migraine 187

Miasmatic Interpretation of Migraine 187

Clinical Tips on Nutrition and Foods 188

PART-V:
MIASMATIC REPERTORY 189-242

Miasmatic Repertory of Mental Symptoms 189-192

Miasmatic Repertory of Vertigo Symptoms 193

Miasmatic Repertory of Head Symptoms 194-196

Miasmatic Repertory of Eye Symptoms 197-198

Miasmatic Repertory of Ear Symptoms 199-200

Miasmatic Repertory of Nose Symptoms 201-202

Miasmatic Repertory of Mouth Symptoms 203-204

Miasmatic Repertory of Facial Symptoms 205-206

Miasmatic Repertory of Respiratory Symptoms 207-209

Miasmatic Repertory of Cardiac Symptoms 210-212

Miasmatic Repertory of Stomach Symptoms 213-216

Miasmatic Repertory of Abdominal Symptoms 217-219

Miasmatic Repertory of Sexual Symptoms 220-223

Miasmatic Repertory of Urinary Symptoms 224-226

Miasmatic Repertory of Rectal Symptoms 227-229

Miasmatic Repertory of Skin Symptoms 230-234

Miasmatic Repertory of Nail Symptoms 235

Miasmatic Repertory of Extremity Symptoms 236-239

Miasmatic Repertory of Sleep Symptoms 240

Miasmatic Repertory of Modality Symptoms 241-242

PART-VI:
MIASMATIC WEIGHTAGE OF MEDICINES 243-254

Leading Anti-Miasmatic Medicines 254-255

Leading Anti-Psoric Medicines 254

Leading Anti-Sycotic Medicines 254

Leading Anti-Syphilitic Medicines 254-255

Leading Anti-Tubercular Medicines..255

Leading Tri-Miasmatics 255

PART-VII:
MODERN CLASSICAL PRESCRIBING – PRACTICAL
APPROACH – CLASSICAL PRESCRIBING 257-260

Approach-A:- Non-Suppressed Cases: Cases with Clarity of Symptoms 257-259

Approach-B:- Contaminated Drug Dependent Cases: Cases without Clarity of Symptoms 260

PART-VIII:
MIASMATIC INTERPRETATION IN PRESCRIBING –
CASE ILLUSTRATIONS...261-287

Case-1:- An Obstinate Long Standing Case of Psoriasis, Completely Cured 261-266

Case-2:- A Diagnosed Case of Atopic Dermatitis..266-271

Case-3:- A Diagnosed Case of Cystic Hygroma on the Neck 271-273

Case-4:- A Case of Baldness, Miasmatic Approach of Prescribing 274-278

Case-5:- A Case of Brain Tumour Completely Cured by Homoeopathy 279-282

Case-6:- A Case of Infertility Associated with Pelvic Inflammatory Disease and
Bilateral Large Ovarian Cysts Completely Cured by Homoeopathy..283-287

PART-IX: LOOK AND
DIAGNOSE THE MIASM 289-290

INDEX 291-294

PART — I
MIASMATIC PRESCRIBING: PHILOSOPHY & UTILITY

INTRODUCTION:

THE UTILITY AND INCORPORATION OF MIASM IN PRESCRIBING:

The consideration of miasms is of paramount importance in effective homoeopathic prescribing particularly in this world of multi-suppressions where perceiving a clear picture of disease is becoming increasingly difficult.

Disease pictures can be complicated for several reasons, and the chart below shows the three pictures which may arise. These pictures are expanded upon within this chapter as an important starting point in understanding the value of miasms and miasmatic prescribing in modern homoeopathic practice.

a) Contaminated Picture: the disease is contaminated or masked (through a lack of expression of symptoms or manifestations due to emotional, physical or iatrogenic suppressions).
b) Conjoint Picture: the original malady exists upon which symptoms of various drugs are superimposed.
c) Scarcity of Symptoms: conditions in which it is difficult to ascertain a totality of symptoms, i.e. one-sided diseases such as insomnia, migraine, fatigue syndromes etc.

a) Contaminated Picture:

The disease picture is contaminated by various forms of suppression, which can be recognised in either of two ways:

i) A lack of expression of symptoms which have been driven inside by heroic suppressive measures.

ii) A contaminated picture formed by the original disease together with a lack of expression caused by physical or emotional suppressions. E.g. an extrovert receives disappointing news and their natural inclination is to sob loudly to recover. Circumstances however forbid this and they are forced to bottle up their feelings — their emotions therefore become suppressed.

b) Conjoint Picture:

In these cases, the symptoms of the original disease are superimposed with symptoms of the artificial drug disease. Conjoint pictures may arise as follows:-

i) The original disease is joined by an artificial chronic disease (due to allopathic medical malpractice §78).	ii) The original disease is joined by an artificial chronic disease (due to homoeopathic medical malpractice, e.g. as in cases of polypharmacy, too frequent repetition of doses or the usage of combinations where the action of such applications has not been proved on healthy human beings).	iii) The original disease is joined by an artificial chronic disease produced by vaccinations and serums.

c) Scarcity of Symptoms:

A scarcity of symptoms will be apparent in cases of *'one-sided disease'*, of which Hahnemann makes us aware in §173 of The Organon. These are diseases with too few symptoms, such as insomnia, anorexia and cases of hyperactive, restless children. They also include the so called modern illnesses such as Chronic Fatigue Syndrome, where there are only one or two symptoms showing on the surface of the case. In a case of insomnia, for example, where loss of sleep is due to anxiety and nothing more, we are unable to make a totality. We cannot prescribe successfully on the basis of one or two symptoms and it is due to suppression that only one or two symptoms are visible. It follows therefore, that the manifestations and expressions of the patient must have been suppressed.

We know that in the modern world, the causes of suppression are many. They do however fall into the three main categories as follows. Examples are given under each category although it should be noted that these examples are by no means exhaustive.

Physical Suppressions
e.g. suppression of perspiration by antiperspirants.
Emotional Suppressions
e.g. broken relationships; disappointments in love; pecuniary embarrassments.
Iatrogenic Suppressions
i) Suppressions by non-homoeopathic remedies e.g. antibiotics, steroids etc. ii) Suppressions by homoeopathic medicines e.g. daily repetition of doses over a prolonged period, polypharmacy, quick alternation of remedies, the use of combinations. iii) Widespread vaccination. iv) Suppressions caused by the use of serums (anti-sera preparations); contraceptive pills and H.R.T.

So we can clearly see that manifestations of one-sided diseases are either contaminated, conjoined with artificial disease symptoms, or hindered and suppressed. Clinical experience of the classical prescribers and my own ancestral wisdom has shown that the best way to open up these cases is from the miasmatic viewpoint. That is to say, we perceive the surface miasm and treat it accordingly. The surface miasm itself being diagnosed by considering the symptoms showing on the surface of the case as presenting complaints.

Uncovering the Layers:

It is apparent therefore, that it is necessary to understand the soil, the very dyscrasia of the person, and the miasm, which represents the stigma, groove or pollution in the system. This stigma/groove/pollution, call it what you will, can only be corrected through constitutional, anti-miasmatic treatment, and through such treatment, the complete annihilation of symptoms and perfect restoration of health will ensue.

In order to make a miasmatic assessment, we need to uncover the layers of predisposing weaknesses, which can be attributed to the different layers of suppressions. These reflect the miasmatic weakness of the individual.

I like to compare these different layers of miasmatic dyscrasia with the lotus flower. The outermost layer or petal reflects the surface miasm, that is, the presenting manifestation of the person. On the basis of the totality of symptoms, together with the miasmatic totality, the constitutional anti-miasmatic remedy is then selected for that presenting totality. This not only removes the surface symptoms but also the corresponding miasmatic dyscrasia, which was being manifested on the surface at that time.

Once the outer layer of the flower is removed the second layer is revealed. This second layer in turn becomes the surface miasm, reflecting a different group of symptoms. Dr. Kent guides us here, stating that there now has to be a change in the plan of treatment. This means that if the previous outermost layer was sycosis (and accordingly an anti-sycotic remedy was given which annihilated all the symptoms of that layer), the next miasmatic layer, which rises to the surface, has also to be addressed by its own presenting symptoms. The totality of the case needs to be reassessed and the next prescription selected on the basis of the totality of symptoms including the miasmatic symptomatology.

The skill of a homoeopathic physician is to recognise the differing layers present as they reveal themselves through the surfacing of symptoms. The remedy they select should not only cover the symptomatic totality as manifested through the surfacing of symptoms in the outermost layer but also the miasmatic totality. In such a way 'layer upon layer of predisposing weakness' can be peeled off, taking with them the layers of suppressions and corresponding miasma, and the miasmatic dyscrasia can be nipped in the bud.

Classical Miasmatic Prescribing:

MTEK is an useful memory aid to arriving at a correct prescription.

M	=	Miasmatic Totality
T	=	Totality of Symptoms
E	=	Essence (should include gestures, postures, behaviours etc)
K	=	Keynotes (which should encompass PQRS symptoms, refer §153 and §209 of Hahnemann's Organon)

When the above criteria are considered and the steps below followed, a correct prescription can be made.

Step I — Make the miasmatic diagnosis of the case i.e. ascertain the surface miasm.

Step II — Assess the Totality of Symptoms + Essence + Keynotes and PQRS (if any) of the case and formulate the indicated remedy.

Step III — Ensure that the indicated remedy covers the surface miasm, as diagnosed in Step I (refer Miasmatic Weightage of Medicines, the last section of this book).

Step IV — Administer the remedy, which encompasses miasm as well as the Totality of Symptoms.

By such a prescription, which covers the miasmatic dyscrasia of the person, the chances of recurrence are eradicated and the axiom of 'rapid, gentle and permanent recovery' (Hahnemann's Organon §3) is encompassed. In cases of one-sided disease with a scarcity of symptoms, the action of the anti-miasmatic remedy is centrifugal, and by bringing the suppressed symptoms to the surface allows a proper totality to be framed.

The miasmatic consideration is therefore of great importance as demonstrated in the following example:-

A person is suffering from features of gastric ulcer, which has been confirmed by radiography. As ulceration is syphilitic, the surface miasm is therefore syphilitic also. Let us say that the totality of symptoms (physical, emotional and essence) of the person reflects towards Kali Bichromicum, an anti-syphilitic remedy. The choice of remedy is therefore simple, as Kali Bich covers both the totality of symptoms and the surface miasm of this gastric ulcer case. Kali Bich will peel away the outer layer and reveal a second layer underneath. This second layer may manifest perhaps through the appearance of warts or moles on the face, an indication of suppressed sycosis and the next assessment of the case should include this new surface totality. Following Kentian ideology we now know that there needs to be a change in the plan of treatment, that is, the previous syphilitic plan needs to change to a current sycotic plan, and a new anti-sycotic medicine needs to be selected based on the presenting totality.

Why Should We Know Miasm?

A thorough dissection and incorporation of miasm in each case will help a homoeopathic prescriber in the following ways:

(i) A deep acting anti-miasmatic medicine by virtue of its centrifugal action will open up such cases (brings to the surface the suppressed symptoms) where the totality of symptoms cannot be framed due to a scarcity of symptoms (i.e. one-sided cases), and those cases with conjoint or contaminated pictures due to various physical, emotional or iatrogenic suppressions.

(ii) Also of importance is the value of selecting an anti-miasmatic medicine, which covers the psychic essence, nature and character of the individual in absence of any recognisable totality. For example, a patient presents with insomnia with no distinguishing modalities or other characters to complete the symptom. By ascertaining that person's psychic essence or character (for instance, suspicious, jealous and exploiting in nature, representing sycosis) we can prescribe an anti-miasmatic medicine to cover the insomnia and open up the case. Thus, the anti-miasmatic medicine covering the essence of the person is capable of surfacing the suppressed symptoms and the totality can then easily be framed.

(iii) To be more confident in prescribing by including the surface miasm of the case in the consideration of the totality; as miasm, the dyscrasia of the person, constitutes a major part of that totality. Miasm and the symptoms are nothing but the two sides of the coin, and one cannot be considered whilst ignoring the other. In fact, the totality of symptoms cannot be said to be total until and unless the selected remedy covers the miasm.

(iv) To evaluate the necessity of a change in the plan of treatment or a change of remedy; when few symptoms have disappeared after the first remedy has been administered, yet the miasmatic totality shows the preponderance of the same miasm on the surface as that which was originally covered by the initial remedy. It indicates that the prescriber can stay with that initial remedy, as can be seen from the following example: a patient came with the presenting symptom of facial wart, for which Causticum was prescribed. As this medicine covers the miasm (here in this case, sycosis) as well as the symptom, the wart has fallen off; and the next suppressed layer, perhaps a profuse yellowish leucorrhoea (which was previously suppressed by cauterisation) comes to the surface. This symptom too is a sycotic manifestation, and is also covered by Causticum, then that remedy will totally eradicate the problem. So knowledge of miasm guides us to stay with the remedy and to allow its full and complete action.

(v) To evaluate the homoeopathic prognosis of the case, as removal of layers of suppression are manifested as clarity of symptoms and also reflected by a quantum jump in the sense of well being. Deep acting anti-miasmatic medicines by virtue of their centrifugal action will remove the layers of suppression which can be evidenced as follows:

- a) A quantum jump in the sense of well being.
- b) Improved energy.
- c) Increased appetite.
- d) Better quality of sleep.
- e) Harmony and tranquillity of temperament.
- f) Stability (in obese people) or weight gain in under weight subjects.
- g) Clarity of the existing or presenting symptoms or even lighter symptoms.
- h) Suppressed symptoms (even of years ago) reappear on the surface and are permanently eradicated. This reappearance can be in a very transient form, which may not even be visible to the naked eye.

(vi) To fulfil Hahnemann's three injunctions of cure: rapid, gentle and permanent.

(vii) Anti-miasmatic medicines help to clear up the suppressions (in relation to the past); clear up the presenting symptoms from their root or origin (in relation to the present); and clear up the susceptibility to get infection and thereby strengthening the constitution (in relation to the prophylactic aspect or future).

And so we return to the key points of this introduction — the utility and incorporation of miasm in prescribing. Miasm represents the past, the present and the future — the past in terms of the layers of suppression and their removal, the present by the removal of these layers, which leads to a clear assessment of the totality of symptoms, and the future where the patient becomes stronger as a whole and is more able to resist morbific influences. Even in this modern world of heroic suppressions, a proper constitutional, anti-miasmatic treatment is capable of achieving the following results:-

PAST

In one-sided cases, the centrifugal action of the anti-miasmatic remedy brings suppressed symptoms to the surface and in so doing allows the proper totality to be framed. A correct anti-miasmatic prescription is also effective in cases where the picture of the disease is either conjoint or contaminated. In such cases, it organises the symptoms and frames a clear picture by removing the blocks.

PRESENT

Removal of the different layers of suppression one after another through changes in the plan of miasmatic treatment according to the presenting surface miasm and corresponding symptomatic totality. Thereby the miasmatic dyscrasias are corrected, which in turn lessen the susceptibility to become sick. Thus we achieve the Hahnemannian ideology of permanent restoration of health.

FUTURE

Clearance of the miasmatic stigmas and dyscrasias serves to improve the immunity and strengthen the constitution.

The proper miasmatic diagnosis of each case can uproot the underlying cause and nip the bud of increased susceptibility to diseases! Miasmatic prescribing is therefore both curative and preventive.

THE PHILOSOPHY OF MIASM:

MIASM — THE CONTAGIUM VIVUM:

Dr. Samuel Hahnemann, the founding father of homoeopathy was the first person to perceive and teach the parasitical nature of such contagious diseases as smallpox, chickenpox, measles, scarlet fever and cholera, a theory first published in 1831 in his article entitled 'An Appeal to thinking philanthropists respecting the mode of propagation of the Asiatic Cholera'. However, it is considered that he must have arrived at such conclusions before 1827 when he expressed his views to his disciples before the publication of his book on Chronic Diseases in 1828. He states in his article on cholera that the cause of the disease was "....composed of probably millions of these miasmatic animated beings....", and thus the idea of Contagium Vivum (the contagious nature of infection and disease) was born. It was not until 1882 that, with the aid of a microscope, Koch discovered the Comma Bacillus of Cholera and confirmed Hahnemann's theory of 50 years before. Whilst it is true that Hahnemann did not have the advantage of a microscope his mind was keen and analytical and he was in possession of phenomenal intuition. Thus equipped he used the terminology of his day to convey the idea of miasm as 'infectious, contagious, excessively minute, invisible, living creatures'.

Hahnemann spent 12 years of intensive study relating the presence of miasms to chronic diseases. He had already discovered and was employing the principles of the Law of Similia and the doctrine of medicine dynamisation to great effect. However, he became perturbed by the seeming recurrence of certain conditions, which appeared previously to have been successfully treated with suitable homoeopathic remedies, and he embarked on his quest to find their cause. His conclusion was that all chronic diseases were the result of the chronic miasms, $7/8^{th}$ of which he termed Psora (conditions arising from the suppression of 'itch-like eruptions' by non-homoeopathic means) and the remaining $1/8^{th}$ being divided between Sycosis (a past suppression of gonorrhoea) and Syphilis (a past suppression of the venereal chancre). Dr. J.H. Allen later added the fourth miasm, Tubercular (conditions arising from the suppression of tuberculous affections by non-homoeopathic means) and it is recognised that many of the manifestations of this tubercular miasm are reflected as a combination of psora and syphilis.

DIFFERENTIATIONS OF PSEUDO-PSORA AND TUBERCULAR MIASMS:

Points	PSEUDO-PSORA	TUBERCULAR
1. SYPHILITIC TAINT (MIASMATIC DYSCRASIA)	The Syphilitic taint is acquired (in the lifetime through sexual exposures)	The Syphilitic taint is hereditary
2. DEVELOPMENT OF MANIFESTATIONS	i) Development of symptoms or manifestations takes place in a galloping or rapid course. ii) If tuberculosis or diseases from the tubercular dyscrasia, the development of the disease will be rapid.	i) Manifestation of symptoms is slow and insidious. ii) Tuberculosis or its dyscrasia will usher its onset in a very slow, insidious way, such as. low grade temperature for months, then dry hacking cough for months, which gradually develop into tubercular manifestations.

KEY WORDS AND CRITERIAS:

BASIC CRITERIA OF THE FOUR GREAT MIASMS:

KEY WORD	MIASM	CRITERIAS
IRRITATION Either physical or mental **Physical** — Physical irritation is characterised by itching e.g. itching all over the body **Mental** — Mental irritation leads to mental turmoil characterised by e.g. anxiety, alertness, apprehension (especially of impending misfortune), which manifests as fear. Psora has the most fears of all the miasms.	PSORA	LACK, SCANTY & ABSENCE e.g. atrophy, anaemia, ataxia, anorexia etc. Therefore any diseased condition characterised by deficiency, scantiness or absence, and all 'hypo' conditions reflect psora So deficient immunity resulting in increased susceptibility to catch infections i.e. 'hyper sensitivity' is a psoric criterion.

KEY WORD	MIASM	CRITERIAS
INCOORDINATION Either physical or mental **Physical** — Incoordination in development Proliferation or excess e.g. tumours, fibroids, warts and any growths. **Mental** — Incoordination in the sensorium or comprehension e.g. absentmindedness Whilst concentrating on studies the mind is abstracted and wanders off elsewhere.	SYCOSIS	HYPER All hypers and excesses are sycotic. e.g. hypertrophy, hyperplasia, hypersexuality, excess working (workaholics).

KEY WORD	MIASM	CRITERIAS
DESCTRUCTION & DEGENERATION Either physical or mental **Physical** Characterised by structural destruction and degeneration i) Ulceration (where there is cellular destruction and degeneration) ii) Pus formation (characterised by degenerated cellular debris) iii) Necrosis (characterised by structural degeneration) **Mental** Characterised by destruction and perversion i) Love for one's own life is destroyed (suicidal tendencies). ii) Perverted sex and sexual cravings.	**SYPHILIS**	**'DYSES' AND IRREGULAR MANIFESTATIONS** e.g. dystrophy, dysplasia, dysphagia Irregular manifestations such as irregular peristaltic movement resulting in dysenteric spasm and stool, or high systolic and low diastolic blood pressure in one individual. Such manifestations reflect irregularity in the circulatory mechanism.

KEY WORD	MIASM	CRITERIAS
DISSATISFACTION Either physical or mental **Physical** i) Person craves sugar but this makes them sick and they become dissatisfied. ii) Perverted sexual cravings or profuse masturbation make the person exhausted (this is from the syphilitic component of the miasm), or the person enjoys sex but exhaustion does not permit so they remain unsatisfied. **Mental** i) Changeable mentality (e.g. wants new clothes, changes occupation, studies, jobs, partners etc. very frequently and is never satisfied). ii) Vagabond mentality (e.g. likes to travel often, cannot stay in one place).	**TUBERCULAR**	**ALTERNATING, PERIODIC, ONE-SIDED AND VAGUE MANIFESTATIONS** i) Alternation — e.g. constipation alternates with diarrhoea. ii) Periodicity — e.g. headache comes on every seventh day. iii) One sided diseases — e.g. insomnia, anorexia, migraine, fatigue etc. iv) Other conditions which present with ill-defined symptoms or too few symptoms. v) All allergic manifestations such as food and dust allergies. vi) All haemorrhages. vii) All recurrent problems.

INFECTION AND IMPLEMENTATION:

MIASMATIC INFECTION AND ITS CRITERIAS:

The Source of Miasmatic Infection:
As Hahnemann states in his article on Cholera published in 1831 that the disease is "... composed of probably millions of [these] miasmatic animated beings", we can conclude that these living organisms are the source of miasmatic infection and that they transmit their miasmatic properties to the infected person provided that the person is susceptible.

Susceptibility: The Precondition:
The precondition of susceptibility to disease is generally caused by underlying psora and without this susceptibility the disease cannot exist. Therefore, a person free from psora is non-susceptible and even if affected with syphilis for example, cannot fall prey to the presence of the bacteria in their system. However, where underlying psora exists in a constitution there will always be a suitable environment for the miasmatic influences from the syphilitic bacteria to infect and manifest.

Transmission of Miasmatic Infection and Dyscrasia: Though Pathologically Sterile:
Miasmatic infections and dyscrasia are transmitted even when a disease is not pathologically present. For example, an infected person may not have the pathological presence of gonococcus but through the latent sycosis in their system they have the ability to transmit the dyscrasia. Therefore, if this sycosis remains untreated, it is transmitted to their offspring who will receive the dyscrasia in the same stage as it is present in the parent host.

Psora is Infectious:
Itch vesicles containing fluid in which the miasm of psora is present transmit infection through touch and within 6 to 14 days, the primary manifestation of psora will become apparent in the newly infected person.

Artificial Chronic Disease: Drug-Miasm:
The prolonged usage of any drug (in a non-homoeopathic way) gives rise to a permanent dyscrasia/stigmata in the system and causes the manifestation of an artificial chronic disease as the criteria of miasmatic states are fulfilled.

Vaccinosis: A Miasmatic Dyscrasia of Sycosis:
A repeated H/O (history of) vaccination leads to the production of a miasmatic state. This state is similar to that which can be produced by gonococcus or cowpox virus and is sycotic in nature.

MIASMATIC INTERPRETATION IN CHRONIC PRESCRIBING:

The most important contribution of Hahnemann's explorations into miasms is the concept that layers of predisposition exist, as has previously been mentioned. The prescriber systematically peels off the layers of predisposing weaknesses by carefully prescribing each remedy based on the totality of symptoms appearing at that moment, in the knowledge that each layer is always the result of the underlying ones and that there is a definite sequence to the presenting layers. Hahnemann states that homoeopathic treatment must be continued until all the layers of predisposition have been removed.

Therefore, if a patient is presenting the features of bronchospasm (asthma) the prescriber has to assess the remedy on the basis of the totality of the presenting surface symptoms, as well as to cover the surface miasm as indicated by those symptoms. The indicated remedy will not only eradicate the presenting symptoms but also by virtue of its miasmatic similarity, will remove the surface miasm too. The next miasm, from the new uppermost layer will manifest through its presenting new group of symptoms and according to Kentian directives, the case will have to be reassessed and a change made in the plan of treatment. The selection of the next remedy should be guided by the then presenting surface manifestations and will therefore cover the surface miasm that has been revealed after eradication of the former miasmatic layer.

Returning again to the analogy of the lotus flower, it is only by this systematic peeling away of layers of predisposing weakness and the removal of differing layers of miasms through changes in the plan of treatment that we can proceed to nip the bud and ensure cure in chronic cases.

IMPLEMENTATION OF MIASMS IN PRESCRIBING: CONCLUSION:

The effective homoeopathic prescription must include the miasmatic totality, manifested by the person. This helps to eradicate the constitutional groove/stigma from the person, failing which, the dyscrasia, the susceptibility to get sick, remains untreated and leads to the future manifestation of disease.

TERMINOLOGIES:

ACUTE MIASM:

In §73, Master Hahnemann mentions those miasms, which are responsible for recurring and non-recurring types of acute specific infectious diseases. Such acute miasmatic diseases are typhus, the itch of wool-workers, purpura miliaris (F.N.§25, 3rd edition of The Organon), smallpox, measles, whooping cough, mumps, plague and Asiatic cholera. These germs have been termed 'fixed' because the diseased conditions produced by them remain almost the same.

Acute miasm: An infecting agent (disease producing dynamic power), which generally has fixed manifestations, capable of producing an acute disease reaction in an organism.

Half-acute miasm: It is denoted by Hahnemann as half-acute because of the possible long period required for the onset of symptoms (i.e. possible long incubation period), but when the symptoms are set forth, it is very rapid in its manifestations, like any acute ailment.

The miasm of rabies (or hydrophobia) is termed half-acute due to the length of time (incubation period) it may take to develop in the system before symptoms begin to manifest, this may be anything from 10 days to 2 years.

CHRONIC MIASM:

By the terminology of chronic miasm Hahnemann meant the infective agent (refer §81, 1st line), which is contagious in nature (refer first ever footnote in the Introduction Chapter; and also §72 last line; §80, 4th line and his book Chronic Diseases), which is responsible for producing chronic diseases or a chronic disease reaction in an organism.

Chronic miasm: Infecting agent capable of producing a chronic disease reaction in an organism. These are the fundamental causes of chronic diseases. A chronic miasm has a tendency to progress and to end only with the life of the patient, if not treated with suitable anti-miasmatic medicines. Hahnemann identified three types of chronic miasms, psora, syphilis and sycosis. Dr. John Henry Allen later added the fourth chronic miasm, the tubercular miasm.

MIASMATIC STATE: DR. BANERJEA'S DEFINITION:

This is a condition, a state of altered or deranged health; resulting after the invisible, inimical infection with the specified miasm. Here miasm is the cause, and the miasmatic state is the effect or manifestation. We do prescribe for the miasmatic state and not for the miasm.

DIATHESIS:

Diathesis is the predisposition to contract (catch) a certain disease, infection or symptom; e.g. a tubercular diathesis is prone to suffer from tubercular manifestations or tuberculosis from the slightest provocation or stimuli.

MIASMATIC DISEASES:

Miasmatic disease = Disease reaction following infection with a miasm.

i) Psora: Derived from the Hebrew word 'tsorat', meaning a groove, a fault, a pollution, a stigma; allied to the Greek word 'Psen', which means to rule, is a disease reaction after infection with the psora (psoric) miasm.

ii) Psoric miasm: Infecting agent capable of producing a 'psora' disease reaction in an organism.

iii) Sycosis: Disease reaction after infection with the sycosis (sycotic) miasm.

iv) Sycotic miasm: Infecting agent capable of producing a sycosis disease reaction (fig wart disease, Ref. Pg. 9 of Chronic Diseases).

v) Syphilis: Disease reaction after infection with the syphilis (syphilitic) miasm.

vi) Syphilitic miasm: Infecting agent capable of producing a syphilis disease reaction (venereal chancre disease, Ref. Pg. 9 Chronic Diseases).

vii) Tubercular miasm: Infecting agent capable of producing a tubercular disease reaction (scrofulous swelling of glands, recurrent tendency to catch cold etc., according to Dr. J.H. Allen). This is also known as Pseudo-psora (pseudo meaning false; so falsely or inappropriately named psoric disease); because there are many symptoms similar to psora, which are caused by 'hypo' or lowered immunity, but they are not exactly similar and so have been classed separately.

viii) Consumptive miasm: A mixed-miasmatic state combining sycosis and psora and also containing certain aspects of the tubercular miasm as follows:

Points	Pseudo-Psora	Syco-Psora
Miasm	Psora ++, Syphilis ++ Syphilo-psora = Tubercular miasm = Pseudo-psora	Psora ++, Sycosis ++ Syco-psora = Consumptive miasm
Manifestations	Psora = hypo Syphilis = destruction The combination of these two miasms causes hypo-immunity leading to total destruction of immunity and recurrent infection. Development of the manifestation may be quick.	Psora = hypo Sycosis = excess Here psora causes hypo-immunity but the manifestation of the same is characterised by profuse or excess secretion of mucus; exudative type. Development of the manifestation may be slow (as sycosis is responsible for slow and insidious onset).

ANTI-MIASMATIC MEDICINE:

Any medicine, which is capable of producing symptoms similar to a particular miasm and hence when administered in the diseased state can annihilate those symptoms as well as eradicate that miasm from the constitution, is defined as an anti-miasmatic medicine. E.g. an anti-psoric medicine is capable of producing psoric symptoms and when administered in the diseased state can eradicate psoric symptoms and thereby the corresponding psoric miasmatic layer.

HAHNEMANNIAN CLASSIFICATION OF MIASMS:

Hahnemann in his Chronic Diseases and Organon made reference to the following miasms:

MIASM	DEFINITION & MANIFESTATION
ACUTE	Acute miasms are responsible for recurring and non-recurring acute infectious diseases and can be divided into three separate categories:
i) Acute Miasms for Specific Diseases	e.g. the miasms of cholera, typhoid, pneumonia, diphtheria etc.
ii) Fixed Miasms	e.g. the miasms of whooping cough, smallpox etc., i.e. those diseases which always appear representing their clinical features more or less in a fixed nature.
iii) Half-spiritual Miasms	e.g. the miasms of measles, pox, scarlet fever etc. which are termed as half-spiritual because the patient either dies, or after completing their parasitical existence in the system the miasms die out leaving the patient to quickly recover.
HALF-ACUTE	The miasm of rabies (or hydrophobia) is termed half-acute due to the length of time it takes to develop in the system before symptoms begin to manifest.
CHRONIC	Responsible for producing chronic diseases or chronic disease reactions in an organism, these miasms can be divided into six separate categories.
i) Marsh Miasm	The miasm of endemic or intermittent fever in marshy land, believed to be due to some 'notorious principle' present there in the atmosphere.
ii) Psoric Miasm	Infecting agent capable of producing a psora disease reaction in an organism. May also be designated as half-spiritual.
iii) Sycotic Miasm	Infecting agent capable of producing a sycosis disease reaction in an organism.
iv) Syphilitic Miasm	Infecting agent capable of producing a syphilis disease reaction in an organism.
v) Drug Miasm	The prolonged use of any medicine or even vaccination in any form may give rise to an artificial chronic disease with a possibility of a permanent dyscrasia. As this satisfies all the criteria of a miasmatic state or disease, such drugs are responsible for producing miasmatic diseases and are termed as the drug miasm.
vi) Accessory Miasm of the Cowpox Vaccine	The cowpox vaccine was believed by Hahnemann to contain an accessory miasm other than the miasm of pox, causing general skin eruptions to appear in the person vaccinated.

THE RATIONALITY OF MIASM:

RATIONALITY OF MIASM: AN EXPLANATION:

Miasm: the expression:

There are many definitions of the word miasm but Hahnemann himself was very precise in his own interpretation — it is an influencing or infecting agent being a particular form of minute, invisible, animated being, specific to a particular form of disease. It is with Hahnemann's guidance we can deduce that the conception of infection or infestation belongs to the dynamic plane. Please also refer to my Ten Principles of Miasm listed at the beginning of the book.

Expressions of miasm by other authors are given below:

i) A heavy vaporous exhalation or effluvium formerly believed to cause disease.
ii) A noxious influence, emanation.
iii) A stigma, a groove or pollution in the system.
iv) A vacuum in the constitution.
v) A fault in the vitality, which invites or helps to maintain disease and fights against the vital force.

The Dynamic Pathology of Hahnemann:

No understanding of homoeopathy is complete without a thorough grasp of the concept of the Vital Force (the autocratic, instinctive, life-preserving dynamic energy of the body). Careful study can reveal to us the mechanics of life — respiration, growth, digestion, how muscles work and how our brains send messages to all parts of our bodies etc., science however has yet to explain life itself. In homoeopathic terms life can be explained by the presence in every living organism of a spiritual vital force, which is autocratic (self-powered), the dynamic energy that animates the material body, rules with unbounded sway, and retains all parts of the organism in harmonious vital operations, as regards both sensations and functions.

Hahnemann believed and states in §11 of The Organon that for disease to develop, the vital force must be primarily deranged by the dynamic influence upon it of a morbific agent inimical to life. The logical conclusion to this is that the material (physical or chemical) properties of the morbific agent are incapable of such derangement and that only the specific dynamic influence of those agents can be responsible. The living pathogenic germs (bacteria and viruses) therefore cannot be taken as anything except physico-chemical carriers of some particular specific dynamic force, corresponding to the vital force of the victims.

So the concept of miasm reduces itself, most significantly, to the different specific inimical forces carried by respective living material bodies or their biological products, or even stigmata. In the word 'miasm' itself, Hahnemann depicted his original philosophic attitude, i.e. the inseparability of matter and spirit. The term miasm however is often employed to denote the cause as well as the effect.

MODUS OPERANDI:

VF Vital Force	+	GMD General Miasmatic Dyscrasia	=	VF + GMD + i.e. VEF Vital Energy Field		DF Disease Force	=	DVF Deranged Vital Force i.e. CEF Complex Energy Field
		i.e. Individual history of miasmatic dyscrasia + Family history of miasmatic dyscrasia						

In the above representation we can see the Vital Force (VF) in its dynamic plane combining with the patient's General Miasmatic Dyscrasia (GMD) i.e. their personal history or personal taint of miasmatic dyscrasia plus their family history of miasmatic dyscrasia (which has been inherited). Therefore the General Miasmatic Dyscrasia (GMD) is always there in the vital dynamic plane, trying to oppose the vital force; being present as two sides of the coin. This energy field in the vital dynamic plane is called the Vital Energy Field (VEF). When the Disease Force (DF) attacks this dynamic field then there are three types of forces : (i) Vital force; (ii) General Miasmatic force or Dyscrasia and (iii) Disease force. It is these three conjoint forces which form a Complex Energy Field (CEF), which then tries to dynamically derange the Vital Force (VF).

MORBIFIC AGENT e.g. micro-organisms, specific nosological agents, pathogens (virus or bacteria) or drugs
Consist of
1. A physical property   2. A chemical property   3. A dynamic property
(Toxin liberated)   (Toxin liberated)   (Through the dynamic aspect the 'miasmatic animated beings' transmit their miasmatic dyscrasia to the dynamic plane of the patient deranging their Vital Force and allowing the manifestation of disease.)

All micro-organisms have a physical (size, shape etc.) and chemical property (chemical nature of protoplasm as well as of the toxin). The physical property allows the release of the toxin from its body and its chemical composition is the chemical property. Our so called 'modern school' friends are interested only in the physical and chemical properties of the micro-organisms whereas homoeopaths have more interest in its dynamic properties through which it transmits its miasmatic dyscrasia or force to the susceptible organism in the environment.

The miasmatic force from the micro-organism (bacteria, virus) is therefore denoted here as the disease force. If a person is susceptible to receive such a force then it enters into the body's dynamic plane and conjoins with the already existing dynamic force. The resultant conjoint, dynamic, inimical force can then attack the vital force in the dynamic plane and dynamically derange the vital force thus causing disease.

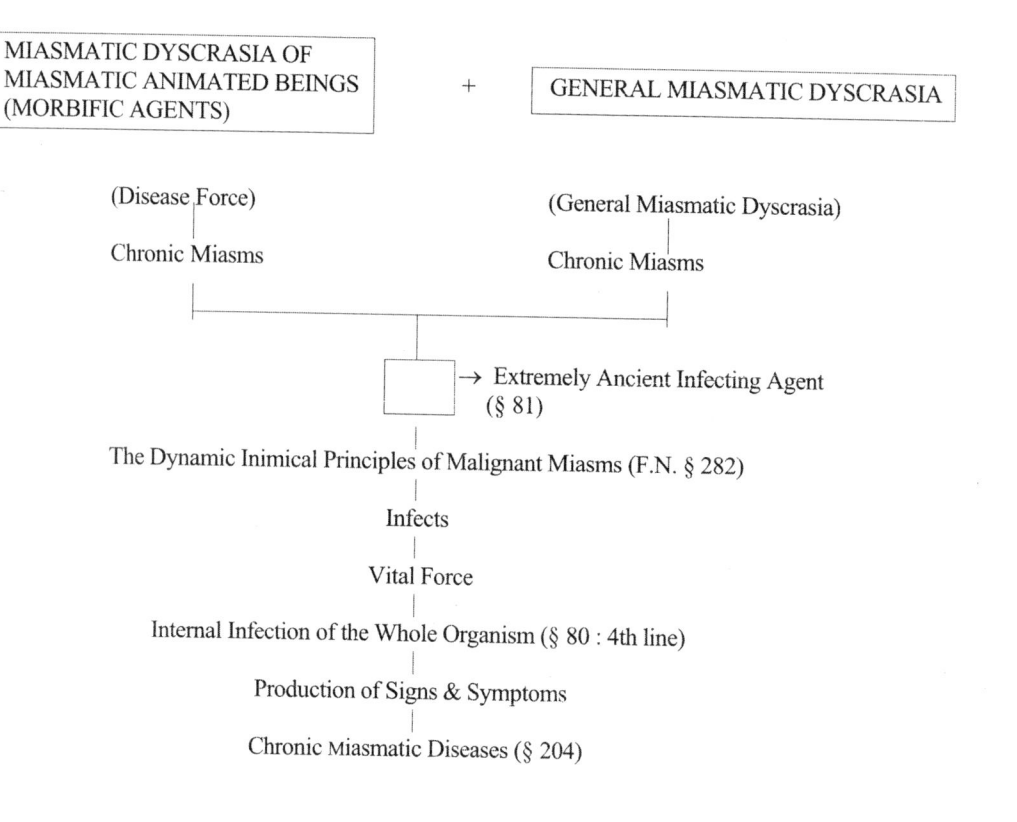

Occurrence of Chronic Disease = Transmission of Miasm = Infection with Chronic Miasm (§72)

```
┌─────────────────────────┐                    ┌─────────────────────────┐
│ MIASMATIC DYSCRASIA OF  │                    │                         │
│ MIASMATIC ANIMATED      │         +          │ GENERAL MIASMATIC       │
│ BEINGS (MORBIFIC AGENTS)│                    │ DYSCRASIA               │
└─────────────────────────┘                    └─────────────────────────┘

        (Disease Force)                           (General Miasmatic Dyscrasia)
              │                                              │
        Chronic Miasms                                 Chronic Miasms
              └──────────────────────┬───────────────────────┘
                                     │
                                     └──→ Extremely Ancient Infecting Agent
                                                     (§ 81)
                                     │
            The Dynamic Inimical Principles of Malignant Miasms (F.N. § 282)
                                     │
                                  Infects
                                     │
                                Vital Force
                                     │
                Internal Infection of the Whole Organism (§ 80 : 4th line)
                                     │
                         Production of Signs & Symptoms
                                     │
                         Chronic Miasmatic Diseases (§ 204)
```

THREE CRITERIAS OF MIASMATIC DISEASE:

i) Miasmatic Diseases of Unknown Causes:

Miasm defined as 'a pollute', 'a noxious effluvium' or 'emanation' was in use as a common medical term during Hahnemann's time, used to indicate the 'unknown cause of disease'.

ii) Miasmatic Disease Terminates with Life:

§79 of The Organon states that chronic miasmatic disease, when uncured, ceases only with the termination of life.

iii) Miasmatic Disease Transmits to the Next Generation:

In §81, Hahnemann confirms the hereditary transmission of miasm from generation to generation.

THE SCIENTIFIC BASIS OF THE MIASM THEORY:

A concept, theory or principle can be granted as scientific, if it fulfils the following criteria:-

i) It is based on clearly observed data, facts and phenomena.

ii) It has been repeatedly confirmed by later observations and experiences under similar conditions.

iii) It gives clear and correct guidance in anticipating and inferring the future events.

The miasmatic concept and approach adheres fully to the above criteria.

THE CLINICAL AND PRACTICAL UTILITY OF MIASMS:

THE PRACTICAL UTILITY OF THE MIASMATIC THEORY:

i) Where there is a contaminated disease picture (i.e. natural disease + suppression of physical or emotional manifestations), an anti-miasmatic prescription reorganises, and thereby arranges, a good symptom picture.

ii) Where the disease picture is conjoint, (i.e. natural disease is superimposed by artificial chronic disease), the miasmatic prescription clears up the ravages caused by medical malpractice, thereby bringing a clear, unadulterated picture of the natural disease back into focus.

iii) In one-sided cases, where on account of a paucity or scarcity of symptoms, it is difficult to ascertain the totality, the anti-miasmatic medicine due to its capability of centrifugal action, brings suppressed symptoms to the surface, allowing the case to be reassessed and the totality more easily ascertained.

iv) In a well-taken case, early development of disease is depicted in the patient's past personal and family histories and any investigation in these spheres without an understanding of the miasmatic approach is akin to navigation in an unfamiliar sea without chart or compass! It is through miasmatic interpretation that a link between the present complaint and the past histories is established and the miasmatic dyscrasia of the person can be perceived. This link or bridge between past and present is known in homoeopathic terms as anamnesis.

v) Even Hering's Law of Cure cannot be assuredly followed without the concept of miasmatic theory. A correct miasmatic prescription will peel off the layers of predisposing weaknesses and thereby clear up the suppressions, with the corresponding improvement ensuing in accordance with Hering's Law of Cure.

REAPPEARANCE OF SUPPRESSIONS & THE CLINICAL UTILITY OF MIASMATIC THEORY:

i) In a permanent cure it is expected that any suppressed conditions will firstly return and then disappear. This is due to the centrifugal action of the medicine bringing the suppressed symptoms to the periphery and allowing the layers of suppression to unfold.

ii) Antecedent miasmatic manifestations are brought back by the similimum prescribed on miasmatic bases allowing a gradual disappearance of the present disorder. The anti-miasmatic medicine by bringing suppressed symptoms to the surface, gradually frees the body from years of different varieties and modes of suppression resulting in an improvement in the health of the patient.

iii) In obstinate cases such as endocrinal diseases and congenital and oncological disorders etc., this progression towards health is often very difficult and sometimes impossible to achieve. In most of these cases the primary miasmatic infection occurred some generations before and the present disorders are the result of hereditary transmission of the intimate combination of the original psora with other miasms, or of all three miasms blended together. Many such cases fall into the incurable category.

iv) Curable cases may be rendered incurable by palliating the antecedent manifestations of the miasm/miasms.

PSORA & ITS STATES:

THE QUALIFYING CONDITION OF PSORA:

To warrant inclusion under the miasm of psora, the disease or pathological condition must bear a definite relationship to a skin eruption of a specific character i.e. a peculiar cutaneous eruption accompanied by intolerable, voluptuous, tickling itching. This is the external manifestation of the monstrous internal chronic miasm of psora. (Ref. Psora and Sycosis in Relation to Modern Bacteriology by Dr. John Paterson, Page Nos.3 & 4).

PRIMARY, LATENT, SECONDARY AND TERTIARY PSORA:

In fact, all the four miasm have four distinct stages. Stage I is the Primary Stage of the original manifestation, e.g. itch eruption in the case of psora; gonorrhoeal condyloma and its discharge in the case of sycosis and syphilitic chancre in the case of syphilis. When suppressed by non-homoeopathic means they progress into Stage II, the Latent Stage. At this point, any exciting cause will bring the latent condition to the surface and this is denoted as Stage III, or the Secondary Stage. When these secondary manifestations are allowed to progress, gross pathological changes ensue and Stage IV, the Tertiary Stage is reached.

i) Primary Psora:

Primary psora shows as a manifestation of the original itch-like eruption.

ii) Latent Psora:

Here the primary manifestation (e.g. itch eruption) has been suppressed by non-homoeopathic measures (e.g. local or topical application), which drive the original eruption inside where it apparently remains dormant or quiescent. The initial disturbance is located in the vital force and manifests through imperceptible, sensorial and functional changes in the body as a whole. Where nosology fails to be applied (i.e. the disease is unable to be named or classified) due to the symptoms not referring to any particular organ or tissue; the patient although showing deviations from a perfectly healthy state, is not termed as specifically diseased. During this period however, the affected person does show an increased susceptibility.

Note: Psora, in its latent state, is suitable for hereditary transmission.

iii) Secondary Psora:

The quiescent or dormant psora when exposed to an exciting or maintaining cause is roused up into activity. In other words the latent or slumbering state is awakened into manifold manifestations. The disharmony of the whole or central life force (vital force) is reflected as disharmony of life in the tissues or organs, and disorders in the case of secondary manifestations are manifested more on the functional plane.

Development of Secondary Psora:
Stage I: Primary psora: The itch-like eruption ↬ suppressed ↬ Stage II: Latent psora. The suppressed state of slumbering psora (no apparent manifestations) ↬ Exciting cause and lowered susceptibility ↬ Stage III: Secondary psora: where with various other manifestations there is the possibility of the original skin eruption being called to the surface of the skin for a second time.

Approach of Treatment: Secondary Psora & Series of Anti-Psorics:
Every other psoric diathesis i.e. the psora that has developed into one of the innumerable chronic diseases springing from it, is very seldom cured by any single anti-psoric remedy, but requires the use of several of these remedies — and in the worst cases the use of quite a number of them, one after the other, allowing each medicine to complete its action in its fullest extent, for its perfect cure.

iv) Tertiary Psora:

The tertiary stage is reached when gross structural changes appear in the tissues or organs. This is a progression from functional changes and is the domain of pathology proper. Nosology becomes relevant at this point.

ORDER OF PROGRESSION IN CHRONIC DISEASE (APPLICABLE TO ALL FOUR MIASMS):

Stage I: Primary psora (the itch-like eruption) or Primary sycosis (the condylomatous wart associated with gleet) or in Primary syphilis (the venereal chancre) or in Primary tubercular miasm (the original pulmonary tuberculosis), are suppressed which leads to:

Stage II: Latent psora, the suppressed state of slumbering psora, Latent sycosis, Latent syphilis or Latent tubercular miasm — Functional changes (affecting the vital force) occur although there are no apparent visible manifestations, and these lead to:

Stage III: Secondary psora/sycosis/syphilis or tubercular state (when the exciting cause and lowered susceptibility arouses the latent state into activity causing the functional changes to progress to the individual tissues or organs with various manifestations and the possibility of the return of the original skin eruption (in case of psora); the condylomatous wart associated with gleet (in case of sycosis), the venereal chancre (in case of syphilis);or the milder manifestation of pulmonary tuberculosis (in case of the tubercular miasm). When these are called upon for a second time they lead to:

Stage IV: Tertiary psora/sycosis/syphilis or tubercular state (when gross structural changes appear in the tissues or organs).

HAHNEMANNIAN DYNAMISM:

HAHNEMANN: THE FATHER OF MODERN BACTERIOLOGY:

Hahnemannian Conception And Modern Bacteriology:

Eighteenth century medicine was dominated by fancies, speculations and loathsome, torturesome therapeutic practices. The discovery of specific micro-organisms for specific diseases seemed to lead to the promised land of scientific medicine to which the practitioners of the time had aspired to for so long. Hahnemann's ideas regarding miasms (in a wider sense), infection, a symptomatic latency of infection, idiosyncrasies and hyper-sensitiveness on the part of the patient, all failed to make an impression on his contemporaries as he was unable to substantiate his claims by experimental verifications — the only kind of evidence which seemed to catch their imaginations. His semi-scientific and semi-philosophical conception of miasms was therefore simply ridiculed.

Kill The Bacteria, Cure the Disease, a Futility:

Since micro-organisms are only one of the many causes of disease, the curative remedy for the disease in the individual must correspond to the combined effects of the various causes. Each and every individual disease varies in its causes and conditions and consequently in its symptoms or effects, and for this reason, it follows that there can be no common specific remedy for a disease. Susceptibility, a pre-condition to acquire the infection, which enables bacteria to enter the body, should be considered and treated accordingly. Mere bacteriology therefore can never serve as a basis for reliable and efficient therapeutics for an individual and the so-called modern scientific school of medicine is slowly but surely beginning to realise the futility of the slogan 'Kill the bacteria and cure the disease'.

Psoric Miasm And Tubercular Bacilli:

With the growth in knowledge of bacteriological science it becomes evident that practically all the diseases known to be due to tubercle bacilli infection are attributed by Hahnemann to psora. Later, Dr. Stuart Close was of the opinion that the causative agent is identical, and that the two terms psora and tuberculosis are synonymous. It is another striking fact that Hahnemann chose leprosy as the typical form of the ancient protean disease, which he classed under psoric diseases. Modern bacteriology confirms that the bacilli of leprosy resemble the tubercle bacilli in form, size and staining reactions and that leprosy sufferers react to the Tuberculin Test and Wassermann Reaction Test.

Stuart Close liked to fix the denotation of the psoric miasm and identify it with Koch's tubercle bacillus. My personal feelings are that the time has not yet come to close the debate. Tubercle bacilli are known to produce skin lesions but there is not yet any experimental or clinical verification that they produce vesicular itching eruptions similar to those said to be produced by Hahnemann's psoric miasm.

LAYERS OF MIASMATIC STATES:

LAYERS OF PREDISPOSITION:

The most important contribution of Hahnemann's explorations into miasms is the concept that layers of predisposition exist. The prescriber systematically peels off the layers of predisposing weaknesses by carefully selecting each remedy based on the totality of symptoms presenting at that moment. Each layer results from an underlying layer, and there is a definite sequence to the layers as they present.

The concept of predisposing layers has considerable practical value in chronic relapsing cases. Let us take an example of a patient who consults a homoeopath for chronic headaches that began after exposure to cold. If the prescriber gives Belladonna he may find that the headaches disappear dramatically and in the case of a constitutionally strong patient, the cure may last for a considerable period of time. However, the vast majority of patients have been weakened through hereditary influence, drugs, or vaccinations, resulting in several layers of predisposition. At the time when the above patient first consults the homoeopath, the totality of symptoms at that moment represents only the uppermost layer of predisposition.

Hahnemann stated that homoeopathic treatment must be continued until all the layers of predisposition have been removed. If the patient and homoeopath were to be satisfied before this stage was reached, then the remaining untreated condition would be likely to slowly degenerate over time into an irreversible pathological process, particularly if further exciting causes occurred.

A miasm is a predisposition towards chronic disease underlying the acute manifestations of illness. It is transmissible from generation to generation, and may respond beneficially to the corresponding nosode prepared from either pathological tissue or from the appropriate drug or vaccine, if the totality for a non-nosodal constitutional medicine is absent.

The degree of chronic weakness of the defence mechanism is a direct result of the intensity of the miasmatic influences. If we contrast two patients with leukaemia, for example, the age at which the disease occurs is a measure of the number of miasms involved. If it were to develop at the age of 70 after a lifetime of good health, it is likely that only the psoric miasm is involved. If, on the other hand, it were to arise in childhood, very likely three or more miasms would be implicated. The number of miasms involved has important prognostic significance; in that the greater the number, the slower will be the response to treatment.

Symptoms of disease develop on the basis of cause and effect and the link between the two is the anamnesis. In other words anamnesis is the bridge which links and traces the sequence of developments between the present complaints with that of the past history and family histories.

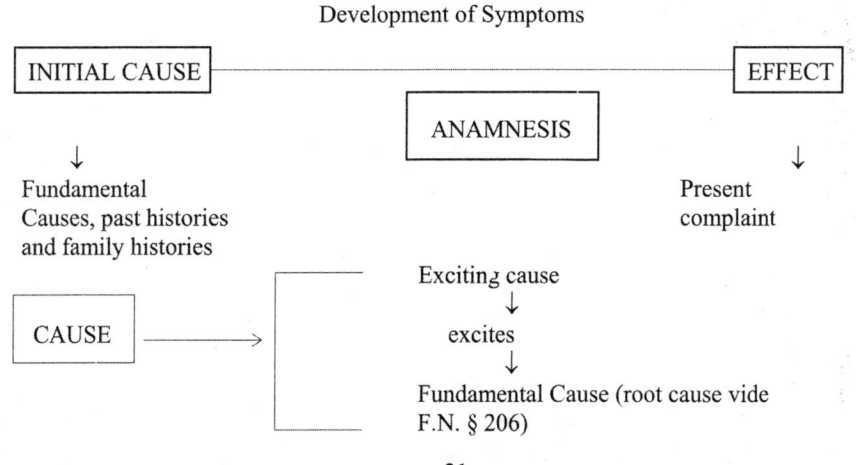

Development of Symptoms

INITIAL CAUSE ——————————————— EFFECT

ANAMNESIS

↓ ↓

Fundamental Present
Causes, past histories complaint
and family histories

CAUSE ——→   Exciting cause
             ↓
             excites
             ↓
             Fundamental Cause (root cause vide F.N. § 206)

Example A:

e.g. SYCOTIC PATIENT (who inherited sycosis from their father is possessed of a fundamental Miasm).
i.e. a CAUSE

The state however remains latent and there is no manifestation of symptoms.

Some exciting cause then excites the latent fundamental cause and symptoms manifest/develop i.e. EFFECT.

So while treating this patient, we generally treat the effect i.e. the present manifestations. Sometimes we try to formulate the totality considering the exciting causes also, but until and unless the fundamental causes are taken into account (which are the root cause vide F.N.§206): we cannot achieve an absolute totality. The absolute totality also comprises the miasmatic totality (vide §209).

Example B :

Belladonna is prescribed for a cold (on the basis of partial-surface totality, i.e. consideration of the effect only) and the cold is removed. From miasmatic consideration however, we know that we have to remove the fundamental cause and may still give Belladonna but keep in mind, perhaps a deep acting anti-tubercular remedy (according to the presence of miasmatic state) with which to finish the case and prevent relapse.

Example C :

A patient has acquired syphilis (fundamental cause) and this has been suppressed by allopathic drugs leading to the development of secondary symptoms. These allopathic drugs obscure the primary symptoms (vide §205) and by treating the present manifestations (i.e. the secondary symptoms) only we are addressing a partial surface-totality and ignoring the fundamental cause.

LAYERS OF PREDISPOSING WEAKNESS:

Example 1:

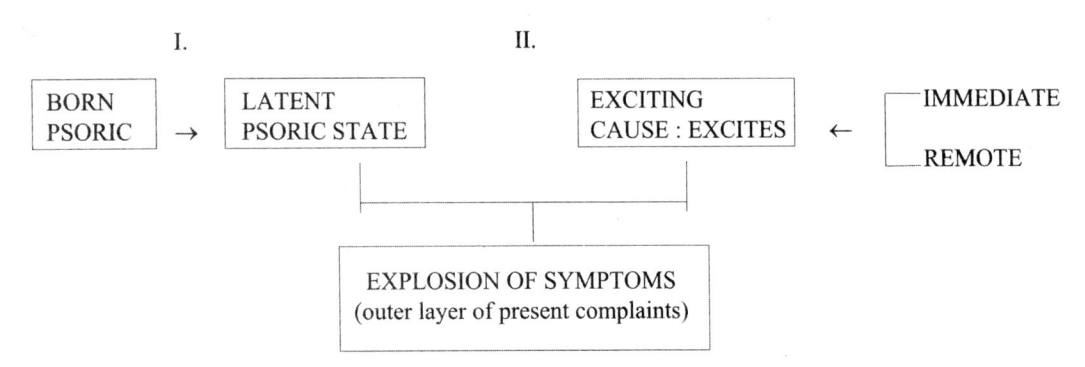

```
        I.                                II.
┌─────────┐     ┌──────────────┐    ┌──────────────────┐      ┌─IMMEDIATE
│  BORN   │  →  │   LATENT     │    │   EXCITING       │  ←   │
│ PSORIC  │     │ PSORIC STATE │    │ CAUSE : EXCITES  │      └─REMOTE
└─────────┘     └──────┬───────┘    └────────┬─────────┘
                       │                     │
                       └──────────┬──────────┘
                                  │
                    ┌─────────────┴──────────────┐
                    │  EXPLOSION OF SYMPTOMS     │
                    │ (outer layer of present    │
                    │         complaints)        │
                    └────────────────────────────┘
```

Example 2:

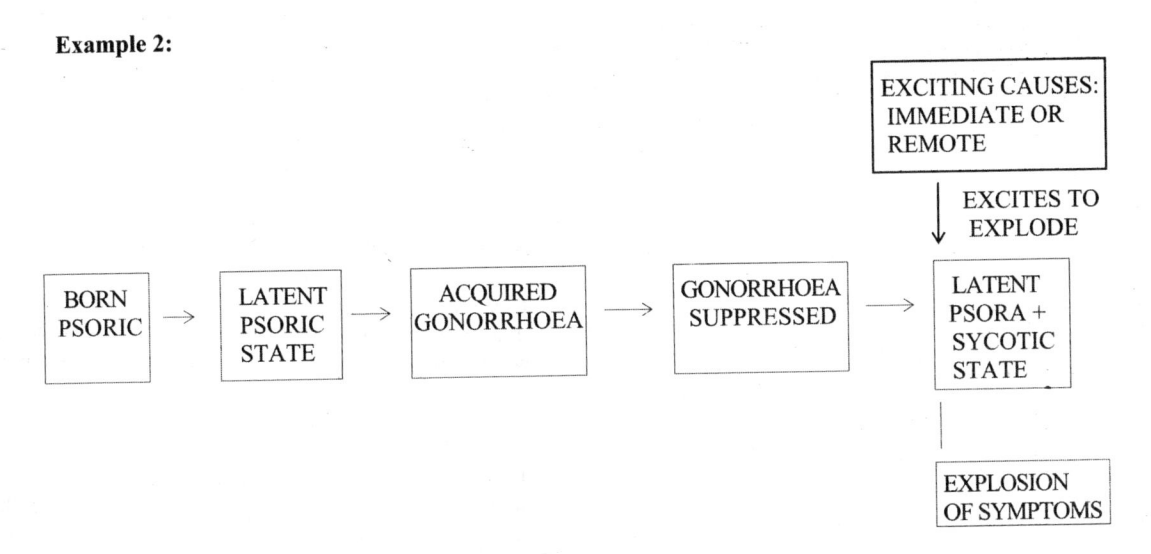

```
                                                              EXCITING CAUSES:
                                                              IMMEDIATE OR
                                                              REMOTE
                                                                    │
                                                                    ▼ EXCITES TO
                                                                      EXPLODE
 ┌────────┐   ┌────────┐   ┌──────────┐   ┌──────────┐   ┌────────┐
 │ BORN   │ → │ LATENT │ → │ ACQUIRED │ → │GONORRHOEA│ → │ LATENT │
 │ PSORIC │   │ PSORIC │   │GONORRHOEA│   │SUPPRESSED│   │ PSORA +│
 │        │   │ STATE  │   │          │   │          │   │ SYCOTIC│
 │        │   │        │   │          │   │          │   │ STATE  │
 └────────┘   └────────┘   └──────────┘   └──────────┘   └────────┘
                                                                │
                                                                ▼
                                                           ┌──────────┐
                                                           │ EXPLOSION│
                                                           │OF SYMPTOMS│
                                                           └──────────┘
```

Exciting Cause: Cause which excites the Latent Psora to explode especially in forming Acute Diseases.

Remote Cause: → Causal Blocks → N.B.W.S. (Never Been Well Since).

e.g. i) Asthma dates from measles or pertussis of childhood.
 ii) Has never recovered from effects of typhoid.
 iii) Chronic sick-headache from some severe disease of youth.
 iv) Bad-effects of mechanical injuries, even if received years ago.

UNFOLDING OF MIASMATIC LAYERS & REMOVAL OF SUPPRESSION:

i) The common chronic diseases of the liver are not diseases, but the localisation of psora in the liver; and should be studied from their beginnings to their ends, i.e. from cause to ultimate. Thereafter, the systematic unfolding of layers will bring suppressed symptoms to the surface.

ii) The return of old symptoms means recovery, so that when discharges return for example, the relief of the secondary manifestations of miasms ensues.

iii) The prescriber *systematically peels off layer upon layer of predisposing weakness* by carefully prescribing each remedy based on the totality.

iv) The important contribution of Hahnemann's exploration into the miasms is the concept that there exist layers of pre-disposition.

The centrifugal action of the anti-miasmatic medicines is capable of opening up those cases in which all the symptoms and their finer modalities have been benumbed or suppressed. Suitable anti-miasmatic medicines will bring the suppressed symptoms from centre to periphery; from inside to the surface, and thereby unfold the layers of the lotus flower!

PLAN OF MIASMATIC TREATMENT:
AMENDMENT TO THE PLAN AS THE SURFACE MIASM CHANGES:

Various views of other authors:

PSORA:

PSORA + SYCOSIS OR PSORA + SYPHILITIC: Treat the surface miasm first →followed by an anti-psoric medicine → then again treat the surface miasm but always finish with an antipsoric.

TRI-MIASMATIC CASES: Start with an anti-psoric → CPT (Change in the Plan of Treatment) → surface miasm → anti-psoric → CPT → surface miasm → an anti-psoric.

PSORA & SUSCEPTIBILITY: Some authors are of the opinion that if the patient does not have the psoric hypersensitivity, the patient would not develop Syphilis even after exposure! So the pre-conditions to the development of Syphilis are: (1) Psoric Susceptibility (main pre-condition); (2) Syphilitic Miasm (exciting cause).

SYCOTIC:

SYCO-PSORIC CASES: Anti-psoric → repeated anti-psoric causes psora to become dormant and sycosis to come to the surface → anti-psoric.

SYCO-PSORA-SYPHILITIC CASES: Anti-psoric → anti-sycotic → anti-syphilitic → anti-psoric.

SYPHILO-SYCO-PSORIC CASES: Anti-Syphilitic → anti-psoric → anti-sycotic.

SYPHILITIC:

SYPHILO-PSORIC CASES: Anti-psoric → anti-syphilitic → anti-psoric → anti-syphilitic.

SYPHILO-SYCOTIC: Anti-sycotic first → anti syphilitic.

SYPHILO-SYCO-PSORA: Anti-psoric first → then surface miasm → CPT and again surface miasm → etc. → to finish treatment with anti-psoric.

DR. BANERJEA'S APPROACH TO A PLAN OF MIASMATIC TREATMENT:

I believe that it is necessary to address the surface symptoms and thereby evaluate the surface miasm, (whatever that miasm may be) and direct treatment considering the totality of symptoms as well as the miasmatic totality present on the surface. For instance in a syphilo-sycotic case it is useless to address the sycotic miasm first, if syphilitic symptoms are on the surface — we must remember that Hahnemann taught us to consider the surface symptoms only.

Hahnemann did however instruct us in his book on Chronic Diseases to address psora first. This may appear to be an anomaly but one must understand that during the Hahnemannian era diseases were present mainly in the simple form that is they were single miasmatic states. Mixed miasmatic states are mentioned in §206 of the Organon and it is to these that we mostly fall pray in this modern world where many layers of suppressions present as different layers of miasmatic states.

To succeed in treatment, we have to address the surface symptoms. These are the outwardly reflected pictures of the internal essence of the disease and it is through these surface symptoms that we are able to clear up the presenting miasmatic state with a proper anti-miasmatic remedy.

THE NATURE OF MIASM:

HAHNEMANN'S CONCLUSIVE EVIDENCE THAT PSORA IS NOT A PREDISPOSITION BUT A DISEASE:

Hahnemann clearly indicates that psora is not a predisposition but a disease brought on by infection with the psoric miasm and that no predisposition (i.e. prior state of altered health) need be present for infection with the psoric miasm to ensue, except the susceptibility to receive psoric infection. He writes:

> "But the miasms of itch need only to touch the general skin, especially with tender children. The disposition of being affected with the miasma of itch is found with almost everyone and under almost all circumstances, which is not the case with the other two miasma. As no other chronic miasma infects more generally, more surely, more easily and more absolutely than the miasma of itch, as already stated, it is the most contagious of all".

The Contagious, Infectious Principle of the Psoric Miasm:

After many years of observation of patients' histories and clinical records of investigations, Hahnemann came to the conclusion that the cause of all chronic non-venereal diseases, is an ancient, almost universally diffused, contagious or infectious principle embodied in some living parasitical micro-organism, with an incredible capacity for multiplication and growth. The sycotic and syphilitic miasms can be safely identified with gonococci and spirochaeta palladium respectively; but a great uncertainty and confusion still exists regarding the denotation of the psoric miasm, in regards to the specific micro-organism responsible.

The Psoric Miasm Was Not Related To Itch-mite Disease Only:

During Hahnemann's time the term 'psora' was used as a general indication for a whole series of varying skin affections and also in the narrow sense of itch proper and scabies. This lead to much confusion particularly following the publication of Hahnemann's book Chronic Diseases. There were those who took the word itch in a limited sense and accordingly jumped at once to the conclusion that itch-mites (e.g. Acarus scabiei or Sarcoptes scabiei hominis) being causally associated with itch and scabies were synonymous with the psoric miasm.

Hahnemann however, meant something very different by his 'psoric miasm' from the ordinary itch mite, with which he had been acquainted for some time, even prior to his homoeopathic days, and although he was not the first to trace all sorts of chronic non-venereal diseases to itch eruptions, his psora theory was much maligned by his contemporaries. When Hahnemann talked of simple itch and itch-mite he advocated external treatment with sulphur lotion without any bad after-effects; but when he was talking of 'psora' and the vesicular type of skin eruptions similar to those of itch proper, he was definitely against all external treatments which he considered would suppress the so-called primary symptoms of psora and lead to the appearance of other chronic diseases over the course of time.

Psora and the Cause of Diseases:

Psora is a symptom syndrome, resulting from long standing non-venereal infection, which shows a skin manifestation. (Ref. A Compend Of The Principles Of Homoeopathy For Students In Medicine by Garth Boericke, Page No.123).

EXTIRPATION OF PSORA:

To elaborate on the revolutionary therapeutic thought of Hahnemann regarding the treatment of skin cases, there are three main points, which deserve consideration:

i) Cessante Cause, Cessat Effectus:

The extirpation of the internal psora disease, which causes the cutaneous eruption, is as necessary as air, and when this is cured, the cutaneous ailment, being the necessary consequence of the internal disease, will naturally disappear — cessante cause, cessat effectus. In other words, treatment or removal of the cause will lead to cessation or annihilation of the effect i.e. the symptoms.

ii) Suppression of Primary Psora:

Destruction of the original cutaneous eruption, which acts vicariously for the internal malady, puts psora in the unnatural position of dominating the internal finer parts of the whole organism in a purely one-sided manner, compelling it to develop its secondary symptoms.

iii) Reappearance of Primary Psora:

Once the original cutaneous eruption has been externally destroyed and secondary chronic ailments have broken out, any reappearance of such an itch-like eruption on the skin will manifest differently to that of before and will not be so easily cured.

THE CURE OF PSORA:

In his book on Chronic Diseases (pages 181-182), Hahnemann makes several references to the use of a series of anti-psoric remedies in the treatment of psora. The following points are of most interest:-

i) "The cure of an old psora that has been deprived of its eruption, whether it may be latent and quiescent or already broken out into chronic diseases, can never be accomplished with Sulphur alone, nor with Sulphur-baths, either natural or artificial".

ii) "Every other psoric diathesis, i.e., the psora that is still latent within, as well as the psora that has developed into one of the innumerable chronic diseases springing from it, is very seldom cured by any single anti-psoric remedy but requires the use of several of these remedies, in the worst cases the use of quite a number of them, one after the other, for its perfect cure".

iii) "Recent itch-disease with its still present cutaneous eruption has been cured at times without any external remedy by even one very small dose of a properly potentised preparation………."

iv) "Psora is a chronic miasma of quite peculiar and especial character, which in several thousands of years has passed through several millions of human organisms, and must have assumed such a vast extension of varied symptoms — the elements of those innumerable, chronic, non-venereal ailments, under which mankind now groans — and could transmute itself into such indefinite multitude of forms differing from one another as it gradually ultimated itself in the various bodily constitutions of individual men who differ from one another in their domiciles, their climatic peculiarities, their education, habit, occupations, modes of life and of diet, and was moulded by varying bodily and psychic relations. It is, therefore, not strange that one single and only medicine is insufficient to heal the entire psora and all its forms, and that it requires several medicines in order to respond, by the artificial morbid effects peculiar to each, to the unnumbered host of psora symptoms, and thus to those of all chronic (non-venereal) diseases and to the entire psora, and to do this in a curative homoeopathic manner".

v) "…….Eruption have been on the skin for some time (although it may not have been treated with external repressive remedies), it will of itself begin to recede gradually from the skin. Then the internal psora has already in part gained the upper hand; the cutaneous eruption is then no more so completely vicarious, and ailments of another kind appear, partly as the signs of a latent psora, partly as chronic diseases developed from the internal psora. In such a case, Sulphur alone (as little as any other single anti-psoric remedy) is usually no longer sufficient to produce a complete cure, and other anti-psoric remedies, one or another, according to the remaining symptoms, must be called upon to give their homoeopathic aid".

PREDILECTIONS:

i) Skin and Psora; Mucus Membranes and Sycosis: Predilections:

In psora the inherent predisposition is towards skin manifestations — a susceptibility to skin disease.
In sycosis, the inherent predisposition is towards catarrh of the mucous membranes and not only of those of the genito-urinary tract. (Ref. Psora And Sycosis In Relation To Modern Bacteriology by Dr. John Paterson, Pg.no.8).
In Syphilis, the inherent predisposition is towards destruction and ulceration.
In the tubercular miasm, the inherent predisposition is towards destruction of the immunity leading to recurrent infection.

ii) Miasm and its Dyscrasias:

Psora	—	Eruptive diathesis.
Sycosis	—	Proliferative; lithic & uric acid; and rheumatic & gouty diathesis.
Syphilis	—	Suppurative diathesis.
Tubercular	—	Allergic; haemorrhagic and scrofulous diathesis.

DR. BANERJEA'S ANCESTRAL & CLINICAL TIPS ON MIASMATIC PRESCRIBING:

There are many key points, some of which I have discovered in my own personal practices and others passed down to me from my predecessors, which I personally find of great benefit when miasmatically assessing a case. They appear below (in no particular order) for your information.

Psora:

i) In this modern world of suppression it is unlikely to find anyone who is totally free from psora. Its highly infectious and contagious nature allows infection of the baby in mother's womb, provided the baby is susceptible to receive such an infection. Most babies therefore, are born psoric and even with treatment by suitable anti-psoric homoeopathic medicines the possibility exists for psora to infect the child again, by virtue of its highly infectious nature and the body's susceptibility to catch such infection.

ii) It is interesting to question who came first in the universe, it is like the question of the chicken or the egg. In the case of homoeopathy we have to ask if it was the susceptibility or the psora which came first into the body.

iii) Even with biblical reference, Adam was susceptible which was the reason he ate the forbidden apple which was psora.

iv) Psora, the deficiency: Psora is the constitutional state of deficiency, of lack in the sense of less inhibition and their consequences. Deficiency or inhibition will bring on a disposition to various immediate disturbances, such as excess (in an attempt to compensate for deficiency) and perversion. Psora is therefore the basic condition of all human pathology. The first reaction to an aggressive agent is inhibition (which relates to psora), the second is fight (which relates to sycosis), and the third is aggression (which relates to syphilis).

v) Desire for cold though aversion to bathing.

Pseudo-Psora:

i) In pseudo-psora the affection is global in distribution and all the components of the intellectual faculty are involved. Perception, attention, concentration, imagination and memory are therefore all under-developed.

ii) While pseudo-psoric affection has global distribution, syco-psora, the other tubercular or consumptive state results in a group of disorders where the subnormality or retardation appear only in certain specific abilities e.g. reading, mathematical calculation, speech and language.

Sycosis:

i) Vaccinations and the use of serums are causes of the sycotic diathesis.

ii) As the barometer's mercury goes up and down, sycosis becomes affected. Aggravation is caused by rising humidity in the atmosphere, from rain, snow and winter cold.

iii) Sycotic patients are predisposed to undue side effects from antibiotics. Dr. O.A. Julian advised a prescription of Medorrhinum in such cases. Undue side effects may also occur from use of the contraceptive pill.

iv) The essence of sycosis is threefold: (i) there is emotional and physical incoordination, (ii) it is hyper in its manifestations (iii) proliferation and excesses occur.

Syphilis:

i) During anti-syphilitic treatment, the patient should follow a simple, nutritious diet and avoid any stimulating foods.

ii) Between 1890 - 1940, the great majority of people living in Central Europe had syphilis.

iii) Penicillin gave the impression that syphilis was cured.

iv) Suppression by penicillin causes syphilis to go deep into the economy and thereby affect the deeper organisms.

v) Emotional mainly and a little expression on the physical.

vi) Alcoholism and general perversion is the fourth stage of syphilis.

vii) An egotistical, selfish element is the final stage of syphilis.

viii) The use of penicillin as a cure for syphilis produced a predisposition to fungal infections i.e. a miasmatic effect.

ix) Patients affected with the syphilitic miasm are apt to become stubborn, obstinate and rigid and have difficulty in adapting to changing circumstances.

Tubercular:

i) Ringworm yields readily to Bacillinum, and Dr. Burnett therefore regarded this cutaneous eruption as a tubercular manifestation (Pg. no.37, Ringworm, Burnett). However, there is also a sycotic component and this enables any syco-tubercular medicine, such as Bacillinum to address the problem.

ii) Any allergic manifestation is predominantly of the tubercular miasmatic dyscrasia.

iii) Constant displeasure and dissatisfaction. Intelligent but whimsical and changeable. The psoric fearfulness develops fully in tri-miasmatic remedies but in the tubercular miasm the fearfulness is extinguished; except for the fear of dogs!

Mixed Miasmatic States:

i) The miasm, psora, will give us psoric expressions, and so on through syphilis and sycosis, but when more than one miasma are combined together, we have a mixed miasmatic expression, either pseudo-psoric or syco-psoric. With regards to the formation of complex diseases, Hahnemann states in a footnote to §40 of The Organon, "that no real amalgamation of the two takes place, but that in such cases the one exists in the organism besides the other only, each in the parts that are adapted for it".

ii) Syco-psoric: Anxious and perplexed. Extremely intelligent but absent-minded. Physical and mental symptoms are aggravated from 3.30 a.m. to 1.30 p.m.

iii) Syphilo-psoric: Dullness of intellect (blunt headed fellow). Melancholic and suicidal with a desire to be in solitude. Likes neither hot nor cold atmosphere or weather.

Miasmatic Characteristics:

1. There are three forms of alteration of cellular function — deficiency, excess and perversion and these relate to the three miasms of Hahnemann as follows:-

    i) Psora = Deficiency

    ii) Sycosis = Excess

    iii) Syphilis = Perversion

2. Thomas P. Paschero relates that "homoeopathy views the constitution as a pathogenic dynamism which the individual inherits and modifies during his life, in three distinct directions: (i) inflammation, (ii) destruction of tissue, or its (iii) proliferation. These dynamic morbid tendencies were called by Hahnemann miasm".

3. The character of the miasm yields the character of the disease or the form of the illness.

4. There are three Dynamis:-

    i) Vital Dynamis

    ii) Disease Dynamis

    iii) Drug Dynamis

Miasm is nothing but a disease dynamis.

5. Miasm is a complex energy field that pervades the organism and predisposes it to certain disorders either acute or chronic, the properties of which are determined by the history of the individual i.e. the miasmatic influences they have been exposed to in their lifetime or through their family or genetic background. Thus we see that:

    i) Disturbances can be transmitted genetically.

    ii) The miasmatic state cannot be auto-cured spontaneously, that is by the body's own defence mechanism.

    iii) The eradication of the miasm is recognised by a quantum jump in the wellbeing of the patient.

6. Giving the remedy indicated at the moment will bring the miasm to the surface.

7. A clear remedy picture hints that the miasmatic condition is light.

8. Any prescription should be based on the miasmatic state, its picture and the diseased condition and not on the miasm itself.

9. Psora is seen as the result of evil thinking and syphilis the result of evil doing.

10. Where syphilis or sycosis is transmitted to offspring; the manifestation of symptoms will be of that transmission stage only.

11. Carriers of miasms may be: (i) Bacteria, (ii) Virus, (iii) Some polluted discharge or fluid, (iv) Poisonous emanation, (v) Contaminated aerial fluid, (vi) a drug or any such medium.

12. Miasmatic influence passes through the organism to the next generation.

Miasm & Bacteria:

1. Diseases such as hypertension, epilepsy, diabetes, mental disorders, cancers and many others are not caused by bacteria, so it cannot be ascertained that Miasm = Bacteria. Moreover as a result of prolonged use of drugs, artificial chronic diseases result from the drug miasm and it is obvious that drugs do not contain bacteria. So miasms and bacteria are not the same. Also, we could not have isolated the bacteria from the fluid of the itch-vesicle of a psoric eruption, but 7/8th of all chronic disease results from the psoric miasm. We are unable to explain psora through bacteria, so there is no sense in the theory that miasm and bacteria are one and the same.

2. All bacteria and viruses contain miasmatic influences. The fluid of the itch vesicle of psoric eruptions for example, contains miasm or miasmatic influences. In other words, this fluid satisfies all the conditions and creates an environment in which miasmatic influence can thrive or survive.

3. Dr. J.H. Allen was probably the first person to recognise drug miasms whereby, the prolonged use of any drug leads to artificial chronic disease, which fulfils the miasmatic criteria.

PHILOSOPHY & MISCONCEPTIONS:

1. HAHNEMANNIAN CONCEPTION: THE ORIGIN OF PSORA: THE ITCH ERUPTION AND ITS SUPPRESSION:

i) "PSORA is the *oldest* miasmatic chronic disease known to us. Just as tedious as syphilis and sycosis, and therefore not to be extinguished before the last breath of the longest human life, unless it is thoroughly cured (*Dr. Banerjea's interpretation: it is quite impossible to fully cure psora and even if it were cured another fresh infection would ensue instantaneously because of its highly infectious nature*), since not even the most robust constitution is able to destroy and extinguish it by its own proper strength, *Psora*, or the Itch disease, is beside this the *oldest* and *most hydra-headed* of all the chronic miasmatic diseases." (Hahnemann's Chronic Diseases).

ii) "The oldest monuments of history, which we possess, show the Psora even then in great development. Moses 3400 years ago pointed out several varieties."

iii) *"Leprosy is similar to an inveterate itch with violent itching. The ancients also mention the peculiar, characteristic voluptuous itching which attended itch then as now, while after the scratching a painful burning follows; among others Plato, who calls itch "glykupikron", while Cicero marks the dulcedo of scabies."* (Hahnemann's Chronic Diseases).

iv) "In consequence of the very much milder form of the Psora during the Fourteenth and Fifteenth centuries, when it appeared as itch, the few pustules appearing after infection made but little show and could easily be concealed. Nevertheless they were scratched continually because of their unbearable itching, and thus the fluid was diffused around, and the Psoric miasma was communicated more certainly and more easily to many other persons the more it was concealed, for the things rendered unclean by the Psoric fluid infected the persons who unwillingly touched them, and thus contaminated far more persons than the lepers, who, on account of their horrible appearance, were carefully avoided." (Hahnemann's Chronic Diseases).

v) Suppression of the 'itch' manifests as follows:

   a) Young people of sanguine temperament develop phthisis.
   b) Generally sanguine persons develop haemorrhoids and renal gravel.
   c) Sanguino-choleric persons develop swelling of the inguinal glands, stiffening of the joints and malignant ulcers.
   d) Obese persons develop catarrh and mucus consumption, inflammatory fever, acute pleurisy and inflammation of the lungs.
   e) Phlegmatic persons develop dropsy and delayed menses.
   f) Melancholic persons may become insane, possibly developing sterility or dying foetus particularly in older women, and deep burning pains in the uterus with cancer of the uterus.

MISCONCEPTION: Do Not Confuse Scabies (Itch) with the Hahnemannian Conception of the Psoric Itch Eruption:

Although many people have assumed Hahnemann to be referring to scabies or itch-mites (e.g. Acarus scabiei or Sarcoptes scabiei hominis) being causally associated with itch and scabies, when he talks of the itch eruption, he never refers to scabies only in relation to psora. This shows clearly that Hahnemann meant something very different by his 'psora' from the ordinary itch (scabies), with which he had been familiar for a long time.

Hahnemann knew of the itch-mite scabious eruption, but never relates in his writings on psora, about its direct association. He mentions other eruptions as representing primary manifestations of the internal psora, and it is obvious that Hahnemann's use of the terms itch, and itch eruption was in a very broad sense (as was in general use at that time), rather than used to describe the specific disease of scabies. This is conclusive evidence that Hahnemann did not associate the itch-mite dependent eruption of scabies with psora.

Dr. Banerjea's Explanatory Logic and Interpretation:

Scabies is not the only state that specifically relates to psora and I have not found any definite evidence that Hahnemann did specifically relate the two. He did however; define psora as characterised by peculiar skin eruptions with an intolerable itch. Itch eruption and psora are therefore different, and we should interpret Hahnemann's writings as follows:

   a) There is something very different in 'psora' compared to the ordinary itch.

   b) Other eruptions represent primary manifestations of internal psora.

   c) The term 'itch' or 'itch eruption' was to be taken in a broad sense (as was in general use at that time), rather than a description of the specific disease of scabies.

2. KENTIAN CONCEPTION: PSORA, THE SPIRITUAL SICKNESS:

i) "If the human race had remained in a state of perfect order, Psora could not have existed".

ii) "It is altogether too extensive, for it goes to the very primitive wrong of the human race, the very first sickness of the human race, that is the *spiritual sickness*, from which first state of the race progressed into what may be called the true susceptibility to psora, which in turn laid the foundation for other diseases. The human race today walking the face of the earth is but little better than a moral leper. To put it another way, everyone is psoric. A new contagion comes with every child. As psora piles up generation after generation, century after century the susceptibility to it increases. This is true of every miasm".

iii) "Man does not seek it, he does not go where it is, he does not associate with those necessarily that have it. He may be exposed; but syphilis is the result of his own action, which is an impure fornication or adulteration which he knows better than to seek, and knows enough from his intelligence to avoid".

iv) "And there is a state prior to it, that state must correspond to that which precedes action, which is thinking and willing".

v) "The will and the understanding are prior to man's action. This is fundamental. The man does not do until he wills; he wills what he carries out."

vi) "The very primitive wrong of the human race, the very first sickness of the human race, that is the *spiritual sickness*. Thinking, willing and acting are the three things that make up the science of the life of the human race".

Initial Immorality → The Primitive Wrong (According to Biblical reference, the bite of the forbidden apple in the garden of Eden)
↓
Spiritual Sickness (which can be referred to Psora)
↓
Thinking → Willing → Acting
resulting in
↓
The manifestation of symptoms which ensues in the following way:

Exciting Causes (excites)
↓
Fundamental Causes
↓
To Explode
↓
Effects (Manifestation of Symptoms)

3. HAHNEMANNIAN & KENTIAN CONCEPTION: PSORA, THE FOUNDATION OF ALL SICKNESS:

i) "Psora has progressed until it has become the most contagious of diseases, because the more complicated it becomes the more susceptible are our children to its beginnings, and its contagion adds to the old disease; and while it goes on, the children become increasingly sensitive to the other miasms". "Psora", says Hahnemann, "became, therefore, the *common mother of man's chronic diseases*. It can be said that *at least seven-eighth's of the chronic maladies existing at the present day are due to Psora*".

ii) "All the diseases of man are built upon psora; hence it is the foundation of sickness; all other sickness came afterwards". (Kent's Philosophy).

iii) "PSORA is that most ancient, most universal, most destructive, and yet most misapprehended chronic miasmatic disease which for many thousands of years has disfigured and tortured mankind, and which during the last centuries has become the mother of all the thousands of incredibly various (acute and) chronic (non-venereal) diseases, by which the whole civilised human race on the inhabited globe is being more and more afflicted". (Hahnemann's Chronic Diseases).

MISCONCEPTION: Psora, The Common Mother

That psora is the common mother of all diseases is an idea totally opposed to Hahnemann's own, yet it is generally taught that psora is the fundamental predisposition, the basic primary cause of all diseases, and that without psora, no illnesses (including syphilis or sycosis), could have developed.

Even Kent holds this view where he writes, "Psora is the beginning of all physical sickness. Had psora never been established as a miasm upon the human race, the other two chronic diseases would have been impossible, and susceptibility to acute diseases would have been impossible. All the diseases of man are built upon psora; hence it is the foundation of all sickness; all other sickness came afterwards".

Dr John H. Allen had views along the same lines and stated that "..... psora is the primary manifestation of primeval sin, of the primary curse, the prophetic fulfilment of thou shalt surely die".

Hahnemann himself however, felt that disease could and did develop in persons totally free of psora, a fact that we must fully comprehend in order to see how this fits into his whole portrait of chronic disease. Hahnemann considered psora itself as a specific disease acquired through infection with the psoric miasm, and that the predisposition to such infection was almost universal. His views that the disposition of being affected with the miasma of the itch is found with almost everyone and under all circumstances are succinctly summed up where he writes, "that no other chronic miasma infects more generally, more surely, more easily and more absolutely than the miasma of itch ... it is the most contagious of all".

Disease can only develop (and manifest) in response to a disease-producing stimulus, regardless of the nature of the stimulus (i.e. chemical, mechanical, dynamic) and such response is dependent on the individual susceptibility to that stimulus. Psora is not a basic predisposition; rather, it is a specific disease, which, in its post-primary stages, results in increased susceptibility (acquired predisposition) of the 'psoric' organism to other more severe and deadly diseases.

"The primary error consisted in regarding psora merely as a dyscrasia or diathesis, as Hahnemann included several of the dyscrasia among the morbid conditions and diseases caused by psora". (Ref. Dr. Stuart Close).

Psora is itself, a disease process and not only a predisposition to disease.

Psora, The Foundation of All Sickness — An inductive Logic:
Dr. Banerjea's Explanatory Logic and Interpretation:

> Diseases could and did develop in people totally free from psora. Hahnemann considered himself to be free from psora but was prone to catching acute epidemic diseases.
> ↓
> Hahnemann stated: "The tendency of being affected or infected with the Psoric Miasm is almost universal, almost sure and mostly everyone and under all circumstances are prone to get infection from the Psoric miasm".
> ↓
> No chronic miasm other than psora infects:
> More generally
> More certainly
> More easily
> More absolutely
> thus psora is the most contagious (a psora-free person may catch the psoric infection at any moment, as it is so contagious and so universal)
> ↓
> So inductive logic, (i.e. inference of a general law from particular instances), clearly demonstrates that according to Hahnemann, psora is most universally present (7/8th or more) amongst almost all diseases
> ↓
> Thus Kent commented that psora was the "Foundation of all sickness"
> ↓
> The common mother of all diseases.

4. ALTHOUGH PSORA CAUSES SUSCEPTIBILITY TO SICKNESS IT IS NOT ONLY A DYSCRASIA BUT A DISEASE PROCESS ITSELF:

i) There must have been some sickness prior to this state, which we recognise as the susceptibility. Therefore, susceptibility is that state prior to any miasmatic or diseased condition, which creates the circumstances suitable for miasmatic or disease force to enter and thrive in the constitution.

ii) *"The three chronic miasms, psora, syphilis and sycosis, are all contagious. In each instance there is something prior to the manifestations, which we call disease. We speak of the signs and symptoms of a disease, we speak of the outcroppings of the symptoms when we speak of syphilis, but remember there is a state prior to syphilis or syphilis would not exist. It could not come upon man except for a condition suitable to its development. In like manner psora could not exist except for a condition in mankind suitable for its development".* (Kent's Philosophy).

Hahnemann's Self-Contradiction: He Was Free From Psora but Prone to Acute Ailments:
Dr. Banerjea's Explanatory Logic and Interpretation:

Susceptibility & Psora: Hahnemann seems to contradict himself when he writes in Chronic Diseases (footnote to page 90), "...It was more easy for me, than for many hundreds of others, to find out and so recognise the signs of the psora as well when latent and as yet slumbering within, as it has grown to considerable chronic diseases, by an accurate comparison of the state of health of all such persons with myself, who, as is seldom the case, has never been afflicted with psora and who has, therefore, from my birth even until now in my eightieth year, been entirely free from (smaller and greater) ailments, enumerated here and further below, although I have been, on the whole, very apt to catch acute epidemic diseases; and have been exposed to many mental exertions and thousand fold vexations of spirit...".

Hahnemann admits then, though indirectly, that there is a state of predisposition prior to infection with the psoric miasm, and seems to distinguish between two kinds of susceptibility on the part of the human being: susceptibility to acute, and susceptibility to chronic infections. Unfortunately he fails to develop his contention, and we must conclude that psora is not only a diathesis or dyscrasia but also a diseased condition in itself. It is the beginning of the morbid dynamic alteration of the vital force, manifesting in and through the organism as altered sensations and functions which may be too trivial to incapacitate someone from following their daily activities and may allow them to consider themselves healthy and to be supposed so by others.

Hahnemann considered the psoric state as a diseased state, which develops following infection with the miasm and held that the miasm was certainly not synonymous with the resultant disease. I have in this text demonstrated Hahnemann's use of the term miasm as an extrinsically derived infecting agent; and that, such views, which represent the foundations of microbiology, were first proposed by Hahnemann, even before the 'discoveries' of Robert Koch.

Homoeopathy has always taught (and modern medicine more recently) that such agents do not 'cause' disease, rather they can only produce (stimulate) disease if the person is susceptible to react in a diseased way to that stimulus. The miasms (infecting agents) have mostly been seen as the cause of disease whilst Hahnemann refers to them as producing (stimulating) a diseased response of the organism through their influence on the life mechanism (vital force).

Psora: is not a Predisposition but a Disease in Itself:
Dr. Banerjea's Explanatory Logic and Interpretation:

```
Infecting Agent (Miasm)
         ↓
Infection with psoric miasm
(extrinsically derived infecting agent)
         ↓
Infectious nature of disease taught first by Hahnemann
         ↓
Person who is susceptible to react in a 'dis-eased' way to that stimulus
         ↓
Resultant disease
         ↓
Named psora
         ↓
In its 'post-primary stages' causes increased susceptibility
(as psora relates to 'hypo', so psora creates hypo-immunity and
that in turn results in hyper-susceptibility)
         ↓
Causes increased predisposition to catch infection
         ↓
So, psora is a disease process which creates an increased predisposition to catch infection
(Hypersensitivity of psora)
```

Stuart Close (Ref. Homoeopathic Philosophy, Pg. 94) is also of the opinion that "the primary error consisted in regarding psora as merely a dyscrasia or diathesis, which is directly opposed to what Hahnemann taught as we now understand it. Instead of regarding Psora as a dyscrasia Hahnemann included several of the dyscrasias among the morbid conditions and diseases caused by psora".

So, Hahnemann calls himself 'Free from Psora' (Pg. 90: F.N. Chronic Diseases) but states that he had the dyscrasia/predisposition to catch acute epidemic diseases. There must therefore be a prior state/predisposition to getting infected with the psoric miasm; and we can conclude that psora is not only a dyscrasia but the diseased condition itself, the beginning of the morbid dynamic alteration of the vital force.

The Prior State or Predisposition is the Susceptibility:
Dr. Banerjea's Explanatory Logic and Interpretation:

> Hahnemann states that he was never afflicted with psora
> ↓
> Whereas he was very apt to catch acute epidemic diseases
> ↓
> So there was a predisposition or dyscrasia in Hahnemann to his catching acute epidemic diseases, though he considered himself free from Psora! But actually he wasn't, as he had that susceptibility to catch infection or acute epidemic diseases, therefore he had lowered immunity, which could have been caused by Psora
> ↓
> Susceptibility is the predisposition, which leads to these infections.
> ↓
> This susceptibility invites psoric disease
> (but whether susceptibility comes first in the body or the psora, that's a "chicken or the egg" question!) Therefore susceptibility can also be inherent.
> ↓
> So psora is not only a dyscrasia but a disease in itself, and tendency to catch infection is one of the manifestation of its diseased state
> ↓
> Therefore, those suffering from psora have increased susceptibility to catch infections
> ↓
> Because psora creates the deficiency in the organism
> ↓
> This deficiency is reflected as lowered immunity (as psora relates to 'hypo'; so psora creates hypo-immunity and that in turn results in hyper-susceptibility)
> ↓
> Thus the patient develops more susceptibility and is prone to catch infections.

Susceptibility is the pre-disposition to invite or be susceptible to change or influence. When life is given or begins there is a pre-structure, which allows it to change, along with processes known as LIFE. Life processes include creation, maintenance and destruction according to the Law of Nature, which are clearly experienced and visible. Susceptibility means vulnerability as opposed to resistance. There is vulnerability to the influences of life processes, which is inevitable. Although a certain amount of resistance is possible, eventually signs of vulnerability or susceptibility become evident, e.g. ageing. It is inevitable that a baby, given appropriate condition, grows into maturity, and then maturity develops into old age. Within the inevitable life cycle there is susceptibility to other influences. One such influence is the miasm psora. Due to its highly infectious nature, any life form (in this case human) will become infected with psora, increasing the vulnerability and influences including emotional, environmental and disease. This infectious psoric influence superimposes onto the already susceptible being and creates another level of vulnerability. Hahnemann explained this as the groove or sigma in the life element, which invites the disease process. It was later that psora was defined specifically by other homoeopaths.

5. PSORA: GENERALLY MANIFESTS FUNCTIONAL DISORDERS BUT CAN ALSO RESULT IN STRUCTURAL CHANGES:

i) A common misunderstanding about the miasmatic theory is that specific pathological condition result from specific miasms. For example, it is often said that eczema is a psoric disease, ulcers are syphilitic, and that cancer, psoriasis and others result from a combination of all three miasms. *In reality, however, all three miasms can result in any pathological change. Cancer, diabetes, insanity, imbecility etc., can all arise from the last stage of any of the miasms, or from any combination of them.*

MISCONCEPTION: Psora is Only a Functional Disease:

Hahnemann listed even the "largest sarcomatous tumours" in the pathology produced in the tertiary stage of psora, together with many other severe, destructive and proliferative disorders.

Largest Sarcomatous Tumour Under Psora in its Tertiary Stage:
Dr. Banerjea's Explanatory Logic and Interpretation:

Primary Psora (Original skin lesion)
↓
Suppressed
↓
Latent Psora
↓
Secondary Psora:
Disharmony of life in the organs reflected in the functional plane
↓
Tertiary Psora:
Gross structural changes in the tissues
(the domain of pathology proper and nosology)
↓
It follows that the Hahnemannian listing under psora of even the 'Largest Sarcomatous Tumours', are apparent at this tertiary stage.

---

6. PSORA LIKE OTHER FUNDAMENTAL MIASMS, TRANSMITS GENERATION TO GENERATION: HERIDITORY TRANSMISSION:

i) "The oldest history of the oldest nation does not reach its origin. Moreover, it is hydra-headed and persists through the last breath of the longest life. Not even the most robust constitution, by its own unaided efforts, is able to annihilate and extinguish psora". (Hahnemann's Chronic Diseases).

ii) "PSORA is that most ancient, most universal, most destructive, and yet most misapprehended chronic miasmatic disease which for many thousands of years has disfigured and tortured mankind, and which during the last centuries has become the mother of all the thousands of incredibly various acute and chronic (non-venereal) diseases, by which the whole civilised human race on the inhabited globe is being more and more afflicted". (Hahnemann's Chronic Diseases).

iii) "PSORA is the *oldest* miasmatic chronic disease known to us. Just as tedious as syphilis and sycosis, and therefore not to be extinguished before the last breath of the longest human life, unless it is thoroughly cured (*Dr. Banerjea's interpretation: it is quite impossible to fully cure psora and even if it were cured another fresh infection would ensue instantaneously because of its highly infectious nature*), since not even the most robust constitution is able to destroy and extinguish it by its own proper strength, *Psora*, or the Itch disease, is beside this the *oldest* and *most hydra-headed* of all the chronic miasmatic diseases." (Hahnemann's Chronic Diseases).

iv) "In the many thousands of years during which it may have afflicted mankind, for the most ancient history of the most ancient people does not reach to its origin, it has so much increased in the extent of its pathological manifestations — an extent which may to some degree be explained by its increased development during such an inconceivable number of years in so many millions of organisms through which it has passed, that its secondary symptoms are hardly to be numbered". (Hahnemann's Chronic Diseases).

MISCONCEPTION: Spontaneous Hereditary Transmission of Psora:

The Hereditary Transmission of Psora is not automatic but through infection only:

The psoric taint cannot be automatically transmitted from parent to child
↓
The transmission of psora from mother to child is possible and does happen
↓
Almost generally, surely, easily and absolutely
↓
As psora is highly contagious
↓
When the mother has psora (infected with psoric miasm and having psoric disease)
↓
The foetus-in-utero (if it is susceptible to receive such psoric infection) will almost surely and absolutely be infected with psora from the mother
↓
So, there are two preconditions which are essential for transmission:
(i) Susceptibility to receive such infection
(ii) Infection with a psoric miasm
↓
Thus the psora, the ancient highly infecting agent, has gradually been passed on through some hundreds of generations (Ref. §81).

---

7. DYNAMIC PATHOLOGY:

i) As dynamic action implies the process whereby one substance is acted off by another substance without communication or actual interchange of the material parts of the substances concerned but rather qualitatively through the qualities inherent in them; so infection is a biological process whereby a living organism is acted upon qualitatively by another living being without communication or interchange of material parts of the beings concerned.

ii) The interaction between a living body with another living one or with a thing falls under a separate category, which is described positively by the term 'dynamic action'.

iii) Modern physiology, pathology and especially bacteriology are busy with discovering the chemico-physical processes underlying this dynamic process in cases of infection by bacteria; and they are equally busy with the discovery of chemico-physical processes underlying each vital process and function. That is why, when Hahnemann asserted that all diseases other than surgical or occupational are of the nature of infection he was stating that in every case of illness, the vital principle of the individual is qualitatively (and not mechanically or chemico-physically) acted on by the exogenous morbific agents and their corresponding dynamic miasmatic force (which is inimical to vital force); and this qualitative derangement of the vital force is described by Hahnemann as the dynamic derangement of the organism manifested by the totality of altered sensation and functions. The dynamic property of a medicine implies this special quality inherent in the medicine by virtue of which, it brings about dynamic derangement of the living organism.

PART – II
MIASMATIC PRESCRIBING:
MIASMATIC DIAGNOSTIC CLASSIFICATIONS

MIASMATIC DIAGNOSIS:
COMPARISON OF THE MENTAL SYMPTOMS

Key Word	*Inconsistent Psoric Mind*	*Avaricious Sycotic Mind*	*Destructive Syphilitic Mind*	*Dissatisfied Tubercular Mind*
1. Introduction	Diversion, perversion and reprobation of the mind to commit evil are the primary manifestations of psora. For this reason the psoric mind is always outwardly manifesting and there can be no deep mental concentration, meditation or sacred thoughts. The 'hypo' psoric state is manifested in the mental sphere as hypo-reasoning, i.e. inconsistent, impractical thoughts and hypo-confidence that results in anxieties and all varieties of fears. Anxiety, inconsistent thoughts, apprehension (especially of impending misfortune) and alertness are therefore the basic criteria of the psoric mind.	The Sycotic taint develops the worst forms of debasement because of its basic suspicion and jealousy. It has the tendency to harm others, even animals (especially mentally in the form of mental torture). Sycotic mental symptoms are either 'hyper', or characterised by incoordination. Examples are: hyper-workaholics, hyper-greedy (avaricious) & hyper-rageous types and those showing an incoordination in behavior like jealousy and/or suspicion. A tendency to exploit may also be present.	The syphilitic miasm has a destructive mentality, which perverts, deforms and vitiates the senses of judgement, the memory and the sharpness of the intellect. The patient can neither realise the symptoms nor can he explain them to the physician. In any such case where the patient cannot explain his symptoms, describe their character, or iterate his desires and aversions, the syphilitic stigmata will be present. Syphilitic mental symptoms are characterised by destruction and even love for one's own life is destroyed leading to suicidal tendencies. There are impulses towards destruction and violence.	Dissatisfaction and lack of tolerance are the innate dyscrasias of the tubercular stigmata. Lack of tolerance leads to anger and irritability, which in time results in depression. The dissatisfied state of the mind makes him changeable both mentally and physically and manifests in the following manners: Persons can never be satisfied in a certain job or place, or with a certain subject or situation. Children desire this or that, especially toys, but when offered, they out rightly reject them and demand something new. Students frequently change their subjects — perhaps studying

41

Key Word	Inconsistent Psoric Mind	Avaricious Sycotic Mind	Destructive Syphilitic Mind	Dissatisfied Tubercular Mind
				science for some time and then changing to arts.
				People continuously desire new jewellery and clothes. They are always finding new passions and cravings, and never find peace or satisfaction in any one object.
				Persons crave and have perversions (this perversion is afforded by the syphilitic component of the tubercular miasm) for the things that will harm them, wanting for example, foods which aggravate their condition.
				Dissatisfaction resulting in changeability is the innate dyscrasia of tubercular miasm.
2. Thoughts & Flow of Words	The psoric attitude towards religion is deceitful and the patient appears as a feigning philosopher due to his inability to concentrate.	This miasm produces the worst forms of cruelty and in this respect is similar to the syphilitic miasm. However, with sycosis there is also cunning deceit and the worst form of manias of all the stigmatas. Men and women who commit suicide are mainly syphilo-sycotic.	Destruction, perversion, dissolution or degeneration are the most significant characteristics of syphilis.	A lack of concentration, and thoughtlessness regarding appearance is representative of the tubercular miasm.
	There may be a passionate craving or indulgence to obtain unnecessary objects and a tendency to build castles in the air!	Sycosis is the most mischievous of all the miasms.	Syphilitics are generally close mouthed and may answer in monosyllables. They lack ideas, expressions and thoughts due to destruction of the intellectual capabilities.	
	Thoughts and words overflow in the mind, and accordingly, words are multiplied.	Sycosis cannot find the right	Suicidal planning and thoughts are syphilo-sycotic but when suicides are committed without	

Key Word	Inconsistent Psoric Mind	Avaricious Sycotic Mind	Destructive Syphilitic Mind	Dissatisfied Tubercular Mind
		words and if he does, he is not sure whether they are right. He has doubts about his spelling and experiences difficulty in narrating his symptoms.	any planning and in a manner devoid of intelligence then the syphilitic miasm is evident on the surface. All the fascists and exploiters of the world are the product of syphilis.	
3. Awareness	Psoric patients are mentally alert, and are quick and active in their motions. They will work like 'Trojans' for a short time, but become easily fatigued both mentally and physically and a profound prostration follows. The fatigue is accompanied by the desire to lie down and extreme fatigue restrains them from performing their duties. Heat of the whole body follows mental impressions or exertions. The patient is sensitive to odours and atmospheric changes and is easily disturbed mentally.	Sycotic patients are always suspicious, a taint which can manifest in a variety of ways. They may be suspicious of their surroundings and of other people. They are even suspicious of their own work and do not trust themselves to the extent that they must go back and repeat what they have previously done or said, and wonder if they have said just what they mean. This suspicion when turned upon others, leads to the worst forms of jealousy. They may be jealous of both their family and friends. In the case of injury, the patient themselves will examine the site of the lesion very carefully and frequently and keep changing physicians.	Mentally dull, heavy, stupid and especially stubborn. Idiocy, ignorance and obstinacy lead to melancholia and gloominess. Mentally slow to react, and if reading for example, they can read only a few lines, which they must read again to fully comprehend. What they read they cannot retain — a kind of mental paralysis.	Tubercular children manifest their traits in the extreme. They may be either slow or dull and experience difficulties in comprehension or they may be very bright, intelligent and alert.

Key Word	Inconsistent Psoric Mind	Avaricious Sycotic Mind	Destructive Syphilitic Mind	Dissatisfied Tubercular Mind
4. Anxiety	Psoric patients are anxious to the point of worry and fear. Anxiety on awakening in the morning which may at times compel them to move about.	Anxiety from changes in the weather and from humidity typifies the sycotic patient.	In syphilis, anxiety occurs at night.	The mental changeability and dissatisfaction of the tubercular patient ends in a depressed state of mind which is striking in the fact that even in this depressed state there is a total absence of disappointment, hopelessness, anxiety or apprehension. Tubercular patients do not worry about anything, even when suffering from the most severe ailments
5. Cruelty	Real cruelty is not typical of the psoric mentality, but there can exist deceitful behaviour with a tendency to make others appear foolish.	Cruelty, mostly in the form of mental tortures, lack of affection, rudeness and vexation are all present in sycosis. Anger from trifles may lead to physical assault. The sycotic patient tries to hurt others emotionally. Sycosis is also present in such instances as where a family suffers because the mother cannot accept her daughter-in-law, and in businesses where employer/employee relations are regularly strained.	Syphilitics are the cold-blooded murderers, the committed criminals and iconoclasts. Physical destruction, bodily assaults, killings and physical tortures are the product of syphilis.	Some cruelty may exist in the tubercular miasm due either to the patient's innate dissatisfaction or from the tubercular combination of psora and syphilis. Tubercular children may exhibit some features of cruelty through physical and mental torture of their friends and/or siblings.

Key Word	Inconsistent Psoric Mind	Avaricious Sycotic Mind	Destructive Syphilitic Mind	Dissatisfied Tubercular Mind
6. Fears	Almost all the fears have a psoric base and these fears manifest as anxiety. Psoric patients are easily frightened, often by trivial things, which lead to trembling and perspiration followed by great weakness. In children there may be fear of darkness, fear of strangers, fear of many fictitious things and fear of animals. They are timid about going to school and their fears become so intrinsically interwoven into their lives that very soon they wear themselves out and become thoroughly exhausted. As a result, mental growth becomes stunted and this in turn affects their physical growth. Adult fears include a fear of death on becoming ill, fear of incurable diseases and fear that they will be unable to accomplish what they attempt. There also occurs sudden anxiety in the region of the heart, particularly when stomach conditions are present.	Sycotic fears are manifested outwardly. There is a fear of making mistakes, so the sycotic patient repeatedly checks what they have done.	The syphilitic patient fears people and conversation due to their own dullness and idiocy. Their gloominess is manifested through anxiety and apprehension and fear is manifested through anguish.	The tubercular miasm is generally fearless although there is an innate fear of dogs.

Key Word	Inconsistent Psoric Mind	Avaricious Sycotic Mind	Destructive Syphilitic Mind	Dissatisfied Tubercular Mind
7. Memory	As psora is 'hypo' in its manifestation so it shows as a weakness of memory.	There is absentmindedness and abstraction of thought in sycosis. A general loss of memory, losing the thread of the conversation, forgetting words and sentences and the previous line just read are characteristic of sycotic incoordination. They often forget recent events but can remember the events of distant past. There may also be momentary loss of thought and slowness of speech.	Syphilitic patients lack a sense of duty and responsibility and often fail to perform family duties due to impaired memory. There is also a lack of self-confidence. Love of one's own life is a natural instinct of man, but the syphilitic patient, due to impaired memory, a lack of self confidence and self-awareness believes there is no way left other than to commit suicide. Syphilis shows forgetfulness and a total destruction of memory. Arithmetical calculation is difficult.	Memory problems, especially in children, result from a lack of tolerance and manifest as a difficulty in comprehension and retaining facts. They are often labelled as problem children, due to their lack of patience and tolerance and their inability or slowness to comprehend. They find it difficult to try again and there is a continued dissatisfaction. On the other hand, tubercular children can also be very bright and show great keenness of intellect.
8. Social Interaction	There is an aversion to people and company, especially unknown people. However, the psoric patient also dreads being alone. Roams in deserted places.	Sycotics are the extroverts but in all cases of deprivation and rudeness sycosis is present. It is the most mischievous of all the miasms for its jealousy, exploiting nature and tendency to mentally torture others. Despite their extrovert nature, sycotic patients show a lack of self-confidence in social interactions.	Syphilitic patients are introvert and have a great desire to escape from both themselves and from others people. Their desire for solitude and aversion to company can lead to suicidal tendencies. Syphilitics lack self-confidence and do not trust others. Due to dullness of intellect, loses the thread of conversation and lacks perception.	Tubercular patients sometimes appear as morose and sullen. They do not like receiving advice from others, especially with regards to their health.

Key Word	Inconsistent Psoric Mind	Avaricious Sycotic Mind	Destructive Syphilitic Mind	Dissatisfied Tubercular Mind
			Syphilitics are close-mouthed and do not worry their friends with their troubles. They regard both the death of an individual and the explosion of a nuclear bomb over a town as appropriate.	
9. Restlessness	Mental restlessness to achieve unnecessary objects is one of the primary manifestations of psora. Psoric anxiety and fears give way to mental restlessness and in turn the patient feels compelled to move about. Psoric patients are not direct thinkers except for a very short time. Thoughts come thick and fast so that they entangle them and they cannot maintain a particular train of thought for any length of time. This mental restlessness causes them to complain they want to do something but they do not know what they want to do. Activities are both started and ended in a dramatic way. Psoric restlessness is particularly noticeable at the new moon and in the case of	The restlessness and dissatisfaction present in this stigmata manifest in a more physical form. Sycotic patients frequently change their posture and cannot keep quiet or still.	Mental restlessness (a psoric component must also be present) drives the patient out of bed and induces symptoms of suicide. Restlessness can be great but is devoid of any realisation or understanding.	Dissatisfaction is the innate dyscrasia of this miasm, which results in changeableness and a restlessness, manifested both mentally and physically. Tubercular patients move home frequently and move from place to place or from town to town, travelling even when strength does not permit. They change occupation, doctors, even their furniture and the arrangements of their rooms, always with a constant desire to do something differently. This constant changeableness results in mental fatigue, which in turn manifests as an apathetic, indifferent state of mind. The patient may, without notice, up and leave to live as a vagrant due to their dissatisfaction with everyday life and the policies of the world. They can be seen

Key Word	Inconsistent Psoric Mind	Avaricious Sycotic Mind	Destructive Syphilitic Mind	Dissatisfied Tubercular Mind
	women, at the approach of the menses. A peculiar characteristic of the mental irritation is that it produces a sense of bodily heat and these patients have flushes of heat while working.			sagging down on pavement with fatigue but will jump up on seeing a dog.
10. Attitude	The psoric miasm shows a selfishness and lack of human conscience. Patients may internally be extremely selfish, but on the outside appear to be very liberal. Rich people, for example, may hide their wealth by dressing down and shrewd people may pretend to be religious and make huge charitable donations. Hide and seek is in the nature of psora. Psoric patients have a tendency to dishonesty and secretiveness; wickedness and impurity will be present.	Sycotic patients have a suspicious attitude towards their surroundings, their family and friends and even to their own work. They are jealous and as a result want to commit detriment and mental torture to other people. Sycotics are the fascists and exploiters of the world. They are possessive and selfish people with a tendency to conceal.	Syphilitics are close-mouthed, melancholic individuals who are continually depressed and constantly dwell on suicide. They are merciless in nature and have no sympathy for anything, including themselves. An urge for destruction seems to be their only emotion. The syphilitic patient lacks a sense of duty and therefore appears unconcerned about their family and relations. However, this is due to the destruction of their sense of realisation, intellect and memory meaning that they cannot realise their duties.	The careless, apathetic, indifferent attitude of the tubercular patient is a reflection of their desire for self-destruction and a suicidal impulse is manifested through this general indifference. They are unconcerned with, or indifferent towards the seriousness of sufferings, and if the suffering is their own, they are always hopeful of recovery. The unrestrained, uncontrollable passions of life, such as masturbation, artificial loss of semen and perverted cravings for sex are adopted by this patient, leading to great debility and the way to an early grave. These unrestrained passions are also characterised by indifference to every thing.

Key Word	Inconsistent Psoric Mind	Avaricious Sycotic Mind	Destructive Syphilitic Mind	Dissatisfied Tubercular Mind
11. Intellect	Thoughts seem to vanish whilst reading and writing. The psoric patient seems unable to control their thoughts, which sometimes seem to disappear altogether.	Sycosis shows an abstraction of memory and an incoordination in thoughts and perceptions.	In the syphilitic miasm, destruction of the intellectual capabilities results in total forgetfulness and a loss of sense of realisation.	With the manifestation of tubercular polarities comes a state of opposites where patients may be either intellectually sharp or totally dull.
12. Behaviour	Indolent patients with an aversion to working and bathing are psoric. They lack discipline, are untidy in appearance and averse to keeping things clean. Time goes either too fast or too slow.	The sycotic patient is always thinking about their own ailments and has difficulty in remaining under the treatment of one physician alone. However, there is also a tendency to suppress their ailments or symptoms. Their behaviour reflects their basic suspicious, jealous, quarrelsome, mischievous, selfish, rude, mean-minded and concealing nature.	The close-mouthed syphilitics are merciless, destructive and violent in their behaviour. Children's minds remain immature and they have a fear of strangers.	Tubercular patients are apt to behave in an indifferent, dissatisfied, changeable, careless or fearless manner. They do not like advice in regards to their health or diet due to their innate dissatisfaction and desire for change.
13. Temperament	Psora shows a change of temperament without any apparent cause. Young people particularly become hysterical especially after acute weakening diseases. Fits of anger alternate with a tearful mood but with this anger there is seldom any desire to harm others. The fits are usually accompanied with trembling followed by great prostration (+++) after which they may	In sycosis, the slightest change of temperature reflects as changes in the mind. Anger is aggravated by changes of weather, particularly from thunderstorms and the sycotic miasm is aptly termed as 'the living barometer'.	Syphilis has fixed ideas, which are not eradicated by any amount of talk or explanations. Perversion and destruction of the intellectual functions result in obstinacy as a marked result of fixed idea and in fixed moods. Depression is always present but syphilitic patients keep their troubles to themselves and sulk	The tubercular patient is extremely irritable and fearful and even becomes frightened and disgusted when looking at their own image. This further fuels their innate desire for change. Patients may be extremely outrageous, foolhardy and impatient which results in quarrelsomeness (syco-tubercular).

Key Word	Inconsistent Psoric Mind	Avaricious Sycotic Mind	Destructive Syphilitic Mind	Dissatisfied Tubercular Mind
	remain sick for quite some time. Psoric patients suffer from a depression of spirits in which they burst out crying to relieve the condition. When in this state, everyone knows of their troubles, as they are unaccustomed to silent grief. However, some psoric patients become so depressed that they are unable to speak. There is a changeableness in psora although the tubercular stigma is usually behind when changeability is manifested to such a large extent. The psoric patient is a chronic complainer, never satisfied with the conditions in their lives.		over them. They remain immersed in melancholia and depression, which leads to an anxious state in which they prefer to be in solitude. Syphilitics are the cold-blooded iconoclasts.	Mental symptoms, especially anger, are worse after sleep and the patient may wake with a feeling of dissatisfaction clearly visible on their face.
14. Criminality	Feigning, deceitful philosopher types are the product of psora.	Sycosis in combination with psora is the basis of most criminal insanities.	A combination of syphilis and sycosis results in sullen, smouldering patients, threatening to break out into dangerous behaviour at any time.	The fearless tubercular patient is unconcerned and indifferent but willing to take risks and undertake ventures.

Key Word	Inconsistent Psoric Mind	Avaricious Sycotic Mind	Destructive Syphilitic Mind	Dissatisfied Tubercular Mind
15. Manias	Psora, with all its anxieties and fears is very likely to develop some manias.	In sycosis there are many manias, which are all, characterised by underlying suspicion. E.g. the patient may check the room again and again to see that no one is hiding behind the cupboard or they may check the lock repeatedly. They may also repeat the same word or sentence, thinking that others cannot understand them, even to the extent of returning to an acquaintance after they have just parted to ensure that they were correctly understood.	Syphilis is characterised by violent and destructive rages and manias.	Even the manias of the tubercular miasm are changeable and patients may change such things as ornaments, clothes, curtains, occupations, household furniture and the arrangement and decor of the room.
16. Modalities	The psoric patient is ameliorated by natural discharges and from the appearance of suppressed skin conditions.	Sycotic mental conditions are aggravated by changes in the weather and humidity and much ameliorated when warts or fibrous growths appear or when old ulcers or sores break open. There is a marked amelioration of all symptoms by the return of suppressed gonorrhoeal manifestations.	In syphilis, the mental symptoms are aggravated at night and ameliorated by unnatural discharges.	All tubercular mental symptoms are aggravated by thunderstorms and ameliorated in open air.

MIASMATIC DIAGNOSIS:
COMPARISON OF CHARACTERISTICS AND NATURE

Key Word	Psora *Sensitising Miasm*	Sycosis *Miasm of Incoordination*	Syphilis *Degenerating Miasm*	Tubercular *Responsive, Reactive Miasm*
1. General Manifestations	i) Psora develops itch.	i) Sycosis develops catarrhal discharges.	i) The syphilitic miasm has virulent open ulcers.	i) The tubercular miasm has haemorrhages.
	ii) Unhealthy skin with burning and itching represents psora.	ii) Oily skin with thickly oozing and copious perspiration, represents sycosis.	ii) Ulcerated skin with pus and blood represents syphilis.	ii) Oily skin with coldness represents the tubercular miasm.
	iii) All 'hypos' are mainly psoric.	iii) 'Hypers' are sycotic.	iii) 'Dyses' are syphilitic.	iii) Allergies are tubercular.
	iv) Hypoplasia is psoric.	iv) Hyperplasia is sycotic.	iv) Dysplasia is syphilitic.	iv) Alternation of 'hypo' and dysplasia is tubercular.
	v) Atrophy, ataxia, anaemia and anoxaemia are psoric.	v) Hypertrophy is sycotic.	v) Dystrophy is syphilitic.	v) Dystrophy with haemorrhage is tubercular.
	vi) Hypotension is psoric.	vi) Hypertension is sycotic.	vi) Irregular, arrhythmic pulse is syphilitic.	vi) Intermittent pulse is tubercular.
	vii) Lack, scanty, less and absence denote psora.	vii) Exaggeration or excess denotes sycosis.	vii) Destruction and degeneration denote syphilis.	vii) Alternation and periodicity is tubercular.
	viii) Weakness is psoric.	viii) Restlessness (especially physical) is sycotic.	viii) Destructiveness is syphilitic.	viii) Changeableness is tubercular.
	ix) An inhibitory tendency is psoric.	ix) An expressive tendency is sycotic.	ix) Melancholic, depressive and suicidal tendencies are syphilitic.	ix) A dissatisfied tendency is tubercular.

Key Word	Psora Sensitising Miasm	Sycosis Miasm of Incoordination	Syphilis Degenerating Miasm	Tubercular Responsive, Reactive Miasm
	x) Dryness of membranes denotes psora.	x) Augmented secretion denotes sycosis.	x) Ulceration denotes syphilis.	x) Haemorrhages and allergies denote the tubercular miasm.
	xi) Psora does not assimilate well.	xi) Sycotics are over-nourished.	xi) Syphilitics have disorganised digestion.	xi) Tubercular types crave the things which make them sick.
	xii) The secretions of psora are serous.	xii) Sycotic secretions are purulent.	xii) Syphilitic secretions are sticky, acrid and putrid.	xii) Tubercular secretions are haemorrhagic.
2. General Nature of the Miasm	Hyper-sensitivity (basically psora is 'hypo' in expression which leads to low immunity resulting in hyper-susceptibility. This manifests as an exalted sensitivity to external allergens and environment). Itching, irritation and burning lead towards congestion and inflammation with only functional changes. The capacity to produce hypersensitivity or in other words the sensitising property of psora is the basic nature. By dint of this property it makes the organism susceptible to all sorts of environmental conditions and diseases, as well as to allergens.	Sycosis produces incoordination everywhere, resulting in over-production, growth and infiltration in the form of warts, condylomata, tumours and fibrous tissues etc.	Syphilis produces destructive disorder, which manifests as perversion, suppuration, ulceration and fissures.	The tubercular miasm produces changing symptomatology and confusing vague symptoms (e.g. dyspepsia, weakness, wasting and fever). Manifestations are variable, shifting in location, alternating in state and contradictory.

		Psora Sensitising Miasm	Sycosis Miasm Of Incoordination	Syphilis Degenerating Miasm	Tubercular Responsive, Reactive Miasm
3.	Key Words and Expressions	Hypo-immunity. Anxiety. Apprehension. Alertness. Fears. Irritation—mental and physical. Sensitivity.	'Hyper' — mental and physical. Hypertrophy; growths; incoordinations.	Destruction — physical and mental. Degeneration. Necrosis and ulceration. Putridity and acidity. 'Dyses'. Irregular; arrhythmia.	Dissatisfaction. Alternation; changeability; migratory. Periodic. Recurrence. Allergic. Vague manifestations. Craves the things which make them sick.
4.	Diathesis	i) Eruptive diathesis.	i) Rheumatic and gouty. ii) Lithic and uric acid. iii) Proliferative diathesis.	i) Suppurative or ulcerative diathesis.	i) Scrofulous diathesis. ii) Haemorrhagic diathesis. iii) Allergic diathesis.
5.	Organs and Tissues Affected	Ectodermal tissues. Nervous system, endocrine system, blood vessels, liver and skin.	Entodermal and soft tissues. Attacks internal organs, pelvis and sexual organs, and the blood (producing anaemia).	Mesodermal tissues. Soft tissues and bones; glandular tissues particularly the lymphatics.	Glandular tissue. Patient is poor in bone, flesh and blood.
6.	Nature of Diseases	i) Deficiency disorders.	i) Deposition and/or proliferation of cells/tissues.	i) Destructive, degenerative disorders, deformities, fragility.	i) Depletion. ii) Drainage and wastage. iii) Alternating disorders.
7.	Pace of Action	i) Hyperactive. ii) Dramatic development of symptoms.	i) Extremely slow, insidious. ii) Silent or even surreptitious in its manifestations.	i) Usually midway in pace, i.e. moderate. Though sometimes rapid and/or sometimes can be insidious. ii) Generally more overt in its manifestations.	i) Depends according to preponderance of psoric or syphilitic miasm.

	Key Word	Psora Sensitising Miasm	Sycosis Miasm of Incoordination	Syphilis Degenerating Miasm	Tubercular Responsive, Reactive Miasm
8.	Constitution	Carbonitrogenoid (excess of carbon and nitrogen).	Hydrogenoid (excess of water).	Oxygenoid (excess of oxygen).	Changeable constitution with alternation and periodicity.
9.	Psychic Manifestations				
	a) The person	The sterile philosopher who has lots of ideas but cannot materialise them. Theoretical persons with no sense of practicality at all. Dishonesty, secretiveness, wickedness and impurity play a large part in the pscric nature.	Deceitful, sullen, cunning persons are sycotic. They are very practical, have a tendency to exploit others and care only for their own benefit and pleasures.	Syphilitic persons seem to have one emotion only–the urge for destruction. They lack any sense of realisation, duty and understanding. Syphilitics are the committed criminals and cold-blooded murderers. They suffer from a vitiated mentality, which impairs their sense of judgement.	The tubercular person is always dissatisfied and changeable. They display both a lack of tolerance and of perseverance.
	b) The nature of the miasm and the person	Psora is the sensitising miasm in that, hyperactivity and hypersensitivity of the mind and body result from increased susceptibility due to hypo-immunity.	Sycosis is the miasm of 'hyper' and incoordinations. These 'hyper' states result in abnormal behaviours and mental incoordinations such as extreme jealousy, loquacity and selfishness.	The destructive syphilitic patient has no love for their own life and either destroys themselves or kills others. They can be both suicidal and cold-blooded murderers. Syphilitics lack mercy and sympathy and may be called iconoclasts.	The changeable tubercular miasm results in dissatisfied patients who are changeable both mentally and physically.
	c) Work	Quickly fatigued with a desire to lie down is characteristic of the psoric miasm. Patients may also be indolent.	Sycotics are hyper-workaholics.	Syphilitic patients show no interest in work due to their lack of realisation and understanding.	The changeable, impatient tubercular types are unable to concentrate on work.

Key Word	Psora Sensitising Miasm	Sycosis Miasm of Incoordination	Syphilis Degenerating Miasm	Tubercular Responsive, Reactive Miasm
d) Behaviour	Psora is fearful, anxious, alert and apprehensive. Nervous persons are psoric.	Sycosis is quarrelsome, jealous, selfish and cunning with a tendency to harm (emotionally) others and to harm animals. The sycotic patient may be ostentatious and fatuous, suspicious of his own work and surroundings. Mischievousness, meanness, and selfishness summarise the essence of sycosis.	Syphilis is cruel, destructive and perverted and may do harm to themselves or others.	Fearlessness and an absolute lack of anxiety are denominating features of the tubercular miasm. Patients are careless, unconcerned and indiffrent about the seriousness of their sufferings and always hopeful of recovery.
e) Memory	Weakness of memory indicates psora.	Absentmindedness is sycotic. Patients lose the thread of the conversation. They are apt to forget the recent events but can remember the events of the past.	Forgetfulness is syphilitic. There is a kind of mental paralysis, the patient may read but cannot retain the information. The mind is slow.	Changeableness of thought and perception is tubercular.
f) Death	Fear of death is psoric. There is also anticipation and anxiety regarding death.	Suicidal patients are mainly syphilo-sycotic. The sycotic patient will plan their death but are unlikely to commit suicide as their attachment to life and will to live is usually too strong.	The syphilitic patient dwells on suicide, has suicidal thoughts and dreams and experiences the urge to commit suicide. Love for their own life is destroyed. When syphilis is coupled with sycosis it becomes the basis of most suicides and criminal inanities, and a preponderance of syphilis results in sullen, smouldering persons likely to break out into dangerous manifestations.	Dissatisfaction with life, changeableness and a vagabond mentality can lead to suicidal impulses. The tubercular instinct for self-destruction is characterised by carelessness.
g) Selfishness & Deprivation	Psora's selfish impulses lead them to deprive others (a trait which is also strongly present in	Sycosis is present in all varieties of deprivation and rudeness. In a factory for	The syphilitic lack of realisation results in patients who are unlikely to deprive others for	Irritable and outrageous behaviour with a lack of tolerance can be reflected as the

Key Word	Psora Sensitising Miasm	Sycosis Miasm of Incoordination	Syphilis Degenerating Miasm	Tubercular Responsive, Reactive Miasm
	sycosis). Deprivation may also manifest in the sense of presenting a false or pseudo-image of themselves. They donate (though not voluntarily), large sums of money to charity, hoping to benefit in some way from their 'generosity'.	example, where labour unrest is common, the sycotic manager tries to deprive the workers out of a concern for his own benefit. A sycotic person will always act in a most selfish way to deprive others.	their own benefit. However, a criminal, for example will not realise the impact that his time in prison will have on his family and is therefore selfish only in the sense of being focussed in one particular direction. The syphilitic patient with their destructive impulses, tends to forget or ignore other responsibilities.	selfish nature of the tubercular miasm.
h) Fear	All varieties of fears are classed under psora and manifest as anxiety, alertness and apprehension of impending misfortune. Mental restlessness is one of the expressions of psoric fear.	As a result of incoordination of thoughts, sycotics manifest some fears. A millionaire for example can develop a constant fear of poverty, which is expressed as selfishness, suspicion and physical restlessness.	Syphilitic fears are not properly manifested due to a lack of realisation and expression. The only possible outward feature one might expect from a syphilitic person is of anguish.	Fearlessness is characteristic of the tubercular miasm and is expressed by the patient as a complete indifference regarding their health e.g. even at the height of fever they will say, "I am fine and don't need the doctor!" There is one fear only and that is of dogs and sometimes other animals.
i) Expression	Psora is full of ideas and philosophical expression. They pile up books and switch from one to another reading only superficially. Psoric patients rarely go into any topic in depth, and although various ideas crowd their minds there is no practicality. This constant flow of ideas is a result of mental restlessness.	Jealousy and suspicion are very evident in sycotic expression, as are the tendencies to suppress and conceal. This innate suspicion means that sycotic patients do not trust anything and repeatedly check everything.	The introverted, close-mouthed syphilitic patient keeps their depression to themselves and it only becomes apparent after they have committed suicide. They have a tendency to suppress and conceal and an inability to realise and express their symptoms. Any true form of expression is lacking. Syphilitics have a desire to	With the tubercular miasm, the mental symptoms, in particular anger, are especially aggravated after sleep. A feeling of dissatisfaction is clearly manifested in their face after sleeping. Changeability, a lack of tolerance and impatience are the expressions of this miasm.

Key Word	Psora Sensitising Miasm	Sycosis Miasm of Incoordination	Syphilis Degenerating Miasm	Tubercular Responsive, Reactive Miasm
10. Key Words of Mental Manifestations	i) Anxious and fearful. ii) Philosophical. iii) Irritability with anxiety. iv) Sadness. v) Nervous. vi) Thoughtful but no practical sense. vii) Lack of concentration and weakness of memory viii) Malicious = psora-syphilo-sycotic. ix) Wariness of life = psora-syphilitic. x) Illusions.	i) Suspicious and jealous. ii) Arrogant. iii) Irritability explodes into anger — the patient may bang the table and throw things and restlessness results. iv) Moaning. v) Chaos = Syco-Syphilo-Psora. vi) Thoughtfulness focussed for their own personal benefits. vii) Incoordination in concentration and absentmindedness. viii) Mischievousness = syco-syphilo-psora. ix) Tendency to exploit everything from life = sycotic. x) Delusions.	escape from themselves as well as from others. Their own idiocy, ignorance and obstinacy lead to melancholia and gloominess. A desire for solitude can lead to depression and melancholia, resulting in suicidal impulses. i) Destructive and melancholic. ii) Close-mouthed. iii) Irritability with cruelty. iv) Lamenting. v) Madness = Syphilo-Syco-Psora. vi) Vanishing of thoughts. vii) Total destruction of concentration; forgetfulness. Dullness is expressed as a weakness in perception. viii) Hatred = syphilo-syco-psora. ix) Loathing of life = syphilo-psora. x) Hallucinations and deliriums.	i) Changeable and fearless. ii) Indifferent. iii) Irritability with impatience. iv) Changeable mood. v) Insanity = Mixed Miasmatic with tubercular. vi) Changeability of thoughts. vii) Changeability of concentration. viii) Indifference = tubercular. ix) Unfulfilling life = tubercular. x) Vacillation of thoughts.

Key Word	Psora Sensitising Miasm	Sycosis Miasm of Incoordination	Syphilis Degenerating Miasm	Tubercular Responsive, Reactive Miasm
	xi) Sadness and depression.	xi) Irascibility, rudeness and ill-manners.	xi) Sentimental and closed-mouthed.	xi) Independent and indifferent.
	xii) Psora initiates many schemes but there are always loop-holes and plans are seldom realised. They may plan a robbery but it is unlikely to happen.	xii) Sycosis is cunning and practical and benefits at the expense of others. They can fill the loopholes and benefit from crime without appearing to be actually present.	xii) Syphilis attacks the guard and is the hired criminal. These patients fail to realise that if they are caught they will be sent to prison and that there will be no one to look after their family!	xii) The tubercular 'criminal' will commit to joining in a bank robbery but change their mind at the last moment and fail to turn up.
	xiii) The psoric memory is poor but the patient is studious and once they have learnt their subject they will remember it.	xiii) Sycotics have an active memory and are able to record everything — the journalist type.	xiii) Syphilitic patients cannot remember recent happenings but can recall past events in chronological order.	xiii) Tubercular patients are intelligent and bright but make careless mistakes.

MIASMATIC DIAGNOSIS:
COMPARISON OF VERTIGO SYMPTOMS

Key Word	Psoric Vertigo	Sycotic Vertigo	Syphilitic Vertigo	Tubercular Vertigo
1. Introduction	Psoric vertigo manifests especially from indigestion or emotional disturbances and may appear in any of the following ways: Vertigo with momentary loss of consciousness when things appear too large or small. Vertigo as if intoxicated, as if floating on air. Vertigo on reading or writing with confusion of the mind; spots or stars before the eyes or a feeling as if there is a veil before the eyes. Vertigo on riding in a boat, car or carriage, sometimes with a sensation of falling, as a result of anaemia of the brain. Vertigo on closing the eyes, disappearing on opening eyes (also sycotic).	Vertigo on closing the eyes, disappearing on opening eyes (also psoric).	Syphilitic vertigo begins at the base of the brain.	Vertigo beginning at the base of the brain can be either tubercular or syphilitic.
2. Modalities	Psoric vertigo is aggravated by movement, warmth, and as the	Sycotic vertigo is aggravated on closing the eyes and	Syphilitic vertigo aggravates at night.	Vertigo in the tubercular patient is ameliorated by rest, from

60

Key Word	Psoric Vertigo	Sycotic Vertigo	Syphilitic Vertigo	Tubercular Vertigo
	sun's rays increase. It is also worse from looking up suddenly and rising from a sitting or lying position and in these cases spots may appear before the eyes. Vertigo also occurs when turning over in bed and on closing the eyes. There is amelioration by rest, lying down and when the sun's rays decrease.	ameliorated on opening them.		being quiet, sleep, eating and from epistaxis.
3. Concomitants	The vertigo of psora is accompanied by temporary loss of vision, nausea and vomiting of mucus only. There is a lightness of the head when stooping. Digestive disturbances may also occur as may frequent eructation and roaring in the ears.	In sycosis, vertigo is associated with restlessness and there may also be sensations of formication (insects crawling over body) or of a living animal moving in the abdomen.	Total forgetfulness accompanies syphilitic vertigo.	In the tubercular miasm, vertigo is associated with impatience and dissatisfaction and redness (flushing) of the face.

MIASMATIC DIAGNOSIS:
COMPARISON OF HEAD & SCALP SYMPTOMS

Key Word	Psoric Head	Sycotic Head	Syphilitic Head	Tubercular Head
1. Headaches a) Introduction	Psoric headaches may result from hunger, exposure to the sun; or from suppressed eruptions. One-sided headaches (also syphilitic). Long standing headaches like migraine. Sharp, severe paroxysmal headache.	Sycotic headaches are characterised by their appearance in the frontal or vertex areas.	In syphilis, constant headaches appear persistently on one side of the brain. They are usually basal or linear.	Tubercular headaches may occur from repelled or suppressed eruptions. They can be extremely painful, persistent and of long standing and are not easily amenable to treatment. In children, tubercular (and syphilitic), headaches may cause the patient to strike, knock, or pound their head with their hands or against some object. Headaches appear periodically and may occur every weekend, Sunday or rest day. They can be seasonal or associated with the new or full moon and appear to be especially painful when on holiday.

Key Word	Psoric Head	Sycotic Head	Syphilitic Head	Tubercular Head
b) Sensation	The psoric headache throbs and there may be a rush of blood to the head with a sensation of heat and flushing.	The sycotic headache appears with a sensation of heaviness.	The syphilitic headache is dull, heavy and persistent. It can often last for days at a time and is so severe as to be unendurable. These feelings may be accompanied by a sensation of bands around the head, a trait also shared by the tubercular miasm.	The tubercular, periodic headaches can be very severe and are sometimes accompanied with a sensation of bands around the head (also a syphilitic manifestation).
c) Modalities	The psoric headache is worse during the morning as the sun ascends and decreases in the afternoon with the sun's descent.	Sycotic headaches are aggravated after midnight, from lying down, and from physical or mental exertion. Amelioration may result from gentle motion.	Syphilitic headaches are aggravated at night, by the warmth of the bed, by rest, while attempting to sleep, riding and exertion.	Tubercular headaches are worse from motion and from preparing for examinations. There is also exacerbation from heat.
	A persistent morning headache constantly returns, usually in the frontal, temporal or tempo-parietal regions.	Headaches in the vertex or frontal regions are aggravated by lying down especially after midnight.	Syphilitic headaches occurring in the occipital or temporal regions are also aggravated at night, by rest and lying down, and during sleep.	Meeting with strangers and entertaining them or the approach of strangers causes or aggravates the tubercular headache.
	Amelioration is from rest, quiet and sleep and hot applications.	Sycotic children have headaches, which are aggravated at night and ameliorated by motion.	Headaches are better in the morning until the evening and worse again at night.	Tubercular headaches are relieved by rest, quiet, sleep, eating and by epistaxis.
	Psoric patients cannot bear much heat about the head although they like heat in general.		Cold applications, changing places, motion, and nose bleeds ameliorate. Head feels better before sleep.	

Key Word	Psoric Head	Sycotic Head	Syphilitic Head	Tubercular Head
d) Concomitants	Psoric headaches may be accompanied by bilious attacks, which come on once or twice a month.	Sycotic headaches are associated with fever, restlessness, sadness, crying, fretting and worrying.	The syphilitic headache is associated with profuse offensive sweat on the head.	Extreme weakness accompanies the tubercular headache. There may also be a deathly coldness of the hands and feet with prostration, sadness and general despondency, or a rush of blood to the head or face with hot hands and feet.
	Headaches with throbbing and redness of the face.	The patient is restless and wants to be constantly on the move, which relieves.	The syphilitic child strikes, knocks or pounds their head with their hands or against some object (a taint also present in the tubercular miasm).	With a tubercular headache comes rolling or boring of the head into the pillow and hunger either before or during the attack.
	There may be great hunger before and during a psoric headache.	Sycotic headaches are also associated with coldness of the body and prostration.		Tubercular headaches may occur with coughs, colds and coryza.
2. Migraine a) Location	Psoric migraines occur mostly in the frontal, vertex or temporal regions or over the whole head. They are often felt only externally (tension headaches).	Sycotic migraines occur in the frontal and vertex regions and occasionally parietal.	Syphilitic migraines are mostly occipital or temporal, although occasionally they occur in the base of brain, the internal head and the meninges.	Tubercular migraines are patchy in their distribution and may be temporal or parietal or occur in the base of the brain or the meninges.

64

Key Word	Psoric Head	Sycotic Head	Syphilitic Head	Tubercular Head
b) Sensation	In psora, migraines may be sharp, severe and paroxysmal. The pain may appear on one side only and is often long-standing and of a functional character.	Sycotic migraines are characterised by a dull aching, heaviness and a reeling sensation.	The syphilitic migraine is constant and persistent and often occurs at the base of the brain on one side only. The pain may be stitching, tearing, boring, digging, maddening, sharp or cutting etc.	Tubercular migraines are extremely painful and occur especially on holidays. They may migrate from the right eye to the left ear and can be caused by the approach of a stranger. There is a sensation of throbbing, or hammering, and a pressive, tightness like a band (with effusion in the meninges).
c) Modalities	The psoric migraine increases and decreases with the sun. There is aggravation in the morning, from motion, cold, hunger and anxiety. Rest, quiet, sleep, warmth (hot applications) and natural eliminations ameliorate.	The sycotic migraine shows aggravation from rest, humidity, lying down and cold. There is also a worsening of symptoms from morning to night and around midnight. Amelioration is from motion, violent exercise, warmth and abnormal discharges.	In syphilis, migraines are aggravated at night, and from evening to morning (during sleep). Hot or warm weather, the warmth of the bed, natural discharges, rest and lying down also aggravate.	In the tubercular miasm, migraines appear worse in the evening and forenoon, from cold and every change in the weather. Patients are averse to having their heads uncovered. Epistaxis, rest, quiet, sleep and eating ameliorate.
d) Concomitants	i) Mental symptoms such as fear, anxiety and apprehension. ii) Red face with throbbing of the carotids. iii) Hot flushes ending with little perspiration.	i) Urogenital symptoms. ii) Crossness, irritability and jealousy. iii) Restlessness.	i) Suicidal tendencies. ii) Imbecility. iii) Migraine may be associated with allied disturbances of the cardiovascular and nervous systems.	i) Red face with throbbing of the carotids (psora offers this symptom to the tubercular miasm). ii) Nose bleed, which relieves symptoms. iii) Migraine with cough, cold and coryza.

Key Word	Psoric Head	Sycotic Head	Syphilitic Head	Tubercular Head
	iv) Sweat on head during sleep.	iv) Vertigo, which appears on closing the eyes and disappears on opening them.	iv) Deficient blood supply.	iv) Hunger during the headache.
	v) Vertigo, aggravated by looking up suddenly, rising from a sitting position or from emotional disturbances.	v) Congestion leads to stagnation causing the arteries to become sluggish.		v) Offensive head sweats.
				vi) Extreme weakness with the migraine.
				vii) Tubercular children suffering from migraine may strike, knock or pound their heads with their hands or against some object.
				viii) Vertigo, which begins at the base of the brain.
				ix) Active congestion leading to pulsation, which shakes the whole body.

Key Word	Psoric Head	Sycotic Head	Syphilitic Head	Tubercular Head
3. Hair	Psoric hair is apt to be thin, dry and lustreless. It appears dead like hemp and is so dry that it must be wet before it can be combed. It can also appear matted and the ends are dry and liable to split.	Sycotic patients may suffer from a fishy odour from both their hair and their scalp.	Syphilitic hair is oily, gluey and greasy, and moist eruptions may appear in the scalp. There can often be a sour, foetid or metallic odour.	As the tubercular miasm is a combination of psora and syphilis, the hair may either be dry, rough and harsh and break and split easily (psoric preponderance) or oily and moist and stick or glue together (syphilitic preponderance). There may be a thick, yellow, heavy crust of pus or it can be moist and greasy with an offensive, musty odour.
	Alopecia can affect the psoric patient and the hair may fall out after an acute illness or fever, or after parturition.	Hair falls out, and alopecia occurs in circular, circumscribed patches. Baldness is a common feature.	In syphilis, the hair has a tendency to fall out in bunches usually on the sides of the head or the vertex.	Tubercular hair is likely to fall out after parturition.
	Hairs grey on the midline of the head, or become white or grey in spots. Greying occurs too early.	In sycosis, there is likely to be an abundance of premature grey hair or immature greyish hair.		
	Bran like dandruff with or without itching.		Dandruff with thick yellow crusts.	

Key Word	Psoric Head	Sycotic Head	Syphilitic Head	Tubercular Head
	Hair may be found over the scapula where psora is joined with sycosis.		Hair falls out from the eyebrows, eyelashes and beard, and the hairs of the beard are often in-growing. Elderly people complain that the eyelashes break and turn inward, causing much irritation to the conjunctiva.	
4. Scalp	In psora, dry eruptions, which become brown and turn into dead scales, appear on the scalp. They are often painful and burn and there is severe itching and dryness. Aggravation occurs in the open air, from the heat of the bed and during the evening. Amelioration is from scratching but burning and smarting follow.	In sycosis, vesicular types of skin eruptions appear in the scalp. There may also be warts, veruccas and tumours.	Syphilitic scalp eruptions have offensive, oozing pus and are aggravated by washing.	In the tubercular miasm, herpetic eruptions occur on scalp. They are aggravated by bathing and in the open air and there is an aversion to having the head uncovered.
5. Shape of Head	In psora the head is generally small in comparison to the rest of the body and there is a dry appearance to the hair and facial skin.	The sycotic head is large and appears over-developed. The top may appear bloated.	In syphilis, the head and ear appear long in comparison to the body. There may be delayed bony developments, open fontanelles and sutures and there is a possibility of glabellar prominence due to defective bone development.	

Key Word	Psoric Head	Sycotic Head	Syphilitic Head	Tubercular Head
6. Perspiration	Sweat on the head smells sour (++) and appears particularly during sleep, or the scalp may be dry and devoid of perspiration.	Sycotic perspiration is sour (++) especially in children and there may be a fishy or musty odour.	Offensiveness and putridity of all the discharges are the general characteristics of syphilis and the perspiration is copious, sour (+) and foetid and may have a metallic smell.	Offensive (++) head sweats occur in the tubercular miasm and there can be a musty odour like old hay.

MIASMATIC DIAGNOSIS:
COMPARISON OF THE EYE SYMPTOMS

Key Word	Psoric Eye	Sycotic Eye	Syphilitic Eye	Tubercular Eye
1. General & Clinicals	Psoric eyes have a great intolerance of daylight and sunlight. Conjunctivitis, iritis and other inflammations are of a functional nature.	Corneal incoordinations and inflammations occur in sycosis. Cataracts (incoordination in the lens), retinoblastoma and other papillomas and glaucoma are sycotic. Tumors, tarsal tumors and styes also occur. Ptosis is syco-syphilitic.	Syphilitic eyes often have scaly red lids. They are subject to all sorts of structural changes, and also to corneal ulceration. Retinal detachment is syphilitic.	Tubercular eyes are characterised by granulations of the lids, haematoma in the eye and all types of inflammation characterised by haemorrhage. Injury to the eyes and black eyes are tubercular.
2. Characteristics	In psora, the vision may be blurred and letters may run together whilst reading. Spots before the eyes are also characteristic of this miasm. The visualisation of various colours and a zigzag appearance around objects is psoric.	Cataracts can be syco-syphilitic, in that opacity of the lens is characterised by incoordination (sycosis) but degenerative changes take place when the syphilitic miasm supervenes.	Cataracts and ulceration of the cornea and lids are characteristic of syphilis. Paralytic weaknesses, deformities and changes in the lens and all refractory changes are syphilitic.	Chronic dilatation of the pupils and sunken eyes occur in the tubercular miasm. Changes in the lens can also be of the tubercular miasm.

Key Word	Psoric Eye	Sycotic Eye	Syphilitic Eye	Tubercular Eye
		Photophobia may occur due to condylomata, and the eyelids are often matted together in the morning.	Photophobia also occurs in syphilis and there can be an intolerance of artificial light.	Styes, photophobia and aversion to artificial lights may also be tubercular.
			Fever of ophthalmic origin.	Disturbances in the glandular structures or in the lachrymal apparatus are tubercular (and also syphilitic).
3. Sensation	In psoric eyes, there is dryness, burning and itching with a constant desire to rub the lids. There may also be a sensation of coldness or of sand-like particles in the eyes and they may be red in appearance. Conjunctival problems occur especially when there is an ardent desire to rub the eyes. Itching in the canthi is not ameliorated by rubbing.	In sycosis, eye pains manifest as dull and aching.	Syphilis shows a sensation of burning and a raw feeling in the eyes.	In the tubercular miasm there is redness in the eyes with a sensation of heat or flushing.
4. Modalities	In psora, functional disturbances are aggravated during the daytime especially in the morning and by sunshine, and are ameliorated by external warmth.	Arthritic troubles of the eye (which are a combination of sycosis and psora), and neuralgias are aggravated by changes in the weather, changes of the barometer and rain.	Syphilitic neuralgia of the eyes is aggravated by warmth and ameliorated by cold.	Tubercular neuralgias are ameliorated by warmth.

Key Word	Psoric Eye	Sycotic Eye	Syphilitic Eye	Tubercular Eye
	There is an intolerance of daylight and sunlight, and general aggravation in the morning, from the rising of the sun to its zenith. All psoric eye problems are ameliorated by heat.	Ophthalmic disorders are aggravated by changes of the season and by rain.	There is a general aggravation of eye symptoms at night and from the warmth of the bed.	Closure of the eyelids during pain ameliorates.

MIASMATIC DIAGNOSIS:
COMPARISON OF THE EAR SYMPTOMS

Key Word	Psoric Ear	Sycotic Ear	Syphilitic Ear	Tubercular Ear
1. Clinicals	In psora, otitis occurs with dryness of the meatus.	In sycotic otitis there is profuse exudation.	Syphilitic otitis is characterised by ulceration. Mastoiditis occurs with degenerative changes in the bones.	In the tubercular miasm, otitis occurs with exudation mixed with blood, cheesy or curdled.
2. Characteristics	In the psoric miasm, the meatus and canal of the ear appear dry and lustreless. Dry scales constantly come out or fall into the canal. Psoric ears may have a dirty appearance. In psora we find functional disturbances of the ear.	Sycotic ears appear swollen and thick about the pinna, and can be oedematous. Growths and anatomical incoordination are apparent about the external ear.	All structural and organic ear problems are syphilitic. Long ears. Degenerative inflammation and destruction of the ossicles of the ear is syphilitic (and can also be tubercular).	In tubercular children the ears often act as a safety valve lessening the severity of other diseases. The appearance of abscesses in the ears of such children indicates a good prognosis as for example in the case of meningitis, the abscesses help to relieve the meningeal pains. Tubercular children may appear well in the daytime but their suffering begins at night and they often awake from sleep screaming with earache. When free of ear problems, these children often suffer from throat infections.

Key Word	Psoric Ear	Sycotic Ear	Syphilitic Ear	Tubercular Ear
	Various noises in the ear are characteristic of the psoric miasm.		In tubercular patients, suppurative otitis media is a good prognosis when suffering from a severe or acute infectious disease. Slight exposure to the cold may result in earache leading to suppurative otitis media with offensive pus. In the tubercular miasm there may be eczematous eruptions and pustules about the ears, humid eruptions, incrustations and fissures (syphilo-tubercular).	
3. Sensation	In psora there is constant itching, a sensation of crawling, dryness and pulsation in the ears.	Sycotic ears have stitching, pulsating, wandering pains.	Burning, bursting, and tearing ear pains are syphilitics.	The tubercular miasm has a sensation of flushing about the ears.
4. Modalities	The psoric patient cannot tolerate noise, due to over-sensitivity and many sounds cause pain in the ears.	Sycotic ear pains are aggravated during day and by changes in the weather.	Otitis media, with offensive discharge of pus is aggravated at night and from warmth.	Suppurative otitis media appearing in measles, chickenpox and scarlet fever when the fever is at its peak, indicates a good prognosis. Recurrent earache with swelling of the glands is aggravated at night and ameliorated during the daytime.

Key Word	Psoric Ear	Sycotic Ear	Syphilitic Ear	Tubercular Ear
5. Concomitant	Nervous restlessness and anxieties may accompany psoric ear symptoms.	In sycosis, pains in the ears make the patient physically restless.	Otitis media is a concomitant with the common cold, eruptions, measles, chicken pox etc. In syphilis, eczemas, which appear behind and about the ears, have thick, foetid pus and cracks.	There may be a peculiar carrion like odour from aural abscesses and any discharges are often cheesy or curdled. There may be eczematous eruptions around the ears, which are humid and pustular. Tonsillitis with earaches. Ears may look flushed and red. Even when there are foetid and copious discharges from the ears, the tubercular child feels alright and says that there is nothing the matter with him.
6. Hearing	The psoric patient has very sensitive hearing and is easily startled by noise.	Incoordination in the sense of hearing causes the patient to hear better in noisy places.	Impairment and total loss of hearing may occur in syphilis.	Loss of hearing with foetid, cheesy, curdled discharge from the ears.

MIASMATIC DIAGNOSIS: COMPARISON OF NASAL SYMPTOMS

Key Word	Psoric Nose	Sycotic Nose	Syphilitic Nose	Tubercular Nose
1. Clinicals	Rhinitis.	Sinusitis.	Degenerative and ulcerative conditions of the nose.	Epistaxis.
		DNS (Deviated nasal septum).		Nasal polyps are tri-miasmatic.
		Swollen adenoids.		
2. Characteristics	In psora we find various olfactory disturbances of functional origin.	In sycosis, there are polyps, growths, moles, papilloma and veruccas in the nostrils. There may also be oedematous swelling of the nasal turbinate.	In syphilis, the nose may be flat or depressed from ulceration or destruction of the nasal septum and ulcers may occur inside the nostrils.	There is a tendency to the recurrent catching of colds in the tubercular miasm.
	Sensation of dryness in the nose.	Bland discharges with a fish-brine smell are characteristic of sycosis.	Clinkers (thick crusts which are dark green, black, or brown), can be offensive and often have to be removed. Manifest with offensive breath.	Epistaxis, which is bright red, may occur from any trivial cause such as over-heating or over-exercise or during fever. Relief comes by cold application but nose bleeds are difficult to stop and recur periodically.
	Psoric colds begin with sneezing, redness and heat. The nose becomes sensitive after it has been blown for some time.	Difficulty in breathing through the nose can be caused by various growths or oedema.		Flushing in the face, eyes and nose is tubercular.
	Discharges are thin and watery and can be acrid.	Moist snuffles with a purulent, scanty discharge with the odour of fish-brine and no formation of crust.		Snuffles are periodic and associated with haemorrhage.

Key Word	Psoric Nose	Sycotic Nose	Syphilitic Nose	Tubercular Nose
	Stoppage of one nostril causes mouth breathing.	Dr. Roberts suggests that sycotic nasal discharges are acrid and corrode the skin. However, acridity of discharges is generally syphilitic.		A thick yellowish discharge with an odour of old cheese or sulphur, ameliorated by cold application is constantly dropping down the throat (post nasal drip).
		There may be a mottled appearance of the mucus membrane.		Nasal polyps (which is tri-miasmatic) are termed as tubercular when characterised by profuse haemorrhage.
		Children born of sycotic parents complicated with gout, take cold easily at the slightest exposure and frequently suffer from acute, copious (+++) watery coryza, which is often excoriating.		Tubercular children haemorrhage from the nose from the least provocation. Blowing the nose, a slight knock, or even washing the face may initiate the nasal bleeding.
3. Modalities	Psoric nasal symptoms are aggravated in the morning, from cold and during sleep; and ameliorated from warmth and by natural discharges.	Sycotic nasal complaints are aggravated by damp and from changes in the weather. Amelioration is from abnormal discharges through various mucus membranes, such as coryza.	In syphilis, nasal symptoms are aggravated at night and from the warmth of the bed, and ameliorated by abnormal discharges.	In the tubercular miasm, nasal conditions are aggravated in a closed room and ameliorated in open air.
				Amelioration by epistaxis is also characteristic of the tubercular miasm.

Key Word	Psoric Nose	Sycotic Nose	Syphilitic Nose	Tubercular Nose
4. Smell	In psora we may find hypo-sensitivity to smell where the sense of smell is weak or lost, or an increased sense of smell due to hyper-susceptibility.	Sycotic incoordination results in the sense of smell being increased profoundly or diminished.	The syphilitic sense of smell may be diminished, lost or perverted.	The tubercular sense of smell is characterised by changeableness and alternation. The patient will alternately smell through each nostril when the other is blocked.
	Psoric patients often cannot tolerate any odours whether good or bad. At times they may become faint, and this hyper-sensitivity may even disturb their sleep; and can induce symptoms, such as nausea, vomiting and headaches.			
5. Septum	Psora suffers from painful boils in the nose or pimples on the septum but there are no malignant manifestations.	In sycosis, burning of the nasal septum can lead to obstruction of the nose	Recurrent boils in the nostrils may result in anosmia.	Tubercular nostrils are narrow and have small openings leading to nasal blockages and thereby mouth breathing.
	There is redness of the mucus membrane of the nasal orifice and a sooty, dirty appearance of the septum.	Thickening of the membranes or enlargement of the turbinate bones due to congestion may cause stoppages.	Destruction of the septum is characteristic of the syphilitic miasm.	
	In rhinitis, the septum is often dry, hot and burning.	Sycotic discharges are either yellow (also tubercular), greenish or greenish-yellow, except in fresh colds where there tends to be copious but thin mucus.		

Key Word	Psoric Nose	Sycotic Nose	Syphilitic Nose	Tubercular Nose
6. Hay Fever	Psoric hay fever is characterised by sneezing, redness and heat and by sensitiveness and a watery discharge.	In sycotic hay fever the discharge is scanty but the patient cannot breathe through the nose or blow any mucus from it. The slightest discharge however relieves the stopped up feeling.	Syphilitic discharges from hay fever are acrid, putrid and offensive.	Tubercular hay fever is periodic and recurrent with much sneezing and various allergic manifestations. The nose may feel clear one hour and be extremely stuffed-up the next. These cases are more difficult to cure and are often characterised by thick and occasionally blood-streaked discharges.

MIASMATIC DIAGNOSIS:
COMPARISON OF THE ORAL SYMPTOMS

Key Word	Psoric Mouth	Sycotic Mouth	Syphilitic Mouth	Tubercular Mouth
1. Clinicals	Stomatitis.	Salivary duct calculi.	Leucoplakia with fungal infection is syphilitic.	Haematemesis.
	Thrush.	Leucoplakia.		
2. Characteristics	Psora does not like to eat highly aromatic or strong smelling substances.	Tumours, warts and papillomas are characteristic of sycosis.	Syphilis is subject to various ulcers in the oral cavity.	In the tubercular miasm we may find various ulcers in the oral cavity, and bright red gums, which may bleed from the slightest touch.
	Ptyalism.		Oozing of blood from the gums, which often comes in the last stage of typhoid fever.	Salivation associated with recurrent hawking and clearing of the throat, due to a sensation of lodged mucus.
	Foetor oris.	Tonsillitis.	Syphilitic saliva is ropy and can be drawn into long threads.	Foetor oris.
3. Taste (All of the miasms may experience either a partial or complete loss of taste.)	All food tastes 'as if burnt', is characteristic of psora. There may be various bad tastes in the mouth, either sourish, an intolerable sweet taste or a bitter taste which is often experienced in the open air.	Sycotic patients are subject to fishy, musty or putrid tastes.	In syphilis there is a metallic, especially coppery taste and the patient always has an unpleasant taste in the mouth.	In the tubercular miasm there is a taste of blood, frequently present in the morning, and of pus. There may also be an occasional bitter where even water can taste unpleasant.

Key Word	Psoric Mouth	Sycotic Mouth	Syphilitic Mouth	Tubercular Mouth
	Perverseness of taste (psora-syphilitic) may occur in which for example, bread tastes bitter or water tastes unusual. Food may sometimes be rejected by the psoric patient who thinks that it tastes abnormal. Psoric eructations taste of recently eaten food or of fat.		Expectoration tastes sweetish,	or salty or of rotten eggs, or may be devoid of taste altogether.
4. Tongue	In psora, there may be burning of the tongue and lips with swelling, or the tongue may be dry and coated or yellow with a bitter taste.	Warts and tumours may be visible on the tongue in sycosis.	In syphilis, imprints of the teeth are visible on the tongue. The tongue may be moist and emit a horribly offensive odour from mouth.	Glossitis is tubercular and there may be a whitish or yellowish coating to the tongue. Ulcers, which look like yoghurt or curd, may also be present.
5. Concomitants	Tartar and other improper substances lodge in the gums, tongue and root of the teeth.	Gum boils without pus formations are sycotic.	In syphilis, gumboils occur with the formation of pus, and there may be loose teeth with offensive saliva.	Tubercular oral symptoms may be associated with gum bleeding, tonsillitis and the recurrent catching of colds with coryza.
6. Teeth	Psoric teeth are painful and bleed easily. Pain from toothache may be intolerable.		Crowns of incisor teeth become crescent shaped. Syphilitic teeth are subject to pathological and structural changes in the dental arch. They are irregular in shape and in order of eruption.	Soft, spongy, receding gums are characteristic of the tubercular miasm. Teeth are irregular and bleed on slightest touch. They also decay as soon as they appear and may be deformed or asymmetrical.

Key Word	Psoric Mouth	Sycotic Mouth	Syphilitic Mouth	Tubercular Mouth
			Syphilitic children suffer every time a tooth comes through and diarrhoea, colds, tonsillitis etc, result.	Teething is painful and accompanied by diarrhoea (sycotic), spasms or convulsions (syphilo-tubercular) and digestive disturbances.
			Asymmetrical teeth, which are decayed and serrated; caries and dental fistulas are syphilitic.	The dental arch is imperfect or irregular.

MIASMATIC DIAGNOSIS:
COMPARISON OF THE FACIAL SYMPTOMS

Key Word	Psoric Face	Sycotic Face	Syphilitic Face	Tubercular Face
1. Characteristics	Usually the psoric face is devoid of perspiration, but conversely can show excessive perspiration.	Sycotic face is swollen and oedematous with reflections of the features of incoordination such as dermoid cysts, tumours and warts.	A greyish, greasy face is characteristic of this miasm and syphilitic children have ashy grey faces, the appearance of marasmus and the general look of a wrinkled, old man.	The tubercular face is characterised by sunken eyes and pallor although flushing of the cheeks appears during the evening. Rise of temperature with flushed face during attacks of cough and cold, during dentition or with wormy complaints.
2. General	Hot flushes to the face appear during the climacteric in the psoric miasm. There may be a hot feeling of the face, especially before periods and periodical hot flushes felt in the face, eyes and ears.	In sycosis, perspiration of the face has a fishy odour.	Syphilitic perspiration of the face and head is often seen as droplets. Syphilitic skin feels cool to touch.	In the tubercular miasm we find red spots on the cheeks with flushes of heat to the head and chest.
3. Appearance	The psoric face has dry, itching pimples and simple acne.	The sycotic face can be pale (psora-sycotic), bluish and dropsical.	In syphilis there is hard acne on the face.	Bloated (syco-tubercular) appearance of face, especially after sleep.

Key Word	Psoric Face	Sycotic Face	Syphilitic Face	Tubercular Face
	There may be a dry, rough, unwashed appearance.	In sycosis we also find a yellow, shallow, puffy, oedematous appearance.	The syphilitic appearance is of high check bones, thick lips and in some cases rough facial skin. The voice may be coarse and deep and is often hollow. The eyelids are red, inflamed and scaly with crusty, broken, stubby and irregularly curved lashes.	Paleness of the face is evident on rising in the morning or after sleep or eating. There may be a cyanotic, blue appearance and a look of anaemic especially as a result of prolonged or profuse haemorrhage.
	The shape of the psoric face is inverted.	Stubby, thick and broken hairs appear in the beard.	A flat, depressed nose is characteristic of syphilis.	Face and head is the shape of a pyramid with the apex at the chin.
	Pale and sallow, sometimes the eyes have a sunken appearance with blue rings (also tubercular).			The tubercular face can also be round, with fair, smooth, clear skin and a waxy complexion. The eyes are bright and sparkling and eyebrows and lashes are soft, glossy, long and silky. The nose is well shaped and the features sharp.
	The psoric patient may have a cyanotic, blue face and an anaemic appearance.			Recurrent, small, painful pimples and boils are characteristic of the tubercular miasm.
4. Lips	Psora has burning, itching lips, which may also be swollen.	In sycosis we find swollen lips with warts and veruccas.	In syphilis there is occasional redness of the lips (like tubercular).	Flushed, red lips, where the blood seems on the point of bursting.

Key Word	Psoric Face	Sycotic Face	Syphilitic Face	Tubercular Face
	Psoric lips are red or blue and congested in patients with poor circulation. Vesicles about the mouth are small, white and transparent, accompanied by much itching.		Deep fissures.	Deep fissures.
5. Facial Expression During Fever	Bright red and shining, and in cases of erysipelas, a sycotic element will also be present.	The sycotic face appears oedematous and heavy during fever.	During fever, syphilitic features are reflective of the dullness and morose feelings of the patient.	The tubercular face is usually pale with circumscribed red spots on the cheeks appearing in the afternoons or evenings in such conditions as dentition, worms, febrile states, colds etc.

MIASMATIC DIAGNOSIS:
COMPARISON OF THE RESPIRATORY SYMPTOMS

Key Word	Psoric Respiratory System	Sycotic Respiratory System	Syphilitic Respiratory System	Tubercular Respiratory System
1. Clinicals	Bronchitis (psora-tubercular).	Pneumonia with consolidation of the lungs.	Ulcerative sore throat.	Pleurisy.
	Pharyngitis.	Emphysema and fibrosis of the lungs.	Quinsy.	Pulmonary tuberculosis.
	Functional diseases of the respiratory system.	Vocal cord nodules.	Lung abscesses.	Tonsillitis, especially recurrent.
2. Structure	In psoric respiratory disorders, the natural curves of the chest remain unchanged.	In sycosis there is an oedematous appearance of the nose, uvula and tonsils with hypertrophy of the nasal turbinate.	In syphilis, there may be a flat, depressed appearance of the nose and irregular depressions in the chest cavity related to collapse of the lungs.	The tubercular chest is often narrow and lacking in width laterally, and in depth antero-posteriorly. The sub-clavicular spaces are hollow.
			Ulcers may be present in the respiratory passage, nose, tonsils and trachea.	The sternum is thin, and flat on the top but protrudes at the lower end and the xiphoid process giving it a barrel shaped appearance — pigeon chest.
			Ulceration, cavities and abscesses may be found especially in advanced lung conditions.	Tubercular shoulders are often rounded and incline forwards infringing on the chest area.
				One lung is larger and better developed than the other, resulting in hyper-functioning of that lung.

Key Word	Psoric Respiratory System	Sycotic Respiratory System	Syphilitic Respiratory System	Tubercular Respiratory System
				Curves and lines in the chest wall are imperfect and certain areas may be sunken and depressed.
3. Sensation	The psoric patient experiences burning pains in the chest and the sensation of a band around the chest.	In sycosis there is a feeling of stitching pains in chest with different types of aching ameliorated by pressure.	Syphilis experiences rawness and soreness in the throat and tonsils.	In the tubercular miasm there is a sensation of mucus constantly stuck in the throat, accompanied by tickling.
4. Location	Psoric respiratory infections generally occur in the upper respiratory tract. There is recurrent catching of colds, and the nose and throat are sensitive.	Sycotic features of incoordination include dilatation of the bronchi and bronchioles as well as the lungs.	Syphilitic respiratory symptoms can manifest anywhere in the respiratory passage, from the nose down to the lung alveoli with features of ulceration, destruction, cavity formation and pyogenic inflammation.	The tubercular patient catches cold easily and therefore always covers up their throat and chest warmly.
5. Modality	All psoric respiratory complaints are aggravated during the winter and from cold, and are ameliorated by warmth in general and the appearance of natural discharges.	Sycotic asthma, pneumonia, bronchitis and coughs and colds are all aggravated in humid moist atmospheres, from changes in the season and during rainy spells. Asthma with profuse expectoration, which is aggravated in the early morning, is characterised by the patient's compulsion to move about. Amelioration comes from lying on the abdomen.	The syphilitic patient feels worse at night and during the morning.	Aggravation of tubercular respiratory complaints comes from cold air and from milk (which builds up lots of catarrh). Symptoms are also worse at night. Amelioration is from open air and epistaxis.

Key Word	Psoric Respiratory System	Sycotic Respiratory System	Syphilitic Respiratory System	Tubercular Respiratory System
6. Concomitants	Anxiety and apprehension of incurable diseases, even when the patient is suffering from trivial ailments, is a characteristic of psora.	Asthma (bronchospasm) is ameliorated by passing stool. Restlessness accompanies sycosis — the patient likes to be constantly on the move. There is a great sense of	Dyspnagia and dyspnoea are syphilitic manifestations but can also be mixed miasmatic. A pus-like putrid expectoration may accompany a syphilitic cough.	Along with tubercular coughs and colds, there is always swelling of the tonsils and of the glands around the neck (cervical lymphadenopathy). exhaustion and the patient tires easily even after sleep. They feel better and regain their strength as the day advances or the sun ascends but weaken again as the sun goes down.
7. Voice	In psora there is huskiness of the voice with dryness of the throat.		Hoarseness occurs in syphilis especially before menstruation.	Voice is coarse and deep with base-like chest tones. There may also be a 'croak' in the voice.
8. Cough	The psoric patient suffers from a dry spasmodic cough resulting from suppression of measles, skin disease etc. which causes the lungs to be affected. In psora, the cough is dry, teasing and spasmodic in type.	The coughs of sycotics are usually bronchial. Hard, racking coughs often in early winter also affect the sycotic patient.	In syphilis we find a short, barking cough. There may be just one or two distinct barks like that of a dog. The syphilitic cough may also be paroxysmal.	The cough of the tubercular patient is deep and prolonged, giving us the lower chest tones. It is worse in the morning and when the patient first lies down in the evening. Teasing cough (which indicates the weakness of the lungs).

Key Word	Psoric Respiratory System	Sycotic Respiratory System	Syphilitic Respiratory System	Tubercular Respiratory System
		A great deal of coughing is required to raise even a tiny amount of mucus; hence the cough is prolonged and teasing.		Quite often the cough of the tubercular patient is deep, ringing and hollow with no expectoration.
				Tubercular coughs are often so dry and tight that they induce headache or the whole body is shaken by their explosive paroxysms.
9. Expectoration	In psora we find haemoptysis, as a result of functional disturbances of the lungs. However, prolonged and persistent haemoptysis can only be possible if the tubercular miasm is present.	The coughs of sycosis have very little expectoration, although there is a large accumulation of mucus in the lungs (this is a feature of incoordination, i.e. large accumulation but little expectoration).	The syphilitic paroxysmal cough is accompanied by a tasteless yellowish/greenish or clear, sticky thread-like discharge.	Mucus, which is viscid, pus-like, sticky, musty or offensive and tastes sweetish or salty, and may sometimes be mixed with blood, is a characteristic indication of the tubercular miasm.
	There is frequent congestion of the throat with the accumulation of much phlegm.	The mucus is usually yellowish or clear (when clear white mucus is expectorated, then the psoric component is also present).		Tubercular expectoration always sinks down and cannot float. It is purulent, greenish-yellow and very often offensive.
	The psoric patient usually expectorates mucus, which is scanty and tasteless.			The tubercular miasms shows a constant desire to hawk or clear the throat from a viscid, scanty mucus.

Key Word	Psoric Respiratory System	Sycotic Respiratory System	Syphilitic Respiratory System	Tubercular Respiratory System
10. **Respiration**	Psoric respiration is slow and sallow. As psoric symptoms are characterised by 'hypo' or less, scanty and absence, so the features of hypoxia, anoxia and anoxaemia are classified as psoric manifestations. Babies which are born pale and cyanosed and in need of resuscitation, due to defective oxygenation and hypoxia caused by the umbilical cord being around the neck during intra-uterine life, can be rescued by treatment from anti-psoric medicines.	In sycosis we find tachypnoea, i.e. accelerated/rapid respiration.	Dyspnoea before going to bed, or while lying down is indicative of the syphilitic miasm. Tubercular patients are poor	In the tubercular miasm, dyspnoea is apparent on ascending stairs. There is weakness and debility, and the breathlessness is often painful. breathers, which results in laboured respiration. They have no desire to take a full breath even though there may be no obstructions in the air passages. As a consequence, the alveoli of the lungs are never fully expanded and do not receive adequate oxygen causing atrophies and the walls to glue together. This can be linked to a dislike of taking in cold air, for fear of being chilled or catching cold. The tubercular patient is unable to expand the chest fully as the expansive power of the lungs is greatly limited.

Key Word	Psoric Respiratory System	Sycotic Respiratory System	Syphilitic Respiratory System	Tubercular Respiratory System
11. Associated Symptoms	In psora there may be frequent stitches in the chest with or without cough.	Sycosis has nasal blockages; and the patient is generally unable to breathe through the nose.	In syphilis, there are destructive changes in the lung parenchyma, lung abscesses, and collapse of the lungs. Advanced pathological changes in the lungs may also occur.	Even with advanced lung conditions, tubercular patients are full of hopes and will never concede that the disease is incurable. They are also likely to say that there is nothing the matter with them. Headache alternates with chest complaints. Cough can induce headache. Glandular swelling and changes in the cervical region may precede lung changes.

MIASMATIC DIAGNOSIS:
COMPARISON OF THE CARDIAC SYMPTOMS

Key Word	Psoric Heart	Sycotic Heart	Syphilitic Heart	Tubercular Heart
1. Clinicals	In psora, cardiac and emotional symptoms alternate (for alternation of symptoms in a recurrent way the tubercular miasm has to be present).	In sycosis, the heart is affected as a result of suppression of rheumatic complaints.	The syphilitic patient is liable to suffer from ulcerative bacterial endocarditis, and heart affections with valvular degeneration.	Palpitations, and a rush of blood to the head and chest with redness of the face and flushed cheeks is characteristic of the tubercular miasm.
	Heart affections may occur from fear, disappointment, loss of friends and over-excitement.	Sycosis has incoordination (such as mitral or aortic regurgitation), dilatation and abnormality of the cardiac valves. RHD (rheumatic heart diseases). Hypertrophy of the heart, and left or right ventricular hypertrophy of the heart.	Syphilis is also subject to congenital abnormalities such as Fallot's tetralogy and PDA (Patent Ductus Arteriosus), which are the cause of structural and/or developmental anomalies.	
	Psoric cardiac symptoms are mostly of a functional nature and accompanied by great anxiety and fear of incurable disease or death.	Sycotic patients are generally fleshy and puffy and their dyspnoea is caused by obesity.		
	Anxiety about the heart with constant worry typifies psora.	A combination of sycosis and psora creates the right soil for valvular and cardiac disturbances.		

92

Key Word	Psoric Heart	Sycotic Heart	Syphilitic Heart	Tubercular Heart
2. Sensation	In psora, there is a feeling of increased circulatory function, congestion and plethora. The precordium may either feel empty or heavy.	In sycosis pain radiates from the precordium to the shoulder or scapular region or vice versa.	In syphilis there is a sensation of heaviness in the precordium with a lack of expression.	Violent palpitations with beating and shaking (for shaking of the frame the sycotic miasm may be present) of the whole body is representative of the tubercular miasm.
	There may be a hammering sensation in the region of the heart, and many other uncomfortable sensations.	Sycotic cardiac pains are like an electric shock, which comes and goes suddenly.		
	The psoric patient may experience a violent rush of blood (in which case the tubercular miasm is likely to be present) to the chest, and a sensation of weakness, goneness, soreness or fullness around the heart.	Soreness or tenderness around the precordium is made worse by the motion of the arms.		
	Sharp, cutting, piercing neuralgic pains about the heart, pulsations of the heart which shake the whole body, and a sensation as if there were a band around the heart are also typical of the psoric miasm.	Sycosis suffers from fluttering, throbbing with oppression and difficulty in breathing at intervals.		

Key Word	Psoric Heart	Sycotic Heart	Syphilitic Heart	Tubercular Heart
3. Modalities	In psora, all heart complaints including cardiac pains and angina are aggravated in the evening, from movement, from coughing, laughing, and after eating. The stitching pains (with which there is generally a sycotic component) of angina almost kill the patient when they make any attempt at movement.	Heat and changes in the weather aggravate sycotic heart conditions.	Syphilitic cardiac problems are aggravated at night, from sunset, perspiration, and extremes of temperature, movement and from the warmth of the bed.	The tubercular patient suffering from a heart condition wants to keep still. They are aggravated by higher altitudes and cannot climb stairs or ascend hills. Breathing on ascending is difficult and sitting up causes the patient to feel dizzy and faint. Aggravation also comes from pressure on the chest and at night.
	Oppression and feelings of anxiety are worse in the morning.	Amelioration is from gentle exercise such as slow walking or riding, except in conditions of rheumatic origin where motion aggravates.	Amelioration occurs during the day (from sunrise to sunset), from changes of position and from cold in general.	Tubercular conditions are ameliorated by lying down and in open air.
	Psoric cardiac symptoms are ameliorated by eructation, and from rest and lying down.	All sorts of abnormal discharges ameliorate and are of good prognostic value in sycosis.		
4. Concomitants	The psoric patient always thinks the heart's action is about to stop and that he will die soon. He keeps his mind on his heart, and is constantly taking his own pulse.	Dyspnoea with pain about the heart; gout and rheumatism of the heart are sycotic manifestations.	Palpitations, which are tuberculo-syphilitic, occur.	Tubercular heart troubles are accompanied by fainting, temporary loss of vision, ringing in the ears, pallor and great weakness.
	In psora, heart problems are accompanied by much anxiety, mental distress, depression and sadness.	Marked anasarca and dropsical manifestations such as cardiac dropsy occur. (Some authors suggest this to be syco-psoric). Gout and rheumatism of the heart are sycotic manifestations.		There is a constant but gradual 'falling away of the chest' and a rush of blood to the chest and face in tubercular conditions.

Key Word	Psoric Heart	Sycotic Heart	Syphilitic Heart	Tubercular Heart
5. Pulse	Bradycardia is psoric. The psoric pulse is full and bounding.	Tachycardia is sycotic. The sycotic pulse is slow and feeble, soft (for soft pulse a psoric component is also present) and easily compressible. The pulse lacks tension.	Irregularity in the pulse is syphilitic. This irregularity can be in rate or rhythm.	The tubercular pulse is feeble but rapid. A small, thread-like but quick pulse is typical of the tubercular miasm.
6. Manifestations	Psoric dyspnoea is painful with features of cyanosis.	Thrombosis (where sycosis is mainly, but not always responsible), embolism (a feature of incoordination) and myocardial infarctions are sycotic. In a cardiac attack, there is imbalance and incoordination in the circulation associated with the formation of embolus or thrombus and sycosis is mainly responsible. In sycosis there may be dropsical swelling and flabbiness after prolonged suffering from cardiac or respiratory complications. There is seldom much pain or suffering in sycotic manifestations unless they are combined with rheumatic difficulties.	Syphilitics may have had heart troubles for years with occasional dyspnoea and pains, which they usually deny. They can drop dead suddenly however from massive cardiac failure (generally sycosis plays a role here too). Due to lack of expression and realisation, syphilitics do not convey their troubles to their friends, family or doctor.	Tubercular dyspnoea is often painful. Persistent emaciation occurs in tubercular cardiac patients.

95

MIASMATIC DIAGNOSIS:
COMPARISON OF THE STOMACH SYMPTOMS

Key Word	Psoric Stomach	Sycotic Stomach	Syphilitic Stomach	Tubercular Stomach
1. Clinicals	Gastritis, oesophagitis with burning, and other functional disorders of the gastro-intestinal tract are psoric. Psora also has acidity, sour eructation, heartburn and nausea with a feeling of faintness.	Meat arouses the latent sycosis and stimulates the formation of uric acid. It is therefore better for the sycotic patient to take meat sparingly and consume more nuts, beans or cheeses as a source of protein. In sycosis there are benign and encapsulated tumours, papilloma and polyps of the gastro-intestinal tract.	Ulcers and degenerative types of cancer result from the syphilitic miasm.	Gastro-intestinal disturbances such as haematemesis and melaena where bleeding predominates typify the tubercular miasm. Milk allergies and allergies to different types of food are tubercular.
2. Sensations & Hunger	Empty, all-gone sensation, especially in the morning, as the patient is unable to assimilate any nutritious substances from the food they eat. The psoric patient may have an excessive hunger for unnatural substances like chalk, clay and other indigestible things especially during fever or pregnancy.	Crampy, colicky pains are sycotic. Children born of sycotic parents often suffer from colic from the moment of birth or colic may be initiated after vaccination. Three month colic in children who become restless, writhe, twist and squirm with pain and draw up the limbs.	In syphilis there are burning, bursting, tearing and ulcerative pains in the gastro-intestinal tract.	The tubercular patient feels like fainting if hunger is not quickly satisfied. Extreme hunger is associated with an all-gone, weak, empty feelings in the stomach (this from the psoric component of the miasm). In the tubercular miasm, patients are constantly hungry and eat beyond their capacity (this is from the sycotic component of the miasm) to digest, or they may have no appetite in morning but feel hungry for other meals.

Key Word	Psoric Stomach	Sycotic Stomach	Syphilitic Stomach	Tubercular Stomach
	Morbid and unnatural hunger (syphilitic component may be present) even after a full meal and at night while sleeping, as if the patient cannot be satiated. Cannot wait for a meal. Hungry especially between 10 a.m. and 11 a.m. The patient has to eat at once or else they become faint.			
	Psoric patients mostly eat beyond their capacity of digestion, which causes various types of diarrhoea, or the patient may be hungry but a few mouthfuls fill them up to the throat.			
	The psoric patient suffers from feelings of distension due to an accumulation of gas, with flatulence, rumbling and gurgling; and sour and bitter eructations which taste of the food just eaten. There is a sensation of fullness, weight and heaviness as if there is a stone or lump in the stomach.			
	All symptoms of acidity and dyspepsia, nausea and vomiting, and pains in the liver and stomach are psoric.			

Key Word	Psoric Stomach	Sycotic Stomach	Syphilitic Stomach	Tubercular Stomach
	There may be a constant gnawing at the pit of the stomach with a cold or hot sensation. Beating, throbbing, constriction and oppression occur especially after eating.			
3. Modalities	In psora, aggravation occurs a few hours after eating. There is aggravation from protein and from being touched, and even the slightest pressure cannot be endured.	Sycotic patients are likely to suffer some discomfort after eating.	Syphilitics are aggravated at night, from extremes of temperature, warmth, and starch.	Tubercular patients suffer aggravation from milk, greasy and oily foods, at night, from any pressure on chest or stomach, and in closed rooms.
	Bilious nausea and vomiting which comes on at regular intervals is ameliorated by rest, quiet and sleep.	Aggravation comes from consuming meat and fat, and it is therefore better to restrict the consumption of meat in rheumatic patients.		Amelioration comes in the open air and in dry weather.
	Temporarily better after eating, but after some time the psoric patient will feel the distension, heaviness and other symptoms return and become aggravated.	In sycosis, amelioration is from lying on the stomach, violent motion, rocking (in case of children), walking, and hot food and drinks.		
	Psoric stomach complaints are generally ameliorated by hot food and drinks, belching and gentle motion.			
4. Concomitants	Shortness of breath, vertigo, giddiness, sweat and anxiety are associated with most psoric gastric symptoms.	Sycosis has loud eructation especially with colicky symptoms.	In syphilis, dullness and depression are associated with gastric manifestations.	In the tubercular miasm, a red face and flushed chin accompany gastric complaints.

Key Word	Psoric Stomach	Sycotic Stomach	Syphilitic Stomach	Tubercular Stomach
				Swelling of the intestinal and mesenteric glands may also occur.
5. Cravings	In psora we find craving for certain items or foods, which are refused when offered, especially in children.	Sycotics (like syphilitics) crave alcohol and tend to abuse it. Beer is preferred as it causes less aggravation than wine.	Syphilitic patients have a perverted craving for alcohol.	Tubercular patients are characterised by a craving for peculiar foods and foods which make them sick.
	Craving for sweet things is followed by vomiting of bile.	There is a craving for rich gravies, table salt, pungent and salty foods, and cold or hot foods.	There may be a craving for cold food.	Meat, potatoes and salt are also craved and salt may be eaten straight from the saucer.
	During fever the psoric patient may have an aversion to sweets and crave acids instead. They may also crave greasy and highly seasoned foods and meat but these do not suit them.			Tubercular patients are extremists and like foods to be either really hot or really cold.
	There is a craving for stimulants such as tea, coffee and tobacco to supply the nerve force.			
	A craving for unusual things during pregnancy but which goes off after the birth, may sometimes be passed onto the child.			

Key Word	Psoric Stomach	Sycotic Stomach	Syphilitic Stomach	Tubercular Stomach
6. Desires	In psora there is a desire for sweets, acids, pickles, sour and indigestible things, meat, ghee (butter oil), hot, spicy and oily foods.	Sycotics desire warm food, coconut and betelnut etc.	As the syphilitic miasm vitiates the mind leading to a lack of expression and realisation; any striking desires and aversions cannot be properly ascertained.	Tubercular patients desire foods, which aggravates their condition. They have an inability to assimilate much starch.
	Psoric patients want everything fried if possible and have a strong repugnance to boiled foods.	Sycotic patients like fat meat well seasoned with salt and pepper and served with rich gravies.	The syphilitic tendency for destruction leads to a desire for stimulants such as tea, coffee, tobacco and wine. There may be a hereditary tendency to alcoholism. Syphilitic patients suffer from nervous weakness and generally feel better for stimulants.	A desire for too warm or too cold food is tubercular and patients thrive better on fat and fat foods. They require plenty of salt and do not easily digest starches.
	A desire for fats, greasy foods, rich pastries and sweet-meats, when satisfied can induce bilious attacks.	A desire for beer is sycotic.	There are desires for very spicy meat (dislikes less spicy preparations), for cold food and drinks, lime and sweet and sour foods. The syphilitic patient also desires milk, which they are unable to assimilate, and indigestible things like chalk, slate, pencil and wine.	There is a longing for stimulants such as beer and wine, and for hot, aromatic foods.

Key Word	Psoric Stomach	Sycotic Stomach	Syphilitic Stomach	Tubercular Stomach
7. Aversions	Psoric patients have both an aversion to and an intolerance of milk. They are also averse to boiled and cold foods.	In sycosis we find an intolerance of spices and aversions to milk and meat. (With regards to meat, there are two different opinions — some authors believe that sycotic patients like fatty meats, and my own belief is that they like meat but that it does not like them). Aversion and/or aggravation from green leafy vegetables; spinach, onion, juicy fruits etc. Any fruit or vegetable, which has a high water content, aggravates the hydrogenoid, sycotic constitution.	The syphilitic patient has a complete aversion to meat and to animal foods.	Milk allergies are present in the tubercular miasm and patients cannot tolerate milk in any form. As the tubercular miasm is changeable, there is a possibility of a strong desire or aversion to rich gravies. Cravings are for potatoes and meat.

MIASMATIC DIAGNOSIS:
COMPARISON OF THE ABDOMINAL SYMPTOMS

Key Word	Psoric Abdomen	Sycotic Abdomen	Syphilitic Abdomen	Tubercular Abdomen
1. Clinicals	Duodenitis, cholecystitis, non-functioning of the gall bladder, colitis and other inflammations of the abdomen, mainly of functional origin and including gastric refluxes are of psoric origin. Ascitis is syco-psoric.	Tumours, papillomas and encapsulated malignant growths in the abdomen and cholelithiasis (gallstones) are sycotic.	Degeneration of the liver cells, including fatty degeneration is of syphilitic origin.	In the tubercular miasm we find swelling of the intestinal and mesenteric glands.
	Constipation is primarily psoric.	Diarrhoea is sycotic (characterised by exaggerated peristalsis).	Dysentery is syphilitic (characterised by irregular peristalsis).	Breakfast diarrhoea or diarrhoea after eating and stool with blood (melaena) is tubercular.
	Dyspeptic symptoms are also psoric in origin.	Appendicitis and appendicular colic are always sycotic.	Cirrhosis of the liver is syphilo-sycotic, as there is incoordination as well as degeneration of the liver cells.	Hernia has a strong psoric element as laxation of the muscles is due to psora but recurrence or persistence is due to the tubercular miasm.
		In children, swelling and protrusion of the umbilicus with a thin, yellowish-green discharge and the odour of fish-brine is characteristic of sycosis.		In tubercular children we find recurrent ulceration of the umbilicus with a yellow discharge.
		Hepato or hepato-splenomegaly (either liver enlargement or liver and spleen enlargement).		Lymphatic involvement of the abdomen is tubercular.

102

Key Word	Psoric Abdomen	Sycotic Abdomen	Syphilitic Abdomen	Tubercular Abdomen
2. Sensation	Sore, bruised, pressive pains in the abdomen are psoric.	Stitching, pulsating and wandering pains in the abdomen are sycotic.	The syphilitic patient is subject to burning, bursting and tearing sensations in the abdomen.	Tubercular patients can feel the beating of the abdominal aorta through the abdominal walls.
	In psora there are sensations of heaviness, fullness with distension of the abdomen; heartburn and waterbrash. There may also be a bearing down sensation.		The stool may contain scrapings of intestine or jelly-like lumps of mucus.	The tubercular abdomen is saucer shaped or may resemble a large plate turned bottom side up.
	An empty, all-gone feeling is characteristic of psora.			
	There may be a stuffed up feeling, which prevents eating, or the psoric patient may experience a sensation of constriction in the abdomen.			
	Rumbling and gurgling occurs in the abdomen as soon as the psoric patient eats or drinks.			
3. Characteristics	Slow peristalsis is psoric.	Accelerated and exaggerated intestinal peristalsis is sycotic.	Dysenteric spasm, especially at night, drives the patient out of bed and may be associated with profuse debilitating perspiration.	In the tubercular miasm we find colic of the lower abdomen, rumbling and gurgling, and flatulence, which causes lower abdominal pain.
	Stitches on stooping or bending the body.	In sycosis, colic is produced by the simplest of foods.	Perverted intestinal peristalsis resulting dysentery is syphilitic.	

103

Key Word	Psoric Abdomen	Sycotic Abdomen	Syphilitic Abdomen	Tubercular Abdomen
4. Modalities	All psoric complaints but especially those of the abdomen are aggravated after eating which causes bloating. The patient cannot bear anything to touch the abdomen.	Children born of sycotic parents often suffer from colic almost from the moment of birth.	Syphilitics are aggravated at night and from warmth.	Tubercular patients experience aggravation from milk and fruits, and from greasy and oily foods.
	Cramps in abdomen from potatoes and beans.	In sycosis, abdominal pains compel the patient to bend forward.	Amelioration for syphilitic abdominal pains is from cold.	Aggravation may also occur when pressure is applied to the abdomen.
	Psoric pains in the abdomen are ameliorated by heat and by gentle pressure, in which case the sycotic miasm must also be present.	Crampy colicky, spasmodic pains, which come on in paroxysms, are ameliorated by hard pressure.		Amelioration is from the open air.

Key Word	Psoric Rectum	Sycotic Rectum	Syphilitic Rectum	Tubercular Rectum
				The tubercular stool is offensive, slimy, and bloody and may have a musty or mouldy smell. or an odour reminiscent of rotten eggs.
7. Worms	Worm symptoms are generally tuberculo-psoric, but when associated with irritation, grinding of the teeth, crawling, creeping and itching of the nose and rectum, then the manifestation is purely psoric. Thread worms.	Wormy symptoms with severe abdominal colic; hyperactive restlessness; excessive dribbling of saliva, and twitching of the muscles are indicative of incoordinations and are sycotic in origin.	Convulsions from worms are a syphilitic manifestation.	All varieties of wormy manifestations are generally recurrent which is characteristic of the tubercular miasm. They may also be associated with allergic manifestations, even allergic dermatitis. Pinworms and many other varieties of intestinal worms are tubercular.
8. Haemorrhoids	Haemorrhoids are generally syco-psoric and are classed under the psoric miasm when they are associated with discomfort and itching.	Rectal haemorrhoids with extreme sensitiveness and pain are sycotic.	Rectal fissures and haemorrhoids with putrid and foetid discharges are syphilitic. They may also ooze pus and sanious fluids.	Strictures, haemorrhoids, sinuses, fistulas and pockets in the rectum are all of tubercular origin and are much aggravated when combined with sycosis and syphilis. Cancerous rectal symptoms are a combinations of the tubercular and sycotic miasms. Bleeding haemorrhoids are tubercular. In this miasm, haemorrhoids, which are suppressed or operated on, may result in asthma-like lung difficulties or heart troubles.

MIASMATIC DIAGNOSIS:
COMPARISON OF THE URINARY SYMPTOMS

Key Word	Psoric Urinary Symptoms	Sycotic Urinary Symptoms	Syphilitic Urinary Symptoms	Tubercular Urinary Symptoms
1. Clinical	Enuresis of functional origin is psoric.	Nephroblastoma, tumours of the kidneys, papillomas of the bladder and nephrotic syndrome where oedema predominates are sycotic.	Destructive and degenerative types of malignant tumours in the kidneys or bladder are syphilitic.	Enuresis, diabetes mellitus (generally tri-miasmatic) and diabetes insipidus (syco-tubercular).
	Nephritis, pyelitis, cystitis and urethritis are psoric in origin because of their infective nature (as all inflammation begins with psora) but strongly sycotic in their manifestations.	Sycosis also has renal dropsy, renal calculi and calculous deposits in other parts of the genito-urinary tract.	Pyaemia with oozing of pus.	Polyps and papillomas of the bladder with haemorrhage are tubercular.
		Hypertrophy of the prostate, and prostatitis from sexual over-indulgence.	Stricture of the urethra.	Haematuria.
2. Characteristics	Phosphaturia after febrile complications occurs in the psoric miasm.	Calculi, complications of the genito-urinary tract and various pains of the urinary tract are generally sycotic in manifestation.	All advanced conditions of the kidneys and genito-urinary tract, with pyogenic inflammations can be associated with structural and pathological changes, and are therefore syphilitic in origin.	The tubercular miasm is responsible for the production of haematuria resulting from different types of pathological manifestations of KUB (kidney, ureter and bladder).
	After fevers and acute diseases, the deposit in the urine is white or yellowish white.			Diabetes mellitus and enuresis are secondary symptoms of the tuberculo-psoric diathesis.

Key Word	Psoric Urinary Symptoms	Sycotic Urinary Symptoms	Syphilitic Urinary Symptoms	Tubercular Urinary Symptoms
3. Sensation	Anuria, oliguria, and stoppage or scanty urine from fright, tension or becoming chilled are psoric manifestations. Psoric patients, especially those advancing in age, experience a sensation of fullness in the bladder. There may also be a feeling of constriction. Smarting and burning in the urinary meatus or in the lumbar area unrelated to any pathological causes might be present.	Stitching and pulsating sensations with wandering pains are sycotic.	Burning and bursting sensations in the bladder or loin area are syphilitic.	A tickling sensation in the urethra is characteristic of the tubercular miasm.
4. Modalities	Psora experiences aggravation from cold. Amelioration of psoric urinary symptoms comes from natural discharges such as urination.	Sycotic urinary symptoms are aggravated in damp, rainy weather and from the changes of the season.	All symptoms of syphilis are aggravated at night, in summer, and from warmth.	Tubercular urinary manifestations are aggravated at night. Amelioration is from the open air.
5. Concomitants	Psoric urinary problems may be associated with anxiety, apprehension and fear of incurable diseases.	Diabetes and albuminuria are tubercular, yet if the conditions are extremely severe, sycosis may also be present, and they can become tri-miasmatic.	In syphilis, all kidney and prostatic symptoms are associated with depression and melancholia.	Restlessness, anxiety and weakness after micturition occur in the tubercular miasm.

111

Key Word	Psoric Urinary Symptoms	Sycotic Urinary Symptoms	Syphilitic Urinary Symptoms	Tubercular Urinary Symptoms
6. Flow	Psoric patients suffer from stress incontinence. The urine passes involuntarily and often frequently, when sneezing, coughing or laughing.	In sycosis, micturition is painful. There may be contraction of the urethra, and children will scream while urinating.	Most urinary complications are of sycotic origin, but when in combination with syphilis the result is diminished flow, and frequent desire for micturition with burning and irritation during the flow.	Colourless, profuse urination, thus diabetes is strongly tubercular.
	There may be burning and smarting while urinating resulting from acidic urine.	Scanty urination (psora is mainly responsible for scanty discharges/excretions), but during the rainy season polyuria is a characteristic of this miasm.	Irritation and burning of the parts, wherever the urine touches, indicates the acridity of this miasm.	The tubercular miasm is responsible for involuntary urination in children. Nocturnal enuresis in children should therefore undergo anti-tubercular treatment.
		In sycosis, there is a frequent desire to urinate before a thunderstorm.		
		Urinary cramps and painful spasms affecting the urethra and bladder may be present in sycosis.		
7. Kidneys	Fibrous changes in the kidneys are psoric in origin.	Sycotic patients suffer from renal calculi with pains, which are stitching and wandering in character.	Fibrous changes with destructive manifestations in kidneys.	In the tubercular miasm there may be recurrent, intermittent and periodic renal spasm with bleeding (haematuria), often noticed particularly during the new and full moon.
	Pain in kidney area, with inflammation of functional origin, nephritis, pyelitis, cystitis and urethritis.	Sycotic tumours of the kidneys or bladder are encapsulated and malignant.		

Key Word	Psoric Urinary Symptoms	Sycotic Urinary Symptoms	Syphilitic Urinary Symptoms	Tubercular Urinary Symptoms
8. Prostate	Psora has prostatitis (which incorporates a sycotic element) with oozing of prostatic fluid.	Enlargement of the prostate gland and complaints arising from it are sycotic.	Syphilitic patients suffer from carcinoma of the prostate with degenerative changes.	Prostate problems with bleeding per urethra are characteristic of the tubercular miasm.
9. Enuresis	In psora, enuresis occurs especially in children as a result of anxiety and fear (particularly a fear of going to school), or from other functional causes.	Enuresis is characterised by the patient waking up during urination due to some discomfort; and enuresis when habit is the only ascertainable cause (features of incoordination), are sycotic.	Syphilitic enuresis is characterised by a complete absence of the sense of realisation. The patient does not remember anything in the morning, lies on the wet bed and cannot be aroused.	The bed wetting of children soon after going to bed is tubercular with a sycotic element unless the patient wakes up during micturition, in which case the sycotic miasm predominates. Bed-wetting of chronic and recurrent character, which may also be periodic and intermittent is also tubercular as is nocturnal polyuria.
10. Urine	Psoric urine is generally dark but can also be yellowish or brownish.	A yellow colour represents sycosis. Sycotic urine may have a fish-brine odour.	Red, the colour of destruction, represents syphilis. Red coloured urine with streaks of pus is characteristic.	Albuminuria, and urine loaded with phosphate, sugar or protein are tubercular. Tubercular urine is pale, colourless and copious. An offensive, musty and putrid, even carrion like odour may be present. Haematuria occurs during sleep.

MIASMATIC DIAGNOSIS:
COMPARISON OF THE SEXUAL SYMPTOMS

Key Word	Psoric Sexual Symptoms	Sycotic Sexual Symptoms	Syphilitic Sexual Symptoms	Tubercular Sexual Symptoms
1. Clinicals	Amenorrhoea.	In general, all varieties of sexual and pelvic disorders (including pelvic inflammatory diseases) come under the purview of sycosis.	Ulcerative and degenerative varieties of tumours are syphilitic.	All varieties of womb infections characterised by profuse bleeding are tubercular.
	Impotency and sterility from lack of sexual desire.	Uterine fibroids and polyps; ovarian tumours and malignancies where the tumour is encapsulated. Polycystic disease of the ovaries, and endometriosis are all sycotic.	Cervical and vulval erosion and ulceration.	Uterine and vaginal polyps with profuse bleeding.
		Leucorrhoea of fish brine odour.	Leucorrhoea, which is acrid, putrid and offensive.	DUB (dysfunctional uterine bleeding), which is characterised by profuse haemorrhage.
		Ectopic pregnancy.	Abortions and stillbirth.	Metastatic and haemorrhagic variety of cancers.
		Genital Warts.		Haemospermia (blood-stained seminal emissions).
		Sterility and infertility from hormonal imbalances.		

Key Word	Psoric Sexual Symptoms	Sycotic Sexual Symptoms	Syphilitic Sexual Symptoms	Tubercular Sexual Symptoms
			Melancholia and fears during menses.	Diarrhoea, fever, visual hallucinations of different colours, auditory hallucinations of different voices, anorexia, nausea, bitter vomiting and epistaxis during menses also typify the tubercular miasm.
				Hysterical manifestations may occur after menses.
				Extremities are cold and often menses can induce general anaemia in young women, and feelings of sadness, gloominess and anxiety.
				Menses is often accompanied by backache and headaches of all kinds.
				Leucorrhoea occurs with palpitations, faintness and loss of vitality in general but with a flushed face, vertigo, a dry, tickling, spasmodic cough and ringing in the ears.

Key Word	Psoric Sexual Symptoms	Sycotic Sexual Symptoms	Syphilitic Sexual Symptoms	Tubercular Sexual Symptoms
6. Discharges	**Female:** Psoric discharges are always bland and scanty. Scanty leucorrhoea. Offensive lochia with small clots. Nightly discharge of genital fluid, in women, with voluptuous dreams. **Male:** Nocturnal passing of semen may occur several times a week or even every night. Night pollution (scanty), easy ejaculation, impotency, and discharge of prostatic fluid during straining at stool or urination are psoric conditions. Semen passes involuntarily during the daytime with little excitation, and often without erection.	**Female:** Sycotic discharges are always profuse, can be yellowish or greenish/yellow. All discharges are of fish-brine smell, which is a characteristic. **Male:** Easy discharge of prostatic fluid with features of prostatitis during straining at stool or urination is characteristic.	**Female:** Syphilitic discharges are always acrid, putrid and offensive. Acrid and putrid leucorrhoea. Nightly discharge of genital fluid, in women, which is acrid and corrodes the part, wherever it touches. **Male:** Azoospermia — dribbling of seminal fluid without the presence of sperm.	**Female:** Tubercular discharges are always profuse and blood-tinged or haemorrhagic, can be associated with clots. Profuse bright red menses with clots. Even leucorrhoeal discharge can be mixed with blood or blood-tinged, can smell musty. **Male:** Semen is emitted during defecation or micturition. Night pollution, a tendency to frequent masturbation, and uncontrolled, unrestrained sexual passion are characteristic of the tubercular miasm. Spermatorrhoea occurs at nightfall and during sleep without dreams.

Key Word	Psoric Sexual Symptoms	Sycotic Sexual Symptoms	Syphilitic Sexual Symptoms	Tubercular Sexual Symptoms
7. Sexual Desire	Female: In psora we find a lack of sexual desire (in both sexes). Male: In psora, the erection may be incomplete, short or lacking.	Female: In sycosis, sexual desire is increased, resulting in various sexual fantasies, voluptuous desires and a nymphomaniac state. Male: Hyper-sexuality is evident in the sycotic miasm.	Female: Syphilitic sexual desires are perverted and can include sexual violence, sadism etc. Male: In the syphilitic male, sexual cravings are perverted or completely destroyed.	Female: Unrestrained, uncontrolled passions including masturbation (in both sexes), and over-indulgence in sex, to the point of perversion, which ultimately leads to exhaustion and becomes detrimental to the health. Male: In the tubercular miasm, masturbation is followed by the loss of all enthusiasm leading to depression followed by weakness of memory.
8. Fertility	Female: In psora there may be sterility or impotence without any organic defect in the sexual parts. There are general or sexual weaknesses and deficient desire or orgasm. Male: The psoric male may suffer from oligospermia (low sperm count).	Female: Sycosis being the miasm of incoordination results in the incapability to conceive due to various factors including hormonal imbalances. In sycosis, sterility and infertility result from pelvic inflammatory diseases and other conditions such as endometriosis.	Female: Possible failure to discharge the ovum at ovulation resulting in infertility is a syphilitic condition. Male: The syphilitic male suffers from azoospermia (complete absence of spermatozoa), which results in infertility.	Female: In the tubercular miasm, infertility results from prolonged menstrual bleeding.

Key Word	Psoric Sexual Symptoms	Sycotic Sexual Symptoms	Syphilitic Sexual Symptoms	Tubercular Sexual Symptoms
9. Menstruation	Scanty (as psora reflects 'hypo'), watery menses.	Sycosis has various menstrual disorders including itching pudenda, pruritus vulvae, mastodynia (breast pain) and polyuria during menses.	In syphilis there is profuse menstrual flow, which is acrid and offensive, and the menstrual blood has a metallic odour.	In the tubercular miasm, menses is exhaustive and prolonged with copious, bright red blood often containing lots of clots.
	In psora, the menses are slow in setting in after puberty and may appear one or more times and then cease for several months or even for a year before returning.	Sycotic menses has the odour of fish-brine, and the stain of the menstrual blood is difficult to wash off.	Irregular periods are syphilitic, with irregularity in both quantity and frequency.	Tubercular menses often appear too soon, perhaps every 2-3 weeks. They may or may not be painful, but are always exhausting. The patient feels poorly a week before menstruation starts.
	Retarded, protracted menses, and retarded menses of short duration are characteristic of psora.	Menstrual pains are spasmodic, extremely sharp and colicky, often coming in paroxysms. The flow may come only with the pains.	Depression and fears during menses are syphilitic.	Flow can also be pale but long lasting, often resulting in anaemia.
	Foetid blood.	Sycotic menses are abundant (tubercular component is present too) and painful.	Syphilitic menses are characterised by bone pains and lumbago.	Tuberculars have profuse and/or long lasting menstrual bleeding.

Key Word	Psoric Sexual Symptoms	Sycotic Sexual Symptoms	Syphilitic Sexual Symptoms	Tubercular Sexual Symptoms
	Dysmenorrhoea may occur at puberty or at the climacteric, and pains are sharp but never colicky.	Menstrual flow is acrid (the acridity component is rendered by syphilis), excoriating and biting, and there may be burning of the pudendum. The discharge is clotted, stringy (stringiness is generally syphilitic, but can be sycotic when it is characterised by the cause, i.e. an incoordination) and yellowish.		Dysmenorrhoea is exhaustive, draining the patient totally.
10. Coition	Female: Psora has weakness of the sexual organs as a result of prolonged suffering from exhaustive diseases. Male: Premature ejaculation is characteristic of psoric males.	Female: In sycosis there is hyper-excitation and frequent sexual arousal. Male: In sycosis, erections are frequent and strong.	Female: In syphilis, an inability to perform coitus, and decreased sexual power can be associated with a burning, acrid, sore feeling in the vagina. Male: In syphilis, erections are troublesome, strong and painful and may occur without any sexual desire.	Female: The tubercular patient suffers from painful coitus due to polyps in the vulva and vagina. Male: The tubercular male suffers from painful erections and coitus, but is still prone to strong sexual indulgence.

MIASMATIC DIAGNOSIS:
COMPARISON OF THE DERMATOLOGICAL SYMPTOMS

Key Word	Psoric Skin	Sycotic Skin	Syphilitic Skin	Tubercular Skin
1. Clinicals	Psora has eczema and eruptions of all kinds in which dryness predominates.	The sycotic patient is subject to warts, veruccas, moles, condylomatas, skin tags, dermoid cysts, fibromas and lipomas. Genital warts may appear in both sexes.	Ulcers and abscesses on different parts of the skin are syphilitic.	Any skin condition characterised by recurrence, periodicity, alternation or haemorrhage. Tubercular conditions are obstinate and difficult to eradicate.
	Pimples with dryness and scurfy scales.	Vesicular eruptions are generally sycotic.	Necrosis, gangrene and bedsores.	Allergic skin manifestations; urticaria.
	Dandruff with bran-like scales.	Herpes of all types.	Deep cracks and fissures in the skin (mainly the palms and soles).	Herpes, which is extremely recurrent and may be periodic.
	Nettle rash is of psoric origin but can only manifest as a combination of two miasms, mainly psora-tubercular (as allergies are tubercular).	Hyperpigmentation of the skin, and melanomas are sycotic.	Depigmentation (desuucuun of pigmentation) of the skin.	Haemangiomas.
		Keloids, corns with thickening of the skin and post-operative scar tumours.	Stitch abscesses.	Recurrent pustular eczemas.
		Radiation hazards resulting in cauliflower-like tumours.	Skin cancer characterised by ulceration and necrosis is syphilitic.	Venous thrombosis and varicose veins with red flushing.

Key Word	Psoric Skin	Sycotic Skin	Syphilitic Skin	Tubercular Skin
		Molluscum contagiosum (syco-psoric).	Burns and scalds with degenerative ulceration.	Petechial haemorrhage, ecchymosis and purpura are tubercular.
		The consequences of vaccinosis.		Ulcerations with haemorrhage.
2. General	Ringworm (more tuberculo-psoric or tuberculo-sycotic, according to the cause and manifestations), itch and eczema are not of psora but the results of psora.	In sycosis, we find disturbed pigment metabolism, resulting in hyper-pigmentation in patches or diffused in different parts.	Ulcerative and degenerative skin conditions are syphilitic.	The tubercular miasm has skin diseases of threatening or destructive natures.
	Tendency of recurrent skin diseases is psoric in origin but psora-tubercular in manifestation (as recurrence is tubercular).	Hypertrophied conditions of the skin are sycotic.	Syphilis has an ulcerous tendency, particularly towards virulent types of open ulcers.	The areas affected tend to be those which are subjected to much use. Eruptions therefore are evident around the fingers and lips, and in or around the mouth.
	In psora, scratching eruptions are followed by dry scales.	Circumscribed or circular patches of hyper-pigmentation in different areas of the skin.	Eruptions, which are slow to heal, are syphilo-psoric.	The tubercular miasm encompasses the state where there is a presence of ringworm or where there has been a past history of the suppression of ringworm.
	Eczemas and eruptions are papular and associated with itching.	Fish scale eruptions can be syco-psoric or tri-miasmatic, combining the dryness of psora, the thickened skin of sycosis and the squamous character of syphilis.	Ulcerated skin with pus and blood represents syphilis.	Recurrent and obstinate boils with profuse pus.

Key Word	Psoric Skin	Sycotic Skin	Syphilitic Skin	Tubercular Skin
	Voluptuous tickling and itching, which is only temporarily relieved by rubbing and scratching.	Painful skin eruptions which are localised and/or in circumscribed spots.		Skin conditions associated with glandular involvement are tubercular.
	Psoric skin diseases are devoid of suppuration and apt to be dry.	Vesicular eruptions which do not heal quickly and urine-coloured patches are sycotic.		
3. Sensation	Sensation of burning.		Syphilitic skin is not itchy but there can be sensations of rawness and soreness.	In the tubercular miasm, a sensation of exhaustion is present with skin diseases.
	Unhealthy skin with itching and burning represents psora.			
	Pruritus is always a manifestation of psora.	Pruritus (is of psoric origin) but manifests in sycosis in the anus, nose and sexual organs with thickening of the skin.		
4. Modalities	In psora, itching often occurs late in the evening before midnight and is most unbearable.	Sycotic skin eruptions are aggravated by the consumption of meat; in humid and rainy weather, and from changes in the weather generally.	All symptoms of syphilis are aggravated at night, in summer, from the warmth of the bed and from warmth in general.	Tubercular skin diseases are aggravated at night, by touch and pressure generally, while thinking of complaints, after undressing, from milk, greasy and oily foods, from the warmth of the bed (syphilitic component), and after itching.
	Psoric skin complaints are aggravated by cold, in winter, and from undressing.			

Key Word	Psoric Skin	Sycotic Skin	Syphilitic Skin	Tubercular Skin
	Amelioration is from natural discharges such as sweat.	In sycosis there is amelioration in dry weather.	Amelioration of the syphilitic miasm comes with any abnormal discharge.	Amelioration is from the open air, and dry weather.
	Relief also comes from the reappearance of suppressed skin eruptions.	When warts or fibrous growths reappear, the sycotic patient feels relieved.		
		Painful skin eruptions are better by pressure.		
5. Concomitants	In psora, when skin diseases are suppressed the mind is directly affected, resulting in anxiety, apprehension, and fear of incurable diseases.	Suppression of sycotic skin diseases affects first the nerve centres of the body and then the heart, liver and reproductive system. Hyperaesthesia, cardiac incoordinations including dropsy; hepatomegaly and various pelvic inflammatory disorders including endometriosis may result.	Leprosy in which liquefaction has already started is tubercular but with syphilis predominating.	When tubercular skin is suppressed, it affects the inner tissues causing destructive and ulcerous tendencies, and the deeper tissues causing debilitated tubercular states such as fatigue syndromes.
		Suppression of ringworm can result in rheumatism, chronic headaches, stomach complaints and chronic bronchitis.	When syphilitic skin is suppressed the intellect is affected, causing dullness, depression and a lack of enthusiasm.	
6. Appearance	Psoric skin appears dirty, dry and harsh and becomes more dry with washing. The skin cannot endure water and often has an unwashed, unhealthy, dingy look.	Small, reddish, flat vesicular eruptions which are slow to heal (in slow healing the syphilitic miasmatic taint must also be present) and recur during the menstrual period are sycotic.	Threatening (ulcerative and destructive) appearance.	Tubercular skin conditions are angry looking and often accompanied by oozing of blood.

Key Word	Psoric Skin	Sycotic Skin	Syphilitic Skin	Tubercular Skin
	Cracks on the hands and feet with extreme dryness.	Warty excrescences, which appear after vaccinations.	Ulcerating moles with hairy tufts are syphilitic.	Skin lesions are red and haemorrhagic in appearance.
		Red pinhead type moles and other moles, warts, wine coloured patches (multi-miasmatic with underlying sycosis), urine coloured patches and other manifestations of unnaturally thickened skin.	Syphilitic eruptions are found around the joints and flexures of the body and are arranged in circular groupings (in all circular and circumscribed manifestations sycosis is also present), rings or segments of circles.	
		Spider web, red capillaries over the centre of the malar bone.	Copper or raw ham coloured eruptions.	
		Acne, which is red in appearance (in red appearance the tubercular miasm is also present), angry looking, papular or vesicular eruptions around the time of the menstrual period, which are isolated and painful.	Putridity and offensiveness of all discharges with ugly looking ulcers, which have a cadaverous base.	
		Sycotic skin looks oily and the tip of the nose appears red. There may be stubby, dead, broken hair in the beard, which falls out due to skin eruptions.		

126

Key Word	Psoric Skin	Sycotic Skin	Syphilitic Skin	Tubercular Skin
7. Colour	Psoric eruptions are not noticeable by their colour but by the roughness of the skin.	Sycosis has a disturbed pigment metabolism producing both hyper and depigmentation, which occurs in patches or is diffused in different parts.	In syphilis, there are copper coloured eruptions, which do not heal fast, but turn to ulceration. The discomfort is aggravated at night and by the warmth of the bed.	Tubercular skin is pale with a bluish tint showing signs of venous stagnation. Varicose veins have a red flushed appearance. Freckles are quite significant especially in fine, transparent, smooth-skinned people.
8. Eruptions	Itching without pus or discharge is characteristic of psora. Warts (syco-psoric) on face, arms and hands, with dryness. Psoriasis has been called "the marriage of all the miasms but its characteristics are predominantly psoric and sycotic". (Dr. Roberts).	Exfoliating eczemas are sycotic. Fish scale eruptions are tri-miasmatic but mainly sycotic in manifestation due to the thickening of the skin and the exfoliative tendency. Herpes (including herpes zoster and genitalis), erysipelas, all sorts of warts and excrescences, barber's itch and other scaly and patchy skin eruptions, which occur in circumscribed spots.	Syphilis has a tendency to develop open ulcers of virulent type. All eruptions are patchy. Ulcers and putrefaction of all tissues devoid of pain and itching. All sorts of ulcers, carbuncles and boils, which do not heal fast (slow to heal is psora-syphilitic) and are characterised by the discharge of offensive and spreading fluid and pus are syphilitic.	Eczema, and ringworm, a history of ringworm and suppression of ringworm are tubercular. Urticaria and herpes (allergic and recurrent varieties e.g. recurrent herpes genitalis). If eruptions are pustular or vesicular the suppuration (coming from the syphilitic component) is marked. Painful eruptions in the vagina during pregnancy are characteristic of a prominent tubercular miasm.

127

Key Word	Psoric Skin	Sycotic Skin	Syphilitic Skin	Tubercular Skin
	Crusts, which are thin, light, fine and small, are present in psora.	Post-operative scar tumours and proliferation of the stitch line after an operation are sycotic.	Stitch abscesses, malignant dyscrasias; gangrenes of the skin and dry gangrene are all syphilitic manifestations.	The formation of pus after insect or fly bites or the slightest injury, which does not heal fast is tubercular.
	Small, sensitive, painful, non-suppurating boils, which may shed scurfy scales.	All sorts of facial skin diseases that may be contracted at the barber's, such as tinea barbae and tinea vesicular, but excluding tinea favosa.	All skin conditions characterised by putridity and offensiveness of discharges.	Recurrent stitch abscesses after an operation or scarring after ulcers are generally associated with bleeding in the tubercular miasm. Recurrent and obstinate boils with profuse pus and fever, heal with difficulty.
		Abnormal growths (a combination of sycosis with the tubercular miasm).	Crusts are always thick (in thickening of the crust, sycosis also plays a role; as thickening is a proliferation or excess deposition) and heavy.	Abnormal growths (with clearness of the skin).
9. Sweat	Scanty, sour smelling sweat, especially on forehead and during sleep is psoric.	In sycosis, sweat appears on the forehead during sleep. The skin has an oily appearance and perspiration is thick and copious.	Syphilitic sweat is offensive and aggravates all complaints.	In the tubercular miasm there is offensive foot or axillary sweat which when suppressed may induce lung trouble or some other severe disease.
10. Parasites	Animal parasites with tickling in the skin and voluptuous itching (voluptuousness is an excessive component rendered by sycosis) are psoric.	Parasitic infestation with thickening of the skin is sycotic.	Parasitic infestation with ulceration of the skin is syphilitic.	Animal parasitic infestations with tickling and bleeding are tubercular.

MIASMATIC DIAGNOSIS:
COMPARISON OF THE NAIL SYMPTOMS

Key Word	Psoric Nails	Sycotic Nails	Syphilitic Nails	Tubercular Nails
1. Nails	Psoric nails have a dry, harsh appearance.	Sycotic nails are thick as a result of hyper or excess deposition of tissue.	Syphilitic nails are thin (as a result of destruction of the cells) and bend and tear easily.	The tubercular miasm has frequent and recurrent brittle nails, which often drop off and then grow again.
	On pressing the tip of the nail, the nail beds present an anaemic appearance.	Ridges or ribs, which can be longitudinal or horizontal, are visible on the nails.	Pitted nails with indentations, or longitudinal or transverse indentations, like grooves or channels in the nails.	Nails with various stains, glossy nails with white specks and scalloped edges, and spotted nails are all tubercular. On pressing the tip of the nail, there occurs red flushing in the nail bed.
		Wavy, corrugated nails with protuberance or bumps are sycotic.	Syphilitic nails have brittle edges, which bend easily.	Asymmetrical nails, which come out easily are tubercular.
		Dome-shaped nails with a convex appearance.	Spoon-shaped; concave nails (the reverse of sycosis).	The natural convexity is often reversed.
		Irregular (feature of incoordination) shaped nails with irregular but thick edges.	Whitlows and panaritium, with pus points at the end or corners of the nails.	Irregular nails, which break and split easily.
		Stitching pains may occur in the nail beds.		Formation of pus at the junction of the nail and flesh, with many hang nails.

129

MIASMATIC DIAGNOSIS:
COMPARISON OF THE EXTREMITY SYMPTOMS

Key Word	Psoric Extremities	Sycotic Extremities	Syphilitic Extremities	Tubercular Extremities
1. Clinicals	Various types of rheumatism, especially of a functional and inflammatory nature; osteitis, osteomyelitis (the initial stage without bone destruction. When the destruction starts, the condition becomes syphilitic); periostitis.	Osteoporosis is syco-syphilitic (the hormonal imbalance is given by sycosis and bone porosis or destruction is afforded by syphilis).	Bone pains, delayed ossification and fragility of the bones; caries and necrosis of the bones and spine are syphilitic.	Rickets are syphilo-tubercular.
	Leg cramps.	Rheumatism, gout and osteoarthritis.	Osteomyelitis with bone destruction and formation of sequestrum.	Nodular growths of glandular origin.
		All joint pains of the small and larger joints are sycotic.	Malignancy of the bones, bone metastasis and sarcoma.	Weakness of the ankle joints.
		Arthritic deformans; tophi and deposits in the joints.	Ulcers and gangrenous inflammations.	Offensive and sweaty palms and soles.
		Oedematous swelling of the extremities.	Paralysis characterised by muscle wasting and degenerative changes (when incoordination and malfunctioning are evident, paralysis is sycotic).	
2. Generals	The extremity pains of psora are generally neuralgic in type.	Incoordination, which may be anatomical or functional, is characteristic of sycosis.	Syphilis shows an extremely irregular development of symptoms.	Pupura and haemorrhagic manifestations are characteristic of the tubercular miasm.

Key Word	Psoric Extremities	Sycotic Extremities	Syphilitic Extremities	Tubercular Extremities
	Sore, bruised and pressive pains are psoric.	The sycotic diathesis is rheumatic and gouty.	Pain in the long bones is syphilitic.	Delayed milestones.
		Sycosis is silent or even surreptitious in its manifestations.		Weakness of the ankle joints is a sure indication of the presence of syphilo-psora, i.e. the tubercular miasm.
		Joints and connective tissues are affected.		
3. Sensation	Sensations of dryness, heat and burning of the hands and feet with sweating of the palms and soles are characteristic of psora.	Rheumatism, numbness and paralytic weakness of the extremities are sycotic.	Burning, bursting and tearing sensations are syphilitic.	Cramps in the lower extremities, legs, feet and toes are tubercular but also found in psora.
	Numbness with tingling sensations; feeling as if parts are going to sleep, which occurs when pressure is brought to bear on the part, when lying lightly on the part or when sitting cross-legged.	Joint pains; stitching, pulsating, shooting, tearing and wandering pains are sycotic. Shooting, and tearing pains may occur in the muscles as well as the joints. Stiffness, soreness, lameness are also characteristic of sycosis.		
	Pricking and tingling in the extremities due to 'hypo' or poor circulation, with coldness of the extremities.	Gouty concretions due to rheumatic affection, with pain in the joints or periosteum with inflammatory deposits.		
	Leg cramps.	Proliferative variety of inflammation or growth of any tissues.		
	Constant chilliness.			

131

Key Word	Psoric Extremities	Sycotic Extremities	Syphilitic Extremities	Tubercular Extremities
4. Modalities	Psoric aggravation occurs in winter. The patient requires warmth both externally and internally.	Pains are worse at the approach of a storm or during a thunderstorm (generally thunderstorm aggravations are predominantly tubercular or syphilo-tubercular; but can also be present in sycosis due to incoordination), from damp humid atmosphere and rainy weather.	Syphilitic pains are worse at night or at the approach of night, and there is general aggravation from sunset to sunrise. The seaside, sea voyages, thunderstorms, summer and warmth, and extremes of temperature also aggravate.	In the tubercular miasm, aggravation comes at night and from thunderstorms.
	Aggravation also occurs between sunrise and sunset, from cold and from standing.	Rheumatic pains are worse from cold and damp, rest, changes in the weather and from meat.	Acute rheumatic pain, osteomyelitis and ulcerous inflammation in the bone marrow with its accompanying pains, are aggravated at night and during stormy weather and changes in the weather.	Milk, fruits, and greasy and oily foods aggravate.
		Stooping, bending and beginning to move also aggravate sycotic conditions.	Movement, perspiration and the warmth of the bed cause aggravation in syphilis. Syphilitic and tubercular pains are similar in character and times of aggravation.	Tubercular patients cannot tolerate any pressure to the chest and feel worse in a closed room.
	Psoric amelioration is evident in the summer, from heat, and by natural discharges such as urine, sweat, menstruation etc. Physiological eliminative processes like diarrhoea, also ameliorate.	Better by moving, from slow motion, stretching and rubbing, pressure, by lying on the stomach and in dry weather.	In syphilis, there is amelioration from sunrise to sunset, in lukewarm climates and during the winter cold. Changes in position also ameliorate.	Neuralgic pains are better by quiet, rest and warmth. Aggravated from motion.

Key Word	Psoric Extremities	Sycotic Extremities	Syphilitic Extremities	Tubercular Extremities
	Psoric conditions are also ameliorated by hot application, scratching, crying and eating, and the appearance of suppressed skin eruptions.	Sycotic conditions are ameliorated by unnatural discharges (which are generally greenish-yellow), and by unnatural elimination through the mucus surfaces, such as leucorrhoea, nasal discharge etc. Physiological eliminations however do not ameliorate.	Syphilitic conditions are better for any abnormal discharges such as leucorrhoea and coryza and from the discharge of pus when old ulcers break open.	Amelioration is from dry weather, open air, and in the daytime.
		The return of suppressed normal discharges such as menses ameliorate, as do the appearance of warts and fibrous growths.		Temporary amelioration comes from offensive foot or axillary sweat which when suppressed induces lung trouble.
		Ameliorated in general from the return or breaking open of old ulcers and old sores, and markedly ameliorated by the return of acute gonorrhoeal manifestations.		Amelioration from nosebleeds is characteristic of the tubercular miasm.
5. Character	In psora there is twitching of the muscles during sleep.	The slightest physical exertion fatigues the sycotic patient.	Aching pains in the bones of the limbs and in the joints are syphilitic.	The tubercular patient is unable to tolerate exertion and lack of exercise leads to flabbiness.
	Various types of rheumatism, especially of functional inflammatory nature without gross structural changes; curvature of the bones, osteitis and osteomyelitis are characteristic of psora.	Easy spraining of the joints while walking; joints and connective tissues which are easily affected, are sycotic.	In syphilis, the ankle joint is weak and the patient stumbles and falls easily.	

Key Word	Psoric Extremities	Sycotic Extremities	Syphilitic Extremities	Tubercular Extremities
		Stiffness, soreness and lameness are characteristic of sycosis, and gouty diatheses have a sycotic base.	The syphilitic stigmata may affect the bony structures causing destructive changes (e.g. osteomalacia).	Profuse perspiration occurs on the palms of the hands and the soles of the feet.
			Burning, bursting and tearing pains are syphilitic, and shooting or lancinating pains may occur in the periosteum or long bones.	Offensive, sweaty palms and soles. Cold, damp, soft and flabby hands, and a **coldness of the hands and feet of which the patient is not always conscious.**
				Tubercular patients have weak wrist and ankle joints and difficulty holding on to objects. They drop things easily, are clumsy in getting about and stumble over the tiniest things.
6. Appearance	The psoric patient suffers from prominent varicose veins in the lower part of the body.	Sycosis has anatomical abnormalities such as six fingers.	The syphilitic patient may be subject to various deformities and atrophy of various organs.	Nodular growths are tubercular.
		Local or generalised oedema or anasarca is characteristic in sycosis.	A marasmic appearance is basically syphilitic because the syphilitic stigma destroys the power of the body to assimilate proper materials from food.	Tubercular patients often have distinctive fingers, which may be either equal and long with blunt or club-shaped tips which do not appear converged, or long and irregularly arranged. The hands are thin, soft and flabby and can easily be compressed. They are also usually very moist, often cold and damp, and perspire profusely.

Key Word	Psoric Extremities	Sycotic Extremities	Syphilitic Extremities	Tubercular Extremities
7. Function	In psora, the patient can walk well and finds it difficult to stand still.	Sycosis infiltrates and corrodes (syphilo-sycosis) by its discharges and smells of fish brine.	Syphilis has paralytic weaknesses caused by destruction or severe impairment of the functions of the nerves and muscles.	Rickets may occur in the tubercular miasm causing soft and curved bones.
		In sycosis, the red blood corpuscles are destroyed through imperfect oxidisation of food. This can lead to anaemic conditions, which may be evidenced by a lack of stamina in the muscles and a pallid, drawn, puffy appearance.		Drop wrists, a weakness and loss of power in the tendons around the joints and tendons and ligaments which sprain easily. The ankles turn easily from the slightest misstep and activities such as playing the piano and typing cause exhaustion and swelling of the fingers and wrist joints.
		Chronic or long-continued inflammation is characteristic especially in the joints.		There is a general lack of energy and a lack of strength in the bones.
		The sycotic miasm is devoid of power. The joints are easily sprained even while walking and there is numbness of the extremities.		The feet are cold and damp and perspire profusely, a fact of which the patient is unaware.
				The slightest physical exertion fatigues the tubercular patient and there is a great sense of exhaustion. As the sun ascends, their strength revives, and as it descends they lose it again. Tiredness comes on at night even after a sleep.

MIASMATIC DIAGNOSIS:
COMPARISON OF SLEEP SYMPTOMS

Key Word	Psoric Sleep	Sycotic Sleep	Syphilitic Sleep	Tubercular Sleep
1. Character of sleep and dream	Sleep: Psoric sleep is unrefreshing with fearful dreams and dreams of anxiety. There is weariness on awakening. Twitching of muscles during sleep. Loud talking and screaming during sleep. Gnashing of teeth during sleep and expulsion of round worms. Somnambulism occurs in psora and there is sleeplessness during the day. Dreams: As soon as the psoric patient closes their eyes, fearful images and distorted faces appear. Dreams are vivid (as if the patient were awake); sad, frightful, anxious and lascivious.	Sleep: The sycotic patient sleeps for a short time, wakes, then returns to sleep again. Restless sleep is characteristic of sycosis. Dreams: The sycotic patient has sexual dreams with fantasies.	Sleep: Rolling the head from side to side during sleep is characteristic of syphilis. Dreams: Sexual dreams with perversions and suicidal dreams are syphilitic. The syphilitic patient dreams of violence; destruction, death and dead bodies, and generally gloomy forebodings.	Sleep: The tubercular patient screams out during sleep. Sleep is accompanied by a sensation of great exhaustion. Dreams: The tubercular patient dreams of travelling.

Key Word	Psoric Sleep	Sycotic Sleep	Syphilitic Sleep	Tubercular Sleep
2. Modalities	Psoric complaints are aggravated during sleep.	In sycosis, sleep is restless in damp, humid weather and during thunderstorms.	Syphilitic sleep is disturbed at the seaside, during the summer, at night and from sweat. Amelioration comes from a change of position.	Tubercular sleep is disturbed in enclosed, stuffy rooms.
3. Concomitants	Psoric sleeplessness is experienced due to an abundance of ideas. Sweating, especially on the head, snoring, salivation, grinding of the teeth, unconsciousness, and passing of stool and urine during sleep are all characteristic of psora.	In sycosis, sleeplessness occurs due to mental and physical disquiet.	The syphilitic patient is sleepless because of tormenting ideas. Sleep is unrefreshing and accompanied by depression and melancholia.	Unrefreshing sleep with great exhaustion is tubercular.

MIASMATIC DIAGNOSIS:
COMPARISON OF MODALITY SYMPTOMS

Key Word	Psoric Modalities	Sycotic Modalities	Syphilitic Modalities	Tubercular Modalities
1. Aggravation	Psora has aggravation in winter and during sleep.	Sycotic aggravation is from rest, damp cold, moist cold, the rainy season, humid atmosphere, from changes in the weather, during thunderstorms and from heat.	In syphilis there is aggravation from sunset to sunrise, from natural discharges such as perspiration, from extremes of temperature, at the seaside and from sea voyages, from thunderstorms, movement, during the summer, from warmth and from the warmth of the bed.	Worse during thunderstorm (like sycosis and syphilis), and at night.
	Wants warmth both internally and externally (aggravation from cold).	Pains in the joints are worse during cold, damp weather.		The tubercular patient cannot tolerate any pressure in the chest.
	Psora is associated with mental restlessness and anxiety. The patient cannot stand still and must walk instead of standing.	The sycotic patient is like a barometer — he has pains when it rains, and when the atmosphere is filled with moisture he suffers.		In the tubercular miasm there is aggravation from milk, fruits, greasy and oily foods and in closed rooms.
2. Amelioration	Sunrise to sunset.	The sycotic patient gains amelioration from motion, during winter, in a dry atmosphere and from any unnatural discharge such as leucorrhoea or catarrh. Natural eliminations do not ameliorate.	Syphilitic amelioration occurs from sunrise to sunset, from a change of position, in lukewarm climates, during winter, from cold and from any abnormal discharge such as leucorrhoea.	In the tubercular miasm, there is amelioration in dry weather, open air and during the daytime.

Key Word	Psoric Modalities	Sycotic Modalities	Syphilitic Modalities	Tubercular Modalities
	In summer, by heat or warmth in general, and from hot applications.	Mental conditions may be much ameliorated when warts or fibrous growths appear, and there is a general amelioration from the return or breaking open of old ulcers and sores. There is also a marked amelioration from the return of acute gonorrhoeal manifestations.	Conditions improve through the discharge of pus (better if old ulcer opens up).	Temporary amelioration is by offensive foot or axillary sweat, which when suppressed, induces lung conditions.
	The psoric patient has a desire to lie down day and night for amelioration of his troubles.	Joint pains are ameliorated in the morning or by stretching, in dry weather and by slow motion.		Amelioration by epistaxis is characteristic of the tubercular miasm.
	Amelioration from natural discharges such as urine and menses, and better through physiological eliminative processes such as perspiration.	Amelioration from lying on stomach, pressure, or return of suppressed normal discharge (e.g. menses).		
3. Process	Psora develops physical irritation, i.e. itch.	Sycosis develops catarrhal discharges.	Syphilis produces open ulcers.	The tubercular miasm produces haemorrhages.

MIASMATIC DIAGNOSIS:
COMPARISON OF CHARACTERISTICS: A SYNOPSIS

Key Word	*Psora* *Sensitising Miasm*	*Sycosis* *Miasm of Incoordination*	*Syphilis* *Degenerating Miasm*	*Tubercular* *Responsive, Reactive Miasm*
1. General Manifestations	i) Psora develops itch.	i) Sycosis develops catarrhal discharges.	i) The syphilitic miasm has virulent open ulcers.	i) The tubercular miasm has haemorrhages.
	ii) Unhealthy skin with burning and itching represents psora.	ii) Oily skin with thickly oozing and copious perspiration, represents sycosis.	ii) Ulcerated skin with pus and blood represents syphilis.	ii) Oily skin with coldness represents the tubercular miasm.
	iii) All 'hypos' are mainly psoric.	iii) 'Hypers' are sycotic.	iii) 'Dyses' are syphilitic.	iii) Allergies are tubercular.
	iv) Hypoplasia is psoric.	iv) Hyperplasia is sycotic.	iv) Dysplasia is syphilitic.	iv) Alternation of 'hypo' and dysplasia is tubercular.
	v) Atrophy, ataxia, anaemia and anoxaemia are psoric.	v) Hypertrophy is sycotic.	v) Dystrophy is syphilitic.	v) Dystrophy with haemorrhage is tubercular.
	vi) Hypotension is psoric.	vi) Hypertension is sycotic.	vi) Irregular, arrhythmic pulse is syphilitic.	vi) Intermittent pulse is tubercular.
	vii) Lack, scanty, less and absence denote psora.	vii) Exaggeration or excess denotes sycosis.	vii) Destruction and degeneration denotes syphilis.	vii) Alternation and periodicity is tubercular.
	viii) Weakness is psoric.	viii) Restlessness (especially physical) is sycotic.	viii) Destructiveness is syphilitic.	viii) Changeableness is tubercular.

Key Word	Psora Sensitising Miasm	Sycosis Miasm of Incoordination	Syphilis Degenerating Miasm	Tubercular Responsive, Reactive Miasm
	ix) An inhibitory quality is psoric in nature.	ix) An expressive quality is characteristic of sycosis.	ix) Melancholic, depressive and suicidal tendencies are syphilitic in nature.	ix) A dissatisfied quality is tubercular in nature.
	x) Dryness of membranes denotes psora.	x) Augmented secretion denotes sycosis.	x) Ulceration denotes syphilis.	x) Haemorrhages and allergies denote the tubercular miasm.
	xi) Psora does not assimilate well.	xi) Sycotics are over nourished.	xi) Syphilitics has disorganised digestion.	xi) Tubercular patients crave the things which make them sick.
	xii) The secretions of psora are serous.	xii) Sycotic secretions are purulent.	xii) The secretions of syphilis are sticky, acrid and putrid.	xii) Tubercular secretions are haemorrhagic.
2. General Nature of the Miasm	Hyper-sensitivity (basically psora is 'hypo' in expression which gives rise to hypo-immunity, in turn resulting in hyper-susceptibility which manifests as an exalted sensitivity to the external environment and allergens). Itching, irritation and burning lead towards congestion and inflammation with only functional changes. The capacity to produce hyper-sensitivity, i.e. the sensitising property of psora is its basic nature.	Sycosis produces incoordination everywhere resulting in over production, growth, and infiltration in the form of warts, condylomata, tumours, fibrous tissues etc.	Syphilis produces destructive disorder everywhere, which manifests as perversion, suppuration, ulceration and fissures.	The tubercular miasm produces changing symptomatology, confusing vague symptomatology (e.g. dyspepsia, weakness, wasting, fever), and conditions which are variable, shifting in location, changing in outlook, alternating in state, and contradictory.
3. Key Words & Expressions	Hypo-immunity.	Hyper — mental and physical.	Destruction — physical and mental.	Dissatisfaction.

Key Word	Psora Sensitising Miasm	Sycosis Miasm of Incoordination	Syphilis Degenerating Miasm	Tubercular Responsive, Reactive Miasm
	Anxiety and apprehension.	Hypertrophy — growths and incoordinations.	Degeneration.	Alternation, changeability, and migratory conditions.
	Alertness.	Necrosis and ulcer	Necrosis and ulceration.	Periodic, recurrent and allergic.
	Fears.		Putridity and acidity.	Vague manifestations.
	Irritation — mental and physical.		'Dyses'.	Craves the things which make them sick.
	Sensitivity.		Irregular and arrhythmic.	
4. Diathesis	i) Eruptive.	i) Rheumatic and gouty.	i) Suppurative or ulcerative.	i) Scrofulous.
		ii) Lithic and uric acid.		ii) Haemorrhagic.
		iii) Proliferative.		iii) Allergic.
5. Organs & Tissues Affected	Ectodermal tissues. Nervous system, endocrine system, blood vessels, liver and skin.	Entodermal tissues — soft tissues. Attacks internal organs, the blood (producing anaemias), and the pelvis and sexual organs.	Mesodermal tissues and bones, and the glandular tissues particularly the lymphatics.	Glandular tissue. The patient is poor in bone, flesh and blood.
6. Nature of Diseases	i) Deficiency disorders.	i) Deposition and/or proliferation of cells/tissues.	i) Destructive, degenerative disorders, deformities and fragility.	i) Depletion.
				ii) Drainage and wasting.
				iii) Alternating disorders.

142

Key Word	Psora Sensitising Miasm	Sycosis Miasm of Incoordination	Syphilis Degenerating Miasm	Tubercular Responsive, Reactive Miasm
7. Pace of Action	i) Hyperactive. ii) Dramatic development of symptoms.	i) Extremely slow, insidious. ii) Silent or even surreptitious in its manifestations.	i) Usually midway in pace, i.e. moderate. Though sometimes may be rapid or insidious. ii) Irregular/arrhythmic pace. iii) Generally more overt in its manifestations.	i) Depends according to preponderance of psoric or syphilitic miasm.
8. Constitution	Carbonitrogenoid (excess of carbon and nitrogen).	Hydrogenoid (excess of water).	Oxygenoid (excess of oxygen).	Changeable constitution with alternation and periodicity.
9. Psychic Manifestations The Person	The sterile philosopher with lots of ideas, which he cannot materialise. Psora is theoretical but has no sense of practicality. Dishonesty, secretiveness, wickedness and impurity play a good part in him.	Sycosis is deceitful, sullen and cunning and has a tendency to exploit others. A very practical person that always cares for their own benefit and pleasures above others.	An urge for destruction seems to be the only emotion of the syphilitic person. They lack a sense of realisation, duty and understanding. Committed criminals and cold-blooded murderers are syphilitic. Their mentality vitiates the sense of judgement.	Dissatisfaction, changeability, and a lack of tolerance and perseverance are tubercular.

Key Word	Psora Sensitising Miasm	Sycosis Miasm of Incoordination	Syphilis Degenerating Miasm	Tubercular Responsive, Reactive Miasm
Nature of the Miasm	Psora is the sensitising miasm for its hyperactive and hypersensitive mind and body, which results from hypo-immunity and increased susceptibility.	Sycosis is 'hyper', and the miasm of incoordinations. This manifests as hyper abnormal behaviours or mental incoordinations such as extreme jealousy, loquacity and selfishness.	Syphilis is the miasm of destruction, destroying the love of one's own life and resulting in self-destruction or the killing of others. Syphilitics therefore have suicidal tendencies or can be cold-blooded murderers. They may be called iconoclasts and have a total lack of mercy and sympathy.	The tubercular miasm is one of changeableness. A dissatisfied state of mind makes the subject changeable both mentally and physically.
Work	Quickly fatigued with desire to lie down is characteristic of psora. The patient is indolent.	The sycotic patient is a hyper-workaholic.	The syphilitic patient is disinterested in work due to their lack of realisation and understanding.	Changeableness and impatience make it hard for the tubercular patient to concentrate on work.
Behaviour	Psora is fearful, anxious, alert and apprehensive.	Sycosis is quarrelsome, jealous, selfish and cunning with a tendency to harm (emotionally) others and animals. Ostentation and fatuousness are sycotic tendencies. The subject is often suspicious of his own works and his surroundings. Mischievous, mean and selfish summarise the sycotic psychic essence.	Syphilis is cruel and destructive and often does bodily harm to himself and others.	Fearlessness and an absolute lack of anxiety are denominating features of the tubercular miasm. There is a careless, unconcerned or indifferent attitude towards the seriousness of their sufferings and they are always hopeful of a recovery.

| Key Word | Psora
Sensitising Miasm | Sycosis
Miasm of Incoordination | Syphilis
Degenerating Miasm | Tubercular
Responsive, Reactive Miasm |
|---|---|---|---|---|
| Memory | Weakness of memory indicates psora. | Absentmindedness is sycotic. The patient loses the thread of the conversation and forgets the recent events although they can remember past events well. | Forgetfulness is syphilitic. There is a mental paralysis where the patient reads but cannot retain the information. The mind is slow. | Changeableness of thought and perception is tubercular. |
| Death | It is only the psoric miasm which fears death. There is often much anxiety and an anticipation towards death. | Men and women who commit suicide today are mainly syphilo-sycotic. Sycotics will plan their own death but too many attachments and an urge to live make it difficult for them to really commit suicide. | The syphilitic patient dwells on suicide, has suicidal dreams and thoughts and an actual urge to commit suicide. Love for their own life is destroyed. | Dissatisfaction with their own life, changeableness and a vagabond mentality lead to suicidal impulses in the tubercular patient. An instinct towards self-destruction is characterised by carelessness. |
| Selfishness & Deprivation | Psora, by dint of its selfish nature has a tendency to deprive others (a characteristic which is also strongly present in sycosis). Deprivation exists in the sense of presenting a false or pseudo image of himself. Psoric patients may donate (although not voluntarily) a large sum of money to charity but they will ensure that they receive some personal benefit from their action. | In all varieties of deprivation and rudeness sycosis is present. The sycotic patient's prime concern is for his or her own benefit, and they will act selfishly to deprive others in order to achieve this end. | Syphilitic patients rarely deprive others as their lack of realisation extends to that of their own benefit. They are selfish only in the sense of being focussed in one particular direction, e.g. with destructive impulse, they forget or ignore everything else around them. | Extreme irritability and outrageousness with a lack of tolerance can be reflected as the selfish nature of the tubercular miasm. |

Key Word	Psora Sensitising Miasm	Sycosis Miasm of Incoordination	Syphilis Degenerating Miasm	Tubercular Responsive, Reactive Miasm
Fear	All varieties of fears are classified as psoric and in this miasm they manifest as anxiety, alertness and apprehension of impending misfortune. Mental restlessness is one of the expressions of psoric fear.	As a result of incoordination of thoughts, sycosis does manifest some fears. A millionaire, for example, may develop a constant fear of poverty, which is expressed as selfishness, suspiciousness and physical restlessness.	The syphilitic lack of realisation and expression means that their fears are not properly manifested. They are close-mouthed and the only possible outward feature one might expect from a syphilitic person is of anguish.	Fearlessness is characteristic of tubercular miasm and this is well expressed by the patient as a complete indifference towards their health. Their only real fear is of dogs or other animals.
Expression	Psora is full of ideas and philosophical expression. There may be piles of books on the table and the person will go from book to book, reading only superficially. There is no depth, various ideas crowd the mind and there is no practicality at all. This constant flow of ideas is as a result of the mental restlessness.	Jealousy and suspicion are very evident in sycotic expression, and there is a tendency to suppress and conceal. This deep suspicion means that the patient does not trust anything and checks everything many times.	The syphilitic patient is an introvert, a close-mouthed fellow who keeps his depression inside and the first thing anyone knows of it is when he has committed suicide. There is also a suppressive tendency to conceal and an inability to realise and express symptoms. These patients want to escape from themselves, as well as from others, and idiocy, ignorance and obstinacy lead to melancholia and gloominess.	In the tubercular miasm, mental symptoms, especially anger are aggravated after sleep and the patient may wake with a look of dissatisfaction clearly manifested on their face. Changeability, lack of tolerance and impatience sum up the expressions of the tubercular miasm.
10. Key Words of Mental Manifestations	i) Anxious and fearful. ii) Philosophical.	i) Suspicious and jealous. ii) Arrogant.	i) Destructive and melancholic. ii) Close-mouthed.	i) Changeable and fearless. ii) Indifferent.

Key Word	Psora Sensitising Miasm	Sycosis Miasm of Incoordination	Syphilis Degenerating Miasm	Tubercular Responsive, Reactive Miasm
	iii) Irritability with anxiety.	iii) Irritability explodes into anger. The subject may bang the table, throw things and become generally restless.	iii) Irritability with cruelty.	iii) Irritability with impatience.
	iv) Sadness.	iv) Moaning.	iv) Lamenting.	iv) Changeable mood.
	v) Nervous.	v) Chaos = Syco-syphilo-psora.	v) Madness = Syphilo-syco-psora.	v) Insanity (recurrent and periodical) = Mixed miasmatic with tubercular preponderance.
	vi) Thoughtful but no practical sense.	vi) Thoughtfulness focussed for their own personal benefit.	vi) Vanishing of thoughts.	vi) Changeability of thoughts.
	vii) Lack of concentration. Weakness of memory.	vii) Incoordination in concentration, absentmindedness.	vii) Total destruction of concentration; forgetful. Dullness = weak perception.	vii) Changeability of concentration.
	viii) Malicious = Psora-syphilo-sycotic.	viii) Mischievous = Syco-syphilo-psora.	viii) Hatred = Syphilo-syco-psora.	viii) Indifferent.
	ix) Wariness of life = Psora-syphilitic.	ix) Tendency to exploit everything from life = sycotic.	ix) Loathing of life = Syphilo-psoric.	ix) Unfulfilling life.
	x) Illusions.	x) Delusions.	x) Hallucinations and deliriums.	x) Vacillation of thoughts.
	xi) Sad and depressed.	xi) Irascible, rude, ill-mannered.	xi) Sentimental and close-mouthed.	xi) Independent and indifferent.

Key Word	Psora Sensitising Miasm	Sycosis Miasm of Incoordination	Syphilis Degenerating Miasm	Tubercular Responsive, Reactive Miasm
	xii) Psora plans a robbery, has plenty of ideas but there are lots of loopholes in the plan.	xii) Sycosis is cunning and practical, fills up the loopholes and appears to hide from the actual site of the crime. He is there however and ends up with the spoils, depriving the others of their share.	xii) Syphilis is the hired criminal at the forefront of the crime. He has the inability to realise that if he is caught he will go to prison and there will be no one to look after his family!	xii) The tubercular criminal is changeable and undependable and although he commits to joining this bank robbery, he changes his mind at the last moment and does not turn up.
	xiii) Psoric memory is poor but the patient is very studious. Once they have learnt a subject they will remember it.	xiii) Sycotics have an active memory and record everything — the journalist type.	xiii) Syphilitics do not remember recent happenings but retain remote incidents in chronological order.	xiii) Tuberculars are careless. They are intelligent and bright but make careless mistakes.
11. Hair	i) Hair falls out after acute fevers.	i) Alopecia in circular spots.	i) Dandruff with thick yellow crusts (can be tubercular also).	i) Breaks, splits and sticks together.
	ii) Dry, lustreless, difficult to comb.	ii) Immature greyish hair.	ii) Falls in bunches. Falling hair from eyebrows, eyelashes and beard.	ii) A thick yellow heavy crust is apt to be tubercular (or syphilitic).
	iii) Splits at ends.	iii) Fishy odour from hair.	iii) Moist, gluey and greasy with an offensive odour.	
	iv) Bran-like dandruff.		iv) Ingrowing hair of eyelashes.	
12. Vertigo	Vertigo from indigestion or emotional disturbances.	Vertigo from closing the eyes, disappearing on opening the eyes.	Vertigo occurring at night.	Vertigo begins at the base of the brain.

Key Word	Psora Sensitising Miasm	Sycosis Miasm of Incoordination	Syphilis Degenerating Miasm	Tubercular Responsive, Reactive Miasm
13. Eye	i) Visualises various colours (spots before the eyes).	i) Aggravated from changes of season and rainy weather.	i) Structural eye changes.	i) Red lids (Psora-tubercular).
		ii) Ptosis.	ii) Deformities of lens; all varieties of refractory changes. Weakness, ptosis (syphilis & sycosis).	ii) Photophobia.
				iii) Aversion to artificial lights.
14. Ear	i) Dry and scaly meatus even in otorrhoea. On looking at the meatus one finds dryness immediately following the discharge.	i) Thickening of the ear (pinna).	i) Long ears.	i) Acute suppurative otitis media developing as a result of some severe disease such as measles or scarlet fever offers a good prognosis in the tubercular miasm.
	ii) Oversensitive to noise.	ii) Growths and anatomical incoordination over the external ear.		ii) Colds and sore throats result in acute suppurative otitis media with offensive pus.
15. Nose	i) Sensitive to odours.	i) Nasal congestion ameliorated even by the slightest amount of nasal discharges (abnormal discharge ameliorates).	i) Ulceration of nasal septum.	i) Epistaxis.

149

Key Word	Psora Sensitising Miasm	Sycosis Miasm of Incoordination	Syphilis Degenerating Miasm	Tubercular Responsive, Reactive Miasm
	ii) Psoric cold begins with sneezing, redness and heat. The nose becomes sensitive to touch when it is continually blown.	ii) A bland or acidic discharge from the nose with a fish-brine smell is characteristic.	ii) Diminution of sense of smell.	ii) Recurrent catching of colds.
	iii) Redness of mucous membranes.			iii) Flushing of nose.
16. Mouth	i) Tartar.	i) Fishy taste.	i) Ulcers in the oral cavity.	i) Taste of pus.
	ii) All food tastes as if burnt is a characteristic.		ii) Asymmetrical teeth.	ii) Bright red, bleeding from gums.
	iii) Refuses highly aromatic substances.		iii) Tongue having the imprint of the teeth.	
	iv) Intolerable sweet taste in mouth.		iv) Saliva is offensive, and can be drawn into threads.	
			v) Coppery or metallic taste.	
			vi) Crowns of incisors are crescentic.	
17. Face	i) Inverted.	i) Dropsical.	i) Oily, greasy face.	i) Sunken eyes and pale face but flushed cheeks.
	ii) Blue — cyanosis due to lack of oxygenation. Blue, the cold colour represents psora.	ii) Yellowish complexion. The colour yellow corresponds to sycosis.	ii) High cheek bones and rough skin.	ii) Round faced with fair, smooth, clear skin and a waxy smoothness of complexion.

Key Word	Psora Sensitising Miasm	Sycosis Miasm of Incoordination	Syphilis Degenerating Miasm	Tubercular Responsive, Reactive Miasm
			iii) Face looks puckered, dried and wrinkled like that of an old person.	iii) The face looks well even in the last stages of disease when the rest of the body has become emaciated.
			iv) Thick lips.	iv) Thin lips.
			v) Eyelids red and inflamed.	v) Eyes are bright and sparkling.
			vi) Scaly, crusty lashes; broken, shabby, irregularly curved and imperfect.	vi) Eyebrows and lashes are soft, glossy, long and silken.
18. Heart & Pulse	i) Psoric heart patients worry about their conditions; take their pulse frequently; fear death; remain quiet.	i) A combination of sycosis and psora provides the right soil for valvular and cardiac disturbances.	i) High blood pressure where the systolic and diastolic pressures are irregularly distributed, e.g. high systolic combined with a low diastolic rate.	i) Palpitations, which are aggravated by higher altitudes. The patient wants to keep still and is unable to climb stairs or ascend hills.
	ii) Bradycardia.	ii) Tachycardia.	ii) Irregular pulse.	ii) The pulse is feeble but rapid.
	iii) Hammering sensation in pericardium.	iii) Rheumatic and valvular heart diseases.		
	iv) Hypotension.	iv) Hypertension.		
		v) Hypertrophy of the heart.		

Key Word	Psora *Sensitising Miasm*	Sycosis *Miasm of Incoordination*	Syphilis *Degenerating Miasm*	Tubercular *Responsive, Reactive Miasm*
19. Abdomen	i) Slow intestinal peristalsis.	i) Accelerated and exaggerated peristalsis. ii) Children born of sycotic parents suffer from colic, almost from the moment of birth. Sycotic children are subject to colic and "three-month's colic".	i) Irregular peristalsis resulting in spasm associated with dysentery.	i) Duodenal ulcers.
20. Stool	i) Constipation is primarily psoric. ii) Offensive stool, not very painful. iii) Stool may be of any colour. iv) Worse from cold, motion, and eating and drinking cold things. Better by warm drinks, hot food, and warm applications to the abdomen.	i) Diarrhoea is sycotic. ii) Diarrhoea gushes and ejaculates forcefully and is colicky in nature. iii) Sour, acrid, grass green stool. iv) Jet like expulsion of faeces, with a sense of insecurity and a constant symptom of griping.	i) Dysentery is syphilitic. ii) Stool is mixed with lots of mucus, scrapings of intestine, and sometimes blood.	i) Morning diarrhoea with extreme prostration and debility is tubercular. ii) Bleeding from the rectum with or without stool.

Key Word	Psora Sensitising Miasm	Sycosis Miasm of Incoordination	Syphilis Degenerating Miasm	Tubercular Responsive, Reactive Miasm
21. Skin	i) Persistent dryness.	i) Painful with pains better by pressure.	i) Ulcerous tendency — open ulcers of virulent type.	i) Skin diseases, which are threatening or destructive in nature.
	ii) Suppression of skin conditions directly affects the mind.	ii) Suppression of skin diseases affects firstly the nerve centres, followed by the heart, liver and reproductive system.	ii) When syphilitic skin is suppressed the intellect is affected causing dullness, depression and a lack of enthusiasm.	ii) Suppression of skin conditions affects the inner tissues causing destructive and ulcerous tendencies; and the deeper tissues causing a debilitated tubercular state.
	iii) Unhealthy skin with itching and burning represents psora.	iii) Oily skin with redness at the tip of the nose and copious perspiration is sycotic.	iii) Ulcerated skin with pus and blood represents syphilis.	iii) Recurrent and obstinate boils with profuse pus are tubercular.
	iv) Eruptions characterised by roughness and unwashability of the skin.	iv) Sycosis has vesicular eruptions.	iv) Copper coloured eruptions are syphilitic. Eruptions are slow to heal (psora-syphilitic).	iv) History of ringworm and the state caused by the suppression of ringworm.
	v) Skin diseases, which spread over the body.	v) Skin conditions appear localised and/or in circumscribed spots.	v) Putridity, acridity and offensiveness of all discharges.	v) Busy and important areas are affected.
		vi) Post operative scar tumours and abscesses.	vi) Stitch abscesses.	

Key Word	Psora Sensitising Miasm	Sycosis Miasm of Incoordination	Syphilis Degenerating Miasm	Tubercular Responsive, Reactive Miasm
		vii) Disturbed pigment metabolism produces hyper-pigmentation and depigmentation in patches or diffused in different parts. Patches may be urine coloured.		
22. Nails	i) Dry, harsh appearance of the nails.	i) Irregular nails, ridged or ribbed, or ridged and corrugated.	i) Spoon-shaped.	i) Fissured, wavy, asymmetrical nails, which come out easily.
		ii) Thick.	ii) Paper-like, thin nails which bend and tear easily.	ii) Irregular nails, break and split easily.
		iii) Pale.	iii) Whitlows are psora-syphilitic (like other periosteal inflammations).	iii) Nails with various stains and spots or with white specks and scalloped edges.
		iv) Convex appearance.	iv) Concave appearance.	iv) Glossy nails.
				v) Formation of pus at the junction of nails and flesh with severe stitching pains.
				vi) The natural convexity is often reversed.
				vii) Hangnails.

Key Word	Psora *Sensitising Miasm*	Sycosis *Miasm of Incoordination*	Syphilis *Degenerating Miasm*	Tubercular *Responsive, Reactive Miasm*
23. Pains	i) Psoric neuralgic pains are usually better by quiet, rest and warmth, and worse by motion.	i) The rheumatic pains of sycosis are worse by cold and damp, and better by moving or stretching.	i) Bone pains are syphilitic.	i) Sense of great exhaustion, patient tires easily and never seems to get rested. As the sun ascends their strength revives a little, as it descends, they lose it again.
	ii) Sore, bruised, pressive pains are psoric.	ii) Joint pains are sycotic and pains are generally stitching, pulsating or wandering.	ii) Burning, bursting and tearing pains are syphilitic.	
24. Malignancy	i) Prone to develop at the age of 40.	i) Prone to develop at any age.	i) Prone to develop at the age of 40.	i) Tubercular malignancies are characterised by metastasis and haemorrhage.
	ii) Prefers tissues of ectodermal origin.	ii) Prefers tissues of entodermal origin.	ii) Prefers tissues of mesodermal origin.	
	iii) Hahnemann says in Chronic Diseases that even large sarcomatous lesions can develop from psora.	iii) Sycotic malignant tumours are encapsulated and grow out of proportion. There is incoordination in cellular proliferation.	iii) Syphilitic malignant tumours break open their capsules causing degeneration, disintegration and cellular necrosis.	

155

Key Word	Psora Sensitising Miasm	Sycosis Miasm of Incoordination	Syphilis Degenerating Miasm	Tubercular Responsive, Reactive Miasm
25. Desires & Aversions	Desires: Sweet, sour, fatty, fried, indigestible, spicy, oily and hot foods.	Desires: Table salt, alcohol, coconut, fatty meat, peppers, pungent, well-seasoned foods and salty foods. The patient craves beer (which causes less aggravation than wine).	Desires: Stimulants — alcohol, tea, coffee, smoking (all signs of destruction), very spicy meat, cold food and sour things. Desires foods, which are either too hot or too cold.	Desires: Indigestible things like clay etc., and fatty, greasy foods on which they thrive. Crave the things, which make them sick. Desires potatoes, tea, tobacco and meat and crave salt which they will eat alone from the saucer. Tuberculars are extremists and like either very hot or really cold things.
	Aversions: Milk, boiled food and cold foods.	Aversions: Meat and wine, which aggravate the sycotic condition, milk, and spices of which they are intolerant.	Aversions: Meat, especially less spicy, and other animal foods.	Aversions: meat (generally desire for meat is strongest but due to the changeability of the miasm, aversion may also occur). The tubercular patient does not digest starches easily.
26. Modalities	Aggravated by standing and from cold. Wants warmth externally and internally and is therefore worse in winter.	Aggravated by rest, damp, rainy, humid atmospheres, during thunderstorms, changes of weather, and from meat.	Aggravated from sunset to sunrise, movement, extremes of temperature, at the seaside, on sea-voyages, and from thunderstorms.	Aggravated from thunderstorm, night, milk, fruits, greasy and oily foods.
	Aggravated between sunrise and sunset.	The sycotic patient is a barometer — when it rains, he has pains and he suffers.	Aggravated by warmth, during the summer, at night, from the warmth of the bed and from sweat (through natural discharges).	Aggravated in closed room. Patient also cannot tolerate any pressure in the chest.

| Key Word | Psora
Sensitising Miasm | Sycosis
Miasm of Incoordination | Syphilis
Degenerating Miasm | Tubercular
Responsive, Reactive Miasm |
|---|---|---|---|---|
| | Ameliorated in summer, from heat, by natural discharges such as urine, menstruation etc. Ameliorated through physiological eliminative processes such as sweat. | Ameliorated from motion, unnatural discharges (which are generally greenish/yellow in colour) and unnatural eliminations through the mucus surfaces, e.g. leucorrhoea, nasal discharge etc. Physiological eliminations do not ameliorate. | Amelioration from sunrise to sunset, change of position, a lukewarm climate, and from any abnormal discharges (such as leucorrhoea, coryza). | Ameliorated in dry weather, open air, and during the daytime. |
| | Ameliorated by hot application, scratching, crying and eating. | Amelioration by slow motion, or by stretching, in dry weather, lying on stomach or by pressure. The return of suppressed normal discharges such as menses also ameliorate. | Amelioration during winter, from cold in winter. | Temporarily ameliorated by offensive foot or axillary sweat which when suppressed induces lung trouble. |
| | The appearance of suppressed skin eruptions ameliorates. | Ameliorated when warts or fibrous growths appear. | Amelioration through the discharge of pus (if old ulcers open up). | Ameliorated by nose bleeding. |
| | | Ameliorated in general from the return or breaking open of old ulcers or sores, and markedly ameliorated by the return of acute gonorrhoeal manifestations. | | Tubercular modalities depend upon the preponderance of the psoric or syphilitic miasm. |

PART — III
MIASMATIC PRESCRIBING:
MIASMATIC DIAGNOSIS OF CLINICAL CLASSIFICATIONS

Key Word	Psoric Clinicals	Sycotic Clinicals	Syphilitic Clinicals	Tubercular Clinicals
1. Psychiatric Clinicals	i) Absorbed, buried in thoughts — focussed.	i) Abrupt.	i) Contemptuous.	i) Discontented.
	ii) Anxiety neurosis.	ii) Absent-mindedness and abstraction of mind.	ii) Depression and melancholia — depressive disorders.	ii) Displeased.
	iii) Alertness.	iii) Anger.	iii) Dullness.	iii) Dissatisfied.
	iv) Apprehensive.	iv) Awkwardness.	iv) Exhilaration.	
	v) Brooding.	v) Busy.	v) Insanity due to mental depression and destructive influences.	
	vi) Company, aversion to.	vi) Cheerful.	vi) Maliciousness.	
	vii) Fear.	vii) Deceitful: exaltation of fancy.	vii) Prostration (+++) of mind.	
	viii) Fright.	viii) Delusion.	viii) Rage & fury.	
	ix) Hypochondriacal.	ix) Despair.	ix) Rudeness.	
	x) Indolent.	x) Hastiness.	x) Sluggishness.	
	xi) Irritable.	xi) Insolence.	xi) Suicidal impulses and other destructive manias.	
	xii) Joyful.	xii) Mistakes in speech.		
	xiii) Nervous.	xiii) Presumptuousness.		
	xiv) Prostration (++) of mind.	xiv) Rashness.		
	xv) Psychic disorders characterised by deficiencies and weaknesses.	xv) Ridiculous.		

Key Word	Psoric Clinicals	Sycotic Clinicals	Syphilitic Clinicals	Tubercular Clinicals
		xvi) Schizophrenia (can be mixed miasmatic according to the preponderance of symptoms).		
	xvii) Startled easily.	xvii) Scornful.		
	xviii) Sulky.	xviii) Selfishness.		
	xix) Thoughtful.			
	xx) Timid.			
	xxi) Weakness of memory.			
	xxii) Note: Superficial transient annoyance is psoric, but when the annoyance precipitates, grows and explodes, we get true irascibility, which is anger, and this is more sycotic.	xix) Note: Psychic disorders are characterised by incoordination and exaggeration. Obsessive neurosis and compulsive neurosis are also sycotic.		
2. Ophthalmo-logical Clinicals	i) Conjunctivitis, iritis and other inflammations of a functional nature.	i) Retinoblastoma and other papillomas and tumours including tarsal tumours.	i) Blindness from destructive processes such as retinal detachment.	i) Haematoma and all types of inflammation characterised by haemorrhage in the eye.
	ii) Photophobia.	ii) Corneal incoordinations and inflammations.	ii) All sorts of structural changes to the eyes and also corneal ulcerations.	ii) Injury to the eyes — black eye.
		iii) Glaucoma.	iii)	iii) Scaly, red lids.
		iv) Ptosis (syco-syphilitic).		
		v) Cataracts (incoordination in the lens).		

160

	Key Word	Psoric Clinicals	Sycotic Clinicals	Syphilitic Clinicals	Tubercular Clinicals
			vi) Styes.		
3.	Clinicals of the Ear	i) Otitis with dryness of the meatus.	i) Otitis with exudation. ii) Tinnitus aureum.	i) Otitis with ulceration in the ear. ii) Mastoiditis with degenerative changes in the bones. iii) Perforation of the ear drum.	i) Otitis with haemorrhage.
4.	Clinicals of the Nose	i) Rhinitis associated with sneezing.	i) Coryza. ii) Sinusitis. iii) D.N.S (deviated nasal septum). iv) Swollen adenoids.	i) All discharges characterised by acridity, putridity and offensiveness. ii) Degenerative and ulcerative conditions of the nose. iii) Ulceration of the nasal septum.	i) Coryza (especially recurrent types). ii) Epistaxis. iii) Nasal polyps are tri-miasmatic.
5.	Oral Clinicals	i) Facial neuralgia. ii) Gingivitis. iii) Stomatitis. iv) Thrush.	i) Gum boils. ii) Leucoplakia. iii) Salivary duct calculi. iv) Tartar.	i) Cleft palate. ii) Leucoplakia with fungal infection. iii) Pyorrhoea. iv) Ulcerations in oral cavity with offensive saliva.	i) Bleeding gums. ii) Haematemesis.
6.	Clinicals of the Respiratory System	i) Anoxaemia. ii) Hypoxaemia.	i) Asthma (hereditary) and catarrhal asthma. ii) Cough and painful hoarseness.	i) Lung abscesses. ii) Quinsy.	i) Allergic bronchospasm. ii) Dry cough especially when aggravated by fever.

Key Word	Psoric Clinicals	Sycotic Clinicals	Syphilitic Clinicals	Tubercular Clinicals
	iii) Bronchitis (psora-tubercular).	iii) Dyspnoea from cardiac incoordination (cardiac asthma).	iii) Sore throat and ulcerative sore throat.	iii) Haemoptysis.
	iv) Hoarseness with burning.	iv) Emphysema.		iv) Pleurisy.
	v) Pharyngitis.	v) Fibrosis of the lung.		v) Pulmonary tuberculosis.
		vi) Pneumonia with consolidation of the lung.		vi) Recurrent cough.
		vii) Vocal cord nodules.		vii) Scrofulosis (glandular enlargement of the cheeks and tonsils).
		viii) Whooping cough.		viii) Tonsillitis especially when recurrent.
7. Cardiac Clinicals	i) Anxiety about the heart with constant worry, typifies psora.	i) Angina pectoris from embolism or thrombus.	i) Patent ductus arteriosus (PDA) where there are structural abnormalities or developmental anomalies.	i) Palpitations and a rush of blood to the head and chest with redness of the face and flushed cheeks is characteristic of the tubercular miasm.
	ii) Bradycardia.	ii) Tachycardia.	ii) Ulcerative bacterial endocarditis.	
	iii) Carditis and pericarditis.	iii) Congestive cardiac failures (CCF).	iii) Congenital abnormalities such as Fallot's tetralogy.	
	iv) Hypotension.	iv) Hypertension.	iv) Hypertensions with irregular distribution of systolic and diastolic pressures.	

Key Word	Psoric Clinicals	Sycotic Clinicals	Syphilitic Clinicals	Tubercular Clinicals
		v) Incoordination (such as mitral or aortic regurgitation, MR or AR); stenosis (such as mitral stenosis) or dilatation or any abnormality of the cardiac valves.	v) Heart affections with valvular degeneration.	
	v) The majority of psoric cardiac symptoms are of a functional nature accompanied with much anxiety and fear of incurable disease and death.	vi) A combination of sycosis and psora provides the right soil for valvular and cardiac disturbances.		
	vi) Cardiac and emotional symptoms alternate.	vii) Hypertrophy of the heart and left ventricular or right ventricular hypertrophy.		
		viii) RHD (Rheumatic heart diseases).		
8. Gastric Clinicals	i) Acidity and sour eructations.	i) Benign and encapsulated tumours.	i) Gastric ulcers.	i) Gastro-intestinal disturbances where bleeding predominates — haematemesis, melaena.
	ii) Nausea with a feeling of faintness.	ii) Papilloma and polyps of the gastro-intestinal tract.	ii) Degenerative varieties of cancer.	ii) Milk allergies and allergies to other different types of food.
	iii) Heartburn. iv) Anorexia. v) Gastritis.			

Key Word	Psoric Clinicals	Sycotic Clinicals	Syphilitic Clinicals	Tubercular Clinicals
	vi) Oesophagitis with burning, and other functional disorders of the gastro-intestinal tract.			
9. Abdominal Clinicals	i) Constipation is primarily psoric. ii) Duodenitis. iii) Cholecystitis, colitis and other inflammations of the abdomen, mainly of functional origin, including gastric refluxes. iv) Dyspeptic symptoms. v) Flatulence.	i) Appendicitis and appendicular colic. ii) Abdominal colic. iii) Cholelithiasis (gallstones) and non-functioning gall bladder. iv) Ascites is syco-psoric. v) Hernia. vi) Hepatomegaly or splenomegaly. vii) Tumours, papillomas and encapsulated malignant growths. viii) Umbilical hernia, and in children, swelling and protusion of the umbilicus with a thin, yellowish/green discharge, smelling of fish brine.	i) Peptic ulcers. ii) Ulcerative colitis. iii) Cirrhosis of the liver is syphilo-sycotic, due to incoordination as well as degenerative changes in the liver cells. iv) Degeneration of the liver cells including fatty degeneration. v)	i) Abdominal tuberculosis. ii) Abdominal worms. iii) Crohn's disease. iv) Haemorrhagic disorders — haemophilia and haemolytic jaundice. v) Infantile liver. vi) Stool with blood — melaena.

Key Word	Psoric Clinicals	Sycotic Clinicals	Syphilitic Clinicals	Tubercular Clinicals
10. Clinicals of the Rectum	i) Constipation. ii) Morning diarrhoeas.	i) Any stool where colic predominates. ii) Diarrhoea characterised by exaggerated peristalsis. iii) Haemorrhoids and polyps (which are blind i.e. non-bleeding). iv) Prolapse of the rectum.	i) Dysentery (characterised by irregular peristalsis) with blood and pus. ii) Fistulas and abscesses. iii) Perineal pyogenic inflammations (perineal abscesses). iv) IBS (Irritable bowel syndrome) where pus and mucus in the stool predominate. v) Ulcers in the rectum.	i) Alternating disorders (e.g. constipation alternating with diarrhoea). ii) Early morning diarrhoeas. iii) Bleeding haemorrhoids and rectal polyps. iv) IBS (Irritable bowel syndrome) where blood predominates. v) Rectal haemorrhage. vi) Recurrent rectal fistulas and abscesses. vii) Bloody stool — melaena.
11. Urinary Clinicals	i) Enuresis of functional origin. ii) Nephritis, pyelitis, cystitis and urethritis.	i) Hypertrophy of the prostate. ii) Nephroblastoma, tumours of the kidney, and papillomas of the bladder. iii) Nephrotic syndrome where oedema predominates.	i) Pyaemia with oozing of pus. ii) Destructive and degenerative varieties of malignant tumours in the kidney or bladder. iii) Stricture of the urethra.	i) Enuresis. ii) Polyps and papillomas of the bladder with haemorrhage. iii) Haematuria.

Key Word	Psoric Clinicals	Sycotic Clinicals	Syphilitic Clinicals	Tubercular Clinicals
		iv) Renal calculi or calculous deposits in other parts of the genito-urinary tract. v) Renal dropsy. vi) Prostatitis from sexual over-indulgence. vii) Urinary ailments with pain.		iv) Diabetes mellitus (generally tri-miasmatic) and diabetes insipidus (syco-tubercular).
12. Sexual Clinicals	i) Agalactea. ii) Amenorrhoea. iii) Impotency and sterility from lack of sexual desire.	i) Ectopic pregnancy. ii) Endometriosis. iii) Diseases of pelvic and sexual organs (uro-genital problems) such as endometriosis, prostatitis, salpingitis, orchitis, ovaritis, etc. iv) Uterine disorders. v) Genital warts. vi) Ovarian tumours and malignancies where the tumours are encapsulated. vii) Leucorrhoea of fish brine odour. viii) Hydrocele.	i) Abortions and stillbirths. ii) Azoospermia. iii) Cervical and vulval erosions and ulcerations. iv) Dysplasia of the cells (in the cervix and other mucosa). v) Offensive menses. vi) Ulcerative and degenerative varieties of tumours. vii) Acrid, putrid and offensive leucorrhoea.	i) Uterine and vaginal polyps with profuse bleeding. ii) Haemospermia (blood stained seminal emission). iii) All varieties of womb infections, which are characterised by profuse bleeding. iv) DUB (dysfunctional uterine bleeding) characterised by profuse haemorrhage.

Key Word	Psoric Clinicals	Sycotic Clinicals	Syphilitic Clinicals	Tubercular Clinicals
		ix) Pelvic inflammatory diseases (P.I.D). x) Polycystic disease of the ovaries (ovarian cysts). xi) Sterility and infertility from hormonal imbalance. xii) Uterine fibroids and polyps. xiii) All varieties of sexual and pelvic disorders are generally sycotic in origin.		
13. Dermatological Clinicals	i) Dandruff with bran-like scales. ii) Dry skin with dermatitis or eczema. iii) Eczema and other eruptions where dryness predominates. iv) Any skin condition characterised by itching. v) Itching dermatitis. vi) Nettle rash. vii) Pimples with dryness and scurfy scales.	i) Herpes of all types, including herpes genitalis. ii) Hyperpigmentation of the skin. iii) Corns with thickening of the skin. iv) Keloids. v) Melanomas. vi) Molluscum contagiosum (syco-psoric). vii) Post-operative scar tumours.	i) Bedsores. ii) Depigmentation of the skin. iii) Deep cracks and fissures in the skin, particularly the palms and soles. iv) Burns and scalds with degenerative ulceration. v) Stitch abscesses. vi) Fungal infections of the extremities and fingers. vii) Necrosis and gangrene.	i) Herpes, which is extremely recurrent or appears periodically. ii) Recurrent pustular eczemas. iii) Allergic skin manifestations such as urticaria (hives). iv) Any skin condition characterised by recurrence, periodicity, alternation or haemorrhage. v) Ecchymosis. vi) Haemangiomas. vii) Acne rosacea.

Key Word	Psoric Clinicals	Sycotic Clinicals	Syphilitic Clinicals	Tubercular Clinicals
		viii) Radiation hazards with cauliflower-like tumours.	viii) Skin cancers with ulceration and necrosis.	viii) Cancer (of metastatic variety).
		ix) The consequences of vaccinosis.	ix) Skin diseases, which ooze offensive pus and fluids.	ix) Obstinate skin conditions, which are difficult to eradicate.
		x) Vesicular eruptions.	x) Ulcers and abscesses on different parts of the skin.	x) Ulcerations with haemorrhage.
		xi) Warts, veruccas, moles, condylomatas, skin tags, dermoid cysts, fibroma and lipomas.		xi) Petechial haemorrhage and purpura haemorrhagica.
				xii) Varicose veins with red flushing.
				xiii) Venous thrombosis.
				xiv) Acute exanthematous diseases.
14. Clinicals of the Extremities	i) Leg cramps.	i) All joint pains.	i) Bone pains.	i) Emaciation without any apparent cause.
	ii) Nervous debility.	ii) Arthritic deformans.	ii) Carbuncles.	ii) Recurrent epilepsy (syphilo-tubercular).
	iii) Neuralgia.	iii) Dermoids.	iii) Caries and necrosis of the bones and spine.	iii) Extreme fatigue with weakness of the lower extremities.
	iv) Periosteitis.	iv) Oedemas	iv) Delayed ossification and fragility of the bones.	iv) Fever of intermittent or enteric types.
	v) Various types of rheumatism, especially when functional and inflammatory in nature.	v) Oedematous swelling of the extremities.	v) Malignancy of the bones; bone metastasis and sarcoma.	v) Nodular growths of glandular origin.

Key Word	Psoric Clinicals	Sycotic Clinicals	Syphilitic Clinicals	Tubercular Clinicals
	vi) Osteitis, and the initial stages of osteomyelitis before bone destruction occurs (once destruction begins the condition becomes syphilitic).	vi) Osteoporosis is syco-syphilitic (the hormonal imbalance is given by sycosis and the bone porosis or destruction is afforded by the syphilitic miasm).	vi) Osteomyelitis with bone destruction and the formation of sequestrum.	vi) Periodic disorders such as new moon and full moon aggravation.
		vii) Hypertrophies and growths anywhere in the body.	vii) Ulcers and gangrenous inflammations.	vii) Recurrent disorders.
		viii) Paralysis characterised by incoordination and malfunction.	viii) Paralysis characterised by muscle wasting and degenerative changes.	viii) Rickets are syphilo-tubercular.
		ix) Rheumatism, rheumatoid arthritis, gout and osteoarthritis.	ix) Rheumatism of the long bones.	
		x) Tophi and deposits in the joints.	x) G.P.I. (General paralysis of the insane).	
		xi) Carcinomas of proliferative and encapsulated varieties.	xi) Carcinomas of destructive and fungative varieties.	

MIASMATIC DIAGNOSIS:
CLASSIFICATION OF MIXED MIASMATIC CLINICALS

Psora-Sycotic Clinicals

1. Abusive.
2. Asthma.
3. Concentration difficult.
4. Confusion.
5. Ecstasy.
6. Fear and anguish.
7. Fleshy growths.
8. Foolish — childish, mania to be ridiculous.
9. Frivolity.
10. Industrious.
11. Irritable.
12. Jealous.
13. Lamenting, moaning.
14. Morose.
15. Propensity to frown.
16. Rheumatic heart diseases.
17. Rheumatism.
18. Stupefaction.
19. Talking to oneself.
20. Tumors.
21. Warts.

Psora-Sycotic-Syphilitic Clinicals

1. Anasarca.
2. Audacity.
3. Bright's disease.
4. Carcinomas with proliferation, ulceration and metastasis.
5. Chilblains.
6. Congenital markings of the skin.
7. Courageous soldier.
8. Dropsy.
9. Eczema exfoliata.
10. Elephantiasis.
11. Erysipelas.
12. Family history of azoospermia, sterility, abortions, death with cerebral and cardiac attacks, insanity, cancer.
13. Fish scale eruptions (dryness of psora + squamous character of syphilis + thickened skin of sycosis).
14. Haughtiness.
15. Herpes zoster.
16. Hypocrisy.
17. Ichthyosis (dryness of psora + squamae of syphilis and moles and warty eruptions of sycosis).
18. Impertinence.
19. Lascivious.
20. Lupus.
21. Madness — chaotic and insanity.

Psora-Syphilitic Clinicals

1. Abrupt.
2. Angina pectoris.
3. Chronic ulceration.
4. Contemptuous.
5. Diabetes.
6. Dullness, imbecility and idiocy.
7. Hatred.
8. Malicious.
9. Scrofulous conditions.

Psora-Sycotic Clinicals	*Psora-Sycotic-Syphilitic Clinicals*	*Psora-Syphilitic Clinicals*
	22. Mental confusion. 23. Mischievous. 24. Naevus. 25. Psoriasis (tri-miasmatic but predominantly psora + sycosis). 26. Rectal carcinoma. 27. Rectal prolapse. 28. Tinea berbae. 29. Tinea vesicular.	

PART — IV
MIASMATIC PRESCRIBING:
MIASMATIC ANCESTRAL TIPS

MIASMATIC ANCESTRAL TIPS:
CLINICAL TIPS ON NATURAL CHARACTERISTICS

Point	Psoric	Sycotic	Syphilitic	Tubercular
1. Mental	i) Anxious.	i) Mischievous = Syco-syphilo-psoric.	i) Anguish = Syphilis + psora.	i) Dissatisfied.
	ii) Arrogance.	ii) Superiority complex.	ii) Inferiority complex.	ii) Vagabond and changeable.
	iii) Memory is poor, but once a subject is learnt the patient will remember it. Very studious but finds concentration difficult.	iii) Absent-mindedness of thoughts. Sycosis has an active memory and records everything — the journalist type.	iii) Difficulty in understanding leads to dullness and weakness of perception. Forgetful, remembers past events in chronological order but does not remember recent happenings. Vanishing of thoughts.	iii) Fickle minded.
	iv) Irritability.	iv) Irascible, rude, ill mannered. Irritability explodes into anger.	iv) Irritability with cruelty. Hatred = Syphilo-syco-psoric.	iv) Impatient.
	v) Madness = Syphilo-syco-psoric.	v) Chaos = Syco-syphilo-psoric.	v) Lamenting. Loathing for life = Syphilo-psoric.	v) Dissatisfaction.
	vi) Malicious = Psora-syphilo-sycotic.	vi) Suspicious and impatient with a tendency to conceal.	vi) Hateful and destructive.	vi) Changeable.
	vii) Sad and timid.	vii) Moaning.	vii) Syphilis makes the mind dull. Depressed.	vii) Mood swings.
2. Grief	Weeps and unburdens themselves to 'safe' people. Moans.	Strange and uncoordinated behaviour follows grief or news of a death. They may dance all night, party or listen to loud music.	Suicidal grief, which they hold in, thus destroying themselves on the inside.	Grief is characterised by changeability and a vagabond attitude towards life.
3. Running	Runs slowly because of anxiety about their own health.	Runs fast because they want to win.	Runs to escape their depressing thoughts. Drops dead before the finish line.	Runs with headphones on with no thoughts as to why they are running and what they want out of it.
4. In the Waiting Room	Appears bashful but wants to talk.	Makes conversation with other patients. Enquires into their condition. Very talkative.	Makes no eye contact with others. Low vibrational energy and a cold expression cause others to feel depressed.	Impatient and constantly asks the nurse how much longer they have to wait!

Point	Psoric	Sycotic	Syphilitic	Tubercular
5. Life in General	Always complains but lives to a ripe old age.	Talk, dance and laugh their way through life but die from the side-effects of overdoing everything.	Never complain but suffer all their life and die at an early age.	Travels the world, is changeable and fickle-minded yet always feels dissatisfied.
6. General Traits	Slowness is psoric. Wariness of life = Psora-syphilitic.	Exploitation and incoordination characterise sycosis.	Syphilitics are destructive, they vex and hurt others.	Tubercular patients are fickle-minded and cannot decide what they want.
7. Ear Infections	Slow onset infections — ear appears a little red; there may be a small amount of fluid and a slight fever. The patient is irritable and clingy.	Sudden high fever, big manifestation, catarrhal discharge and pain.	Corrosive infections, smelly, inside the ear, and smouldering, destructive infections.	Haemorrhage from the ear.
8. Nose	Clear nasal mucus.	Colds and sinusitis.	Acrid and offensive coryza.	Hay fever and blood-stained discharges.
9. Secretions	Serous.	Purulent.	Acrid, putrid and offensive.	Bloody.
10. Teeth	Poor teeth, often small.	Teeth visibly rotten above the gum-line.	Teeth rot below the gum-line. Often jammed together, malformed or have gaps in between. Orthodontic treatment is required to make room in the mouth for the teeth as they come through.	Bleeding gums.
11. Strep Throat	Red and painful.	Very swollen with green/yellow pus.	Fever occurs during the night. Pus is grey and blood-streaked and lots of crypts appear in the tonsils.	Recurrent infections, which vary in location.
12. Lung Inflammation	Slow appearance, mild fevers and coughing that will not go away. Lung infections are underdeveloped and weak in their manifestation.	Sudden inflammation, high fever and loud coughing. Discharge is green/yellow.	Sudden onset; infections followed by a healing crisis or death.	Haemorrhage results in haemoptysis.
13. Abdomen	Distension soon after eating and there is a tendency to defecate undigested stool. Psora eats hastily and perspires profusely while eating, they must loosen their garments after a meal and often suffer from drowsiness, headaches, palpitations, heartburn, etc.	Meat aggravates sycotic conditions.	Perverted cravings characterise syphilis.	Tubercular cravings are changeable.
14. Hunger	Intermittent hunger accompanied by an all-gone sensation in abdomen, or constant, ravenous hunger. Psora does not assimilate well, craves sweet and sour (although the sweet craving disappears during fever) and usually desires warm food (hot meals).	Sycosis desires cold food, and subjects are often over-nourished.	Syphilis craves potatoes and meat and prefers luke-warm food. The digestion is disorganised.	The tubercular miasm craves the things which make them sick. They loose flesh while eating well and often show an aversion to cow's milk.

MIASMATIC ANCESTRAL TIPS: CLINICAL TIPS ON DEMENTIAS

		Psoric	*Sycotic*	*Syphilitic*
Terminal Dementia		1. Emotional disability and loss of control (emotional incontinence) occur early and the intellectual deficit is less conspicuous. The psoric terminal dementia patient is therefore easily provoked to anger and tears, although, alternatively they may become foolish or flippant.	1. Suspicious of others, jealous, fault finding and quarrelsome are the characteristics of the sycotic patient suffering from terminal dementia. They become increasingly secretive. May commit sexual or other offences.	1. Syphilitic terminal dementia patients are self-centred, depressed hypochondriacal and indifferent to the feelings of others. At times they may lose all interest in life and dwell on suicidal thoughts or even commit suicide. 2. The intellectual deficit worsens progressively — the initial memory loss is of recent events but extends in due course further backwards in time (retrograde amnesia). There is an inability to grasp, to understand, to retain and to recall new impressions.
Senile Dementia		1. Interferes with the person's well-being. 2. Irritable and difficult. 3. The patient tires easily and finds it difficult to comprehend.	1. Interferes with the person's adjustment. 2. Memory of recent events is impaired while the person retains the ability to remember remote experiences (also syphilitic). 3. The patient has difficulty in grasping and comprehending due to absentmindedness. 4. Judgement is defective and the patient may become deluded. Thoughts that someone is stealing their property or possessions are common delusions in sycotic patients suffering from senile dementia.	1. There is a decrease of interest and the person becomes increasingly egocentric.

MIASMATIC ANCESTRAL TIPS:
CLINICAL TIPS ON BRONCHOSPASM

	Psoric Bronchospasm		*Sycotic Bronchospasm*		*Syphilitic Bronchospasm*		*Tubercular Bronchospasm*
1.	Hypersensitivity of the tracheo-bronchial tree to any allergen is psoric.	1.	Sycotic asthma is devoid of any allergic history.	1.	No nasal allergies are present in the syphilitic patient.	1.	Tubercular patients are always tired, catch cold easily, and are debilitated and often anaemic. They suffer from painful dyspnoea.
2.	Often associated with a family history or a past history of allergy such as rhinitis, eczema or urticaria. Food allergies may also have been indicated.	2.	Hereditary bronchial asthma is generally sycotic.	2.	F/H (family history) of syphilis.	2.	F/H (family history) of tuberculosis.
3.	Nasal allergies lead to sneezing followed by cough, dyspnoea and expectoration.	3.	Dyspnoea starts with a cough, which is followed by expectoration. There is no nasal allergy or rhinitis.	3.	Bronchial conditions begin with dyspnoea (nasal allergies are not initially present).	3.	Nasal blockages lead to mouth breathing and tubercular patients are poor breathers in general. There is no desire to take a full respiration and the patient cannot fully expand the chest which is often narrow (pigeon chest), lacking not only in width laterally but also in depth antero-posteriorly. The sub-clavicular spaces are hollow, one lung is larger than the other and there is a constant desire to hawk.
4.	Asthma, which starts in winter, is psoric.	4.	Starts or aggravates in rainy weather.	4.	Asthma, which starts in the summer, is syphilitic.	4.	The tubercular patient is subject to recurrent colds despite their great desire to be in the open air.
5.	The psoric patient is averse to open air and suffers aggravation during the early morning and in the evening. Amelioration comes from sweating.	5.	Open air and early morning or late morning aggravation. Amelioration is from movement and lying on the abdomen, although some author's suggest that sycotic asthma is better by lying on the back. The patient is compelled to move, a sycotic characteristic, and asthma, pneumonia, bronchitis, coughs and colds are all aggravated in humid, moist atmospheres and during the rainy season. Stitching pains in the chest with different types of aching are ameliorated by pressure.	5.	Summer, warmth, midnight, sweat, lying down and the period of time before going to bed all aggravate. Dyspnoea occurs before going to bed or while lying down.	5.	Dyspnoea occurs on ascending stairs.

Psoric Bronchospasm	Sycotic Bronchospasm	Syphilitic Bronchospasm	Tubercular Bronchospasm
6. There is frequent congestion of the throat with the accumulation of much mucus or phlegm. Expectoration is usually mucus, which is scanty and tasteless.	6. Discharge and expectoration are yellow or greenish/yellow and there is profuse expectoration with asthma, which is worse during the early morning.	6. Ulcers are present in the respiratory passage.	6. Expectoration is yellowish and smells of sulphur or has the odour of old cheese.
7. A dry spasmodic cough results from the suppression of measles, skin diseases etc. and leads to affection of the lungs.	7. The coughs of sycosis are usually bronchial.	7. There is a paroxysmal cough with tasteless, yellowish, greenish or clean, sticky, thread-like discharge.	7. Teasing cough with expectoration, which is sticky, viscid, pus-like, offensive and tastes sweetish or salty.
8. The overall prognosis is favourable.	8. Asthma alternates with skin symptoms but the prognosis is favourable.	8. The overall prognosis is unfavourable.	8. The overall prognosis is unfavourable.

MIASMATIC ANCESTRAL TIPS: CLINICAL TIPS ON CANCER

TEN SYMPTOMATOLOGICAL ENUNCIATIONS OF CANCEROUS MANIFESTATIONS AND THEIR CORRESPONDING MIASMATICS:

Lesion/Indication	Symptomatic Illustrations	Miasmatic Interpretation
1. Ulceration	i) Ulceration of any mucus membrane such as that of the mouth or cervix, which is chronic and does not tend to heal easily.	Syphilo-psoric.
2. Growths	i) A tumour, growth or malformation of the glands, which is chronic in nature and may be either painful or painless.	Syco-syphilitic or mixed miasmatic.
3. Swallowing	i) Long-standing dysphagia.	Syco-psoric.
4. Hoarseness	i) Chronic hoarseness. ii) Unexplained, nagging cough.	Syphilo-psoric or tubercular.
5. Haemorrhage	i) Persistent haemorrhage from any part/orifices. ii) Haemorrhage during intercourse.	Tubercular.
6. Bowel/bladder habit	i) Any sudden change in bowel and/or bladder habit. ii) Chronic indigestion with anorexia can be a concomitant.	Psora-sycotic. Psora-tubercular.
7. Warts & moles on the skin	i) Crops of warts, moles and birthmarks in which there is a sudden and progressive colour change. ii) Blackish discolouration of the skin.	Syco-psoric.
8. Emaciation, anaemia & insomnia	i) Sudden and progressive weight loss with anaemia and insomnia.	Tubercular (syphilo-psoric).
9. Psychic anxieties	i) Unexplained and excessive fear, anxieties or apprehension. ii) Fear of death or diseases (esp. incurable ones). iii) Contradictory states of mind, modalities, desires and aversions.	Psora-tubercular.
10. Repeated history of infective illnesses	i) Repeated history (more than three at least) of infective diseases in a short space of time.	Psora-tubercular.

Psoric Cancer	Sycotic Cancer	Syphilitic Cancer	Tubercular Cancer
Psora is responsible for deficiency, which leads to deficiency in immunity (i.e. hypo-immunity). The cancer is caused by continuous physical and/or emotional irritation and it is the lowered immunity which makes the person vulnerable to such irritation.	Sycosis is responsible for proliferation and growth. There is hypertrophy, the cells proliferate and tumours are formed. Initially these tumours are benign and encapsulated but become malignant as the cells proliferate out of proportion.	Syphilis is responsible for destruction, disintegration and degeneration. Cells break, disintegrate and degenerate, as do the capsules of the tumour. The malignant property of the cells leads to necrosis followed by pus formation and fistulous openings in the tumour.	Tubercular miasm is responsible for the migration and haemorrhage. Disintegrated and degenerated cells haemorrhage and then migrate resulting in metastasis.

PROPHYLACTIC ASPECT OF HOMOEOPATHIC MEDICINE IN CANCER:

The prophylactic aspect of homoeopathic medicine allows us to treat cancer miasmatically. In the case of a tumour in its benign sycotic state, the application of the correct anti-miasmatic remedy serves to fill the vacuum in the constitution, and in cases where anti-syphilitic and anti-tubercular constitutional medicines are applied the degenerative, haemorrhagic and migratory properties of that tumour are negated thereby preventing degeneration of the cells as well as metastasis.

MIASMATIC ANCESTRAL TIPS: CLINICAL TIPS ON RHEUMATISM

MIASMATICS OF RHEUMATIC MANIFESTATIONS:

Psora	*Sycosis*	*Syphilis*	*Tubercular*
1. Various types of inflammatory rheumatism, e.g. osteitis.	1. Rheumatism with numbness and paralytic weakness of extremities. Anatomical abnormalities like six fingers may be evident.	1. Pain in the long bones aggravated at night. Aching pain in bones of limbs. The syphilitic stigmata can affect the bony structure, which may be changed. Various deformities (arthritis deformans) and atrophy or emaciation of the extremities may occur.	1. Lack of strength of bones. Delayed milestones. Sense of great exhaustion, easily made tired, never seems to get rested. Tired even after a sleep. As the sun ascends, their strength revives a little, as it descends they lose it again. Rickets, marasmus and delayed walking in children.
2. Psoric rheumatic pains are generally associated with neuralgic pains which are sore, bruised and pressive in character.	2. Joint pains are Sycotic. Easy spraining of joints while walking. Joints and connective tissues are affected.	2. Bony pains (esp. in the long bones) are syphilitic.	2. Tubercular rheumatic pains are recurrent and periodic, often associated with new moon and full moon phases.
	3. Stitching, pulsating and wandering pains are sycotic. Pallid, oedematous, puffy. Stiffness, soreness and lameness are characteristic. The gouty diathesis is sycotic.	3. Burning, bursting and tearing pains are syphilitic. There is a lack of nutrition of the bones.	

MIASMATICS OF RHEUMATIC MODALITIES:

Psora	*Sycosis*	*Syphilis*	*Tubercular*
Acute inflammatory rheumatic pain, which is better by quiet, rest, and warmth and worse by motion. Aggravated in winter — wants warmth externally and internally. Aggravated between sunrise to sunset, by cold and from standing. Ameliorated in summer, from heat, by natural discharges such as urine, sweat, menstruation etc. and through physiological eliminative processes such as diarrhoea. Also ameliorated by hot application, scratching, crying, eating and the appearance of suppressed skin eruptions.	Aggravated by rest, damp, rainy, humid atmosphere, during thunderstorms, changes of weather and from meat. Ameliorated by motion, unnatural discharges through the mucus surfaces, such as leucorrhoea and nasal discharge (which are generally greenish/yellow). Physiological elimination however does not ameliorate. Amelioration by slow motion, or by stretching, in dry weather, lying on stomach or with pressure and the return of suppressed normal discharges (e.g. menses). Ameliorated when warts or fibrous growths appear, and from the return or breaking open of the old ulcers or sores. Markedly ameliorated by the return of acute gonorrhoeal manifestations. The sycotic patient is a barometer — when it rains, he has pains, and he suffers.	Acute rheumatic pain, osteomyelitis, degenerative and ulcerous inflammations, necrotic and carious changes in the bone with burning pains, all are aggravated from sunset to sunrise, perspiration (through natural discharges), seaside, and sea-voyage, and from thunderstorms. Also aggravated by warmth, during the summer, at night, from the warmth of the bed, movement, sweat, and extremes of temperature. Amelioration occurs between sunrise and sunset, from a change of position, in lukewarm climates, and from any abnormal discharges (such as. leucorrhoea or coryza). Amelioration during the cold of winter, and through the discharge of pus (if old ulcers open up).	Aggravated by thunderstorms, at night and by milk, fruits, and greasy or oily foods. Aggravation also occurs in closed rooms, and the patient is unable to tolerate any pressure to the chest. Ameliorated in dry weather, open air and during the daytime. Temporarily ameliorated by offensive foot or axillary sweat which when suppressed induces lung trouble. Tubercular manifestations are always ameliorated by nose bleeding. Other modalities depend upon the preponderance of the psoric or syphilitic miasm.

MIASMATIC ANCESTRAL TIPS: CLINICAL TIPS ON ECZEMA

	Psoric		*Sycotic*		*Syphilitic*		*Tubercular*
1.	Eczema is not psora but the results of psora.	1.	Sycotic eczemas are exfoliating in nature and occur only in circumscribed spots.	1.	Syphilitic skin shows all sorts of ulcers and boils, which heal slowly and are apt to discharge offensive fluid and pus.	1.	Tubercular skin produces eczema, which affects mainly the busy and important areas of the body.
2.	Psoric eczema is dry and the skin appears dirty and harsh.	2.	Sycotic eruptions are small, reddish, flat and vesicular.	2.	The ulcers that develop are open and virulent in type.	2.	Eczema in the constitution with a past history of ringworm. Suppression of eczema and of ringworm leads to respiratory diseases.
3.	Itching occurs without any pus or discharge.	3.	The skin is oily with thick copious perspiration.	3.	The ulcers are devoid of pain and itching (due to destruction of the sensory receptors) but become aggravated at night and from the warmth of the bed.	3.	Recurrent and obstinate boils occur with profuse pus and fever. These boils heal only with difficulty.
4.	There is a sensation of burning with scaly eruptions and a tendency to recurring colds.	4.	The eczema is painful and the circumscribed patches may be localised. Pain is better by pressure.	4.	Burning pains in eczema without associated ulcers < at night and from the warmth of the bed.	4.	Allergic eczemas.

MIASMATIC ANCESTRAL TIPS: CLINICAL TIPS ON AIDS

MIASMATIC INTERPRETATION OF THE VARIOUS SYMPTOMATIC MANIFESTATIONS OF AIDS:

	Point	Aids Psoric Taint	Aids Sycotic Taint	Aids Syphilitic Taint	Aids Tubercular Taint
1.	Fatigue & Debility	i) Psoric patients are mentally alert and are quick and active in their motions. Short bursts of hard work cause both physical and mental fatigue and this is followed by profound prostration and a desire to lie down. Extreme fatigue prevents the patient performing their normal duties. ii) Indolence, an untidy appearance, a general lack of discipline and an aversion to work, bathing and keeping things clean are the innate dyscrasia of psora. In AIDS however, the manifestation of fatigue does not belong to psora alone.			i) Unrestrained and uncontrollable passions such as masturbation, artificial loss of semen, and a perverted craving for sex cause debility in the tubercular patient. These unrestrained passions are characterised by indifference. ii) Weak wrist and ankle joints, difficulty in holding objects and clumsiness affect the tubercular patient. There is a sense of great exhaustion, they are easily made tired and never seem to get rested. Tiredness is particularly evident at night and they feel tired even after a sleep. As the sun ascends, their strength revives a little but as it descends, it diminishes again. iii) Skin suppression affects the inner tissues resulting in destructive and ulcerous manifestations which proceed to affect the deeper organs leading to a debilitated tubercular state.
2.	Lymph-adenopathy	i) The sensitising property of psora causes the organism to become susceptible to all kinds of environmental conditions, diseases and allergens. The glands swell from the least exposure and from the least cold.	Glands enlarge out of propotion.	Glands: Ulcreate, degenerate and tends to necrosis. Fistulas opening from glands with oozing of offensive pus.	i) Glandular swellings, (scrofulosis) are of tubercular preponderance with a psoric background. Cervical lymphadenitis is also tuberculo-psoric and these patients are apt to catch cold easily. ii) Nasal polyps (tri-miasmatic) occur and when characterised by profuse haemorrhage can be deemed as more tubercular.

Point	Aids Psoric Taint	Aids Sycotic Taint	Aids Syphilitic Taint	Aids Tubercular Taint
				iii) The tubercular miasm is responsive and reactive and a rapid response to any stimulus such as the slightest change of weather can be seen in tubercular patients.
				iv) Any suppression of skin diseases directly affects the respiratory system and result in asthma, TB or tonsillitis.
				v) Swollen glands and tonsils always accompany coughs and colds.
3. Dermatitis & Fungal Infections	i) Dirty, dry, harsh skin with itching and burning is characteristic of psora.		i) In syphilis there are all sorts of ulcers and boils, which heal slowly with the discharge of offensive and spreading fluid and pus. There is also a tendency to develop open ulcers of the virulent type.	i) The tubercular miasm has eczemas and ringworm, or a history of ringworm and its suppression.
	ii) Psoric eruptions are not noticeable by their colour but by their roughness of skin.		ii) All fungal infections are predominantly syphilitic.	ii) The busy and important areas of the skin are affected, such as the lips, the tips of the fingers, heels etc. The threat of ulceration is more prominent even than in syphilis.
	iii) Suppression of skin diseases affects the mind manifesting as anxiety and anguish.		iii) Skin suppressions affect the intellect resulting in dullness, depression and a lack of enthusiasm.	iii) Skin suppressions affect the inner tissues and result in destruction and ulceration of the deeper organs.
4. Allergy	i) Psora is often present in the background of allergic reactions by virtue of its 'hypo' manifestations which lower the immunity and result in an increased susceptibility to allergens.			i) Any allergic manifestation has a prominence of the tubercular miasmatic dyscrasia.
5. Diarrhoea & Recurrent Gastro-enteritis	i) In psora, diarrhoea is painless and is often due to gluttony or fright.	i) Diarrhoea is primarily sycotic and all the intestinal features of sycosis are severe in nature.	i) In syphilis, lienteria, diarrhoea and dysentery all occur with pus and a bloody stool due to perversion of the digestive power and system.	i) Tubercular diarrhoeas come on from the least exposure to cold. Breakfast diarrhoeas and diarrhoeas after food are characteristic.
	ii) Painless, offensive morning diarrhoea with rumbling and gurgling in the abdomen occurs after taking cold things. The psoric stool may be of any colour.	ii) Sycotic diarrhoea is characterised by a sour, acrid, grass green and corrosive stool, which gushes and ejaculates forcefully and has the odour of fish-brine. Symptoms come on from getting wet and changes	ii) In syphilis, extreme weakness (destruction of all strength) follows any loose motions. The stool is black and extremely offensive and may be accompanied by colic, which is aggravated at night.	ii) The tubercular stool is slimy, greasy and bloody, with a musty, mouldy smell or with the odour of rotten eggs. Nausea and gagging often precede the stool and prostration with a desire to be left alone follow.

Point	Aids Psoric Taint	Aids Sycotic Taint	Aids Syphilitic Taint	Aids Tubercular Taint
		in the weather or seasons. Colic and a constant sensation of gripping may also be present.		Morning diarrhoea occurs with extreme prostration and debility. Bleeding per rectum is also characteristic of the tubercular miasm.
	iii) Diarrhoea comes on from preparation for an unusual event.	iii) The sycotic patient suffers from a sense of insecurity, which causes them to rush to the toilet.	iii) Diarrhoea occurs at the seaside and ulcers are often present in the rectum.	iii) Rectal diseases alternate with heart, chest or lung complaints, esp. in asthma and respiratory conditions. Tubercular manifestations of the brain may sometimes alternate with a bowel difficulty and any brain symptoms which appear or disappear during diarrhoea are a sure indication of the presence of the tubercular miasm.
	iv) Aggravation occurs in the morning, from cold and motion and after eating. When bloating occurs the patient cannot endure any touch to the abdomen. Amelioration is from pressure and warmth and from warm drinks and hot food.	iv) Diarrhoea is aggravated by changes in the weather and the seasons, and by cold. In cases of abdominal pain the patient will bend forward as hard pressure ameliorates.	iv) Syphilitic patients suffer nighttime aggravation.	iv) Aggravation occurs from cold, at night or in the early morning, driving the patient out of bed.
	v) All symptoms of acidity, dyspepsia, nausea and vomiting, and liver and stomach pains are psoric.	v) Crampy pains in the lower abdomen are characteristic of sycosis.	v) Perverted intestinal peristalsis leads to dysenteric spasm. Dysentery is syphilitic.	v) Abdominal colic occurs in the lower abdomen, and flatulence causes lower abdominal pain with rumbling and gurgling.
6. Mental Symptoms	i) The psoric mind manifests outwardly and is incapable of any deep mental concentration, meditation or sacred thought. Thoughts therefore tend to be inconsistent and fictitious. The psoric patient cannot materialise what he thinks and is totally theoretical with little or no practicality at all.	i) The sycotic mentality is suspicious, mischievous, mean, selfish and forgetful.	i) The syphilitic miasm perverts, deforms, and vitiates the senses of judgement, the memory and the sharpness of the intellect. The patient is unable to realise his symptoms or relate them to the physician. Desires for and aversions to foodstuffs are also lost.	i) Dissatisfaction and a lack of tolerance are the innate dyscrasia of the tubercular stigmata.
	ii) In psora there is an inability to concentrate.	ii) In all varieties of deprivation and rudeness sycosis is present.	ii) The syphilitic patient is mentally dull, heavy, stupid and particularly stubborn. Idiocy, ignorance and obstinacy lead to melancholia and gloominess. Slowness of the mental powers mean that anything the patient reads has to be re-read before they can begin to comprehend.	ii) The tubercular lack of tolerance leads to anger and irritability, which in time results in depression.

Point	Aids Psoric Taint	Aids Sycotic Taint	Aids Syphilitic Taint	Aids Tubercular Taint
	iii) Anxiety is another psoric characteristic and the patient will become anxious to the point of worry and fear.	iii) Absent-mindedness, loss of memory and losing the thread of conversation are characteristic of sycosis. The patient forgets recent events but has a good recollection of the distant past.	iii) The syphilitic patient lacks any sense of duty or responsibility due to their impaired memory. This results in low self-esteem and an inability to accept normal family responsibilities.	iii) The dissatisfied state of the tubercular mind makes the patient changeable, both mentally and physically.
	iv) Weakness of memory indicates psora; forget-fullness indicates syphilis, and absent-mindedness indicates sycosis.	iv) The narrow-minded sycotic patient feels inferior to others and has a tendency to hide from them. They experience turmoil in their memorizing powers.	iv) In syphilis, a desire for solitude and an aversion to company can lead to suicidal tendencies. Patients are introverts with a desire to escape from themselves as well as others.	iv) Changeableness and dissatisfaction ends in a depressed state of mind, which is characterised by a total absence of disappointment, hopelessness, anxiety or apprehension.
	v) Psoric patients are mentally restless and unable to focus for any length of time. They complain that they want to do something but they do not know what. Activities are started and ended in a very dramatic fashion.	v) Sycotic mental functions are uncoordinated. There is incoordination in memory, forgetfulness, absent-mindedness, slowness of speech and an inability to find the right words.	v) Lack of self-confidence results from impaired memory and the patient may come to feel that the only way out is by suicide.	v) Mental fatigue is responsible for the tubercular patient's apathetic, indifferent state of the mind.
	vi) Changes of temperament may be experienced without any apparent cause, and young people in particularly may become hysterical esp. after acute, weakening diseases.	vi) Incoordination in behaviour leads to failure to speak the truth, excessive suspicion, jealousy, crossness, irritability and secretiveness.	vi) Dullness of intellect causes the patient to loose the thread of the conversation and to lack perception.	vi) The carelessness, apathetic, indifferent attitude of the tubercular patient is a reflection of self-destruction.
	vii) Psoric patients are prone to depression of spirits but unaccustomed to silent grief so that everyone knows of their troubles. The act of bursting into tears is liable to relieve the whole condition.		vii) Syphilitic patients are always depressed but keep their troubles to themselves and brood over them. This depression is likely to end in an anxious state where the patient likes to be in solitude and the first thing anyone knows of it is when the patient has committed suicide.	vii) A suicidal impulse is manifested by an indifference to everything, which eventually ends in self-destruction.
			viii) Syphilitic mental symptoms are ameliorated by unnatural discharges.	viii) Tubercular mental symptoms esp. anger are worse after sleep and a feeling of dissatisfaction is clearly manifested on the face on awakening.

MIASMATIC ANCESTRAL TIPS: CLINICAL TIPS ON MIGRAINE

MIASMATIC INTERPRETATION OF MIGRAINE:

Point	Psoric Migraine	Sycotic Migraine	Syphilitic Migraine	Tubercular Migraine
1. Location	Headache mostly frontal, temporal, of the vertex or may be of the whole head.	Frontal, vertex and occasionally parietal.	Mostly occipital or temporal. Occasionally in the base of the brain, the internal head and the meninges.	Headaches are temporal, in the base of the brain, parietal or in the meninges. They are patchy in distribution.
2. Sensation	Sharp, severe, paroxysmal headaches. One-sided headaches are often psoric, as are long standing headaches such as migraines, esp. when of a functional character.	Dull, aching, heaviness and reeling.	Stitching, tearing, boring, digging, maddening, sharp, cutting sensations. Headaches are often persistent and may occur constantly to one side at the base of the brain.	Extremely painful headaches, esp. when the patient is on holiday, which migrate from right eye to left ear. Headaches when approaching a stranger. Throbbing, as if hammering and pressive, tightness like a band (with effusion in meninges) is characteristic.
3. Modalities	Headache from hunger and headache, which increases and decreases with the sun. Aggravation occurs in the morning, from motion, cold, anxiety and the sun. Amelioration is from rest, quiet, sleep, warmth (hot applications) and natural eliminations.	Rest, humidity, morning to night time, midnight, lying down and cold aggravate; whilst motion, violent exercise, warmth and abnormal discharges ameliorate.	Night time, evening to morning (during sleep), rest, lying down, the warmth of the bed, hot or warm weather, natural discharges and exertion, all aggravate.	There is an aversion to having the head uncovered and aggravation occurs in the evening and forenoon, from changes in the weather and from cold. Nose bleeds, rest, quiet, sleeping and eating, all ameliorate.
4. Concomitants	i) Red face and throbbing carotids. ii) Mental symptoms such as anxiety, apprehension and fear appear as a secondary manifestation to the headache. iii) Hot flushes which end with little perspiration. iv) Sweat on head during sleep. v) Vertigo, which is aggravated by looking up suddenly, rising from a sitting position or from emotional disturbances.	i) Urogenital symptoms. ii) Cross, irritable and jealous behaviours. iii) Restlessness. iv) Vertigo, which appears on closing the eyes and disappears when the eyes are opened.	i) Suicidal tendencies. ii) Imbecility. iii) There may be an association with allied disturbances of the cardiovascular and nervous systems.	i) Red face and throbbing carotids (psoric component). ii) Nose bleeds which relieve the headache symptoms. iii) Coughs, colds and coryza. iv) Hunger during the headache. v) Offensive head sweats. vi) Extreme weakness.

Point	Psoric Migraine	Sycotic Migraine	Syphilitic Migraine	Tubercular Migraine
				vii) In the tubercular headaches of children, they strike, knock or pound their heads with their hands or against some object.
				viii) Vertigo, which begins at the base of the brain.
		Congestion leads to stagnation and causes the arteries to become sluggish.	Deficient blood supply.	Active congestion leads to pulsation, which shakes the whole body.

MIASMATIC ANCESTRAL TIPS: CLINICAL TIPS ON NUTRITION AND FOODS

	Food	Aggravation +++	Aggravation ++	Aggravation or Amelioration
1.	Fats	Sycosis	Syphilis & psora	Syphilis & psora
2.	Proteins	Psora	Syphilis & sycosis	Syphilis & sycosis
3.	Starch	Syphilis	Sycosis & psora	Sycosis & psora

PART — V
MIASMATIC PRESCRIBING:
MIASMATIC REPERTORY

MIASMATIC DIAGNOSIS: MIASMATIC REPERTORY OF MENTAL SYMPTOMS

Mental Symptoms	Rubric	Psora	Sycosis	Syphilis	Tubercular	Mixed Miasms
Abrupt						Psora-sycotic
Absent-minded			✓			
Abusive						Syphilo-sycotic
Active			✓			
Active	then fatigued mind	✓				
Advice	rejects, health, regarding				✓	
Affection	lack of					Syphilo-sycotic
Alert						Psora-tubercular
Alone	dreads to be	✓				
Anger	alternating, tears, with				✓	
Angry	change, of weather, on		✓			
Anguish						Psora-sycotic
Anxiety		✓				
Anxiety	heart, felt in	✓				
Anxiety	move, compelled to					Psora-sycotic
Anxiety	night, at					Psora-syphilitic
Anxiety	waking, on	✓				
Anxiety	weather, from change of					Psora-sycotic
Appearance	change, likes to				✓	
Appearance	thoughtless				✓	
Apprehension		✓				
Apprehension	of impending misfortune	✓				
Arithmetic	difficult, calculation			✓		
Audacity						Syco-syphilitic
Avaricious			✓			
Aversion	people, to	✓				
Bright					✓	
Brooding		✓				
Busy			✓			
Changeable						Tuberculo-psoric
Chaotic						Syphilo-syco-psoric
Checks	everything done			✓		
Checks	everything said			✓		
Cheerfulness				✓		
Cold-blooded	murderer			✓		
Company	aversion to	✓				
Company	without notice, leaves			✓		
Comprehension	difficult					Syphilo-tubercular
Comprehension	slow					Tuberculo-psoric
Conceals	feelings		✓			
Conceals	ideas		✓			
Conceals	own personality					Sycotic or syphilitic
Concentrate	cannot	✓				
Concentration	difficult					Psora-tubercular
Confidence	lack of					Psora-syphilitic

Mental Symptoms	Rubric	Psora	Sycosis	Syphilis	Tubercular	Mixed Miasms
Confidence	lacking, totally			✓		
Conversation	thread of, loses		✓			
Courageous (audacious, rash)						Psora-syphilo-sycotic
Courageous soldier						Syco-syphilitic
Craves	new things				✓	
Craves	things which make him sick				✓	
Cruelty	mental		✓			
Cruelty	physical			✓		
Cruelty	physical and mental				✓	or Syphilo-sycotic
Danger	threatening					Syphilo-sycotic
Deceitful				✓		
Deceitful	in religion	✓				
Degeneration of mind				✓		
Desires	objects, to obtain unnecessary	✓				
Despair			✓			
Destroyed	for one's own life, love			✓		
Destruction				✓		
Destruction	self, of					Syphilo-tubercular
Destructive				✓		
Disappointment	none				✓	
Discipline	lacking	✓				
Dissatisfaction					✓	
Dissatisfaction	after sleep, worse				✓	
Disturbed	easily	✓				
Disturbed	mentally, easily	✓				
Diversion	thought, of	✓				
Dullness						Psora-syphilitic
Duties	due to exhaustion, cannot perform	✓				
Duty	sense of, lack of			✓		
Ecstasy						Psora-syphilitic
Exaltation of fancy			✓			
Exhaustion	duty being performed, prevents	✓				
Exhilaration					✓	
Explain	cannot, symptoms			✓		
Explain	cannot, thoughts			✓		
Exploit	to, tendency		✓			
Exploits			✓			
Expression	difficult			✓		
Extrovert			✓			
Fatigue	easily	✓				
Fatigue	total prostration, followed by	✓				
Fear		✓				
Fear	children in, of animals	✓				
Fear	completion, of task	✓				
Fear	death, of	✓				
Fear	disease, of	✓				
Fear	dogs, of				✓	
Fear	in children, of darkness	✓				
Fear	in children, of strangers	✓				
Fear	to converse with, of people					Psora-syphilitic
Fearless					✓	
Fears						Psora-sycotic
Fears	a mistake, of making					Psora-sycotic
Fixed	ideas					Syphilo-sycotic
Foolish	with ridiculous behaviour, childish					Psora-sycotic; or can be syphilitic
Forgetful						Syphilo-sycotic
Forgetfulness	total			✓		
Forgets	events, recent		✓			
Forgets	say, what he is about to					Syco-tubercular

Mental Symptoms	Rubric	Psora	Sycosis	Syphilis	Tubercular	Mixed Miasms
Forgets	words		✓			
Frightened	by trivial things	✓				
Frightened	easily	✓				
Frightened	perspiration, followed by	✓				
Frightened	trembling, followed by	✓				
Frightened	weakness, followed by	✓				
Frivolity						Syco-psoric
Gloomy				✓		
Hatred						Syphilo-syco-psoric
Haughtiness						Syco-psora-syphilitic
Hopeful					✓	
Hopeful	recovery, of				✓	
Hopeless	not				✓	
Hurry			✓			
Hurtful			✓			
Hypocrisy						Syco-syphilitic
Iconoclast				✓		
Ideas	of, overflow	✓				
Idiocy						Syphilo-psoric
Imbecility						Psora-syphilitic
Impatient					✓	
Impertinence						Syphilo-sycotic
Impetuous			✓			
Impulsive						Syco-syphilitic
Impulsive	destructive			✓		
Indifferent					✓	
Indolent		✓				
Industrious			✓			
Insanity						Syphilo-psora-sycotic
Insolence			✓			
Introvert					✓	
Irritability						Syco-psoric
Jealous						Syco-psoric
Joyful		✓				
Lamenting (moaning)						Syco-psoric
Lasciviousness						Syco-psora-syphi
Madness						Syphilo-psoric
Malicious						Syphilo-psoric
Mean			✓			
Meditation	difficult	✓				
Melancholy				✓		
Memory	destroyed			✓		
Memory	impaired	✓				
Mental conditions	discharges, ameliorated by	✓				
Mental conditions	discharges, unnatural, ameliorated by	✓				
Mental conditions	gonorrhoea, ameliorated by	✓				
Mental confusion						Mixed miasmatic
Mental exertion	exhaustion, followed by	✓				
Mental exertion	heat in the body, followed by					Psora-tubercular
Mischievous						Syphilo-psora-sycotic
Mistrust				✓		
Monosyllabic				✓		
Morose						Psora-sycotic
Obstinate						Tuberculo-syphilitic
Paralysis	mind, of			✓		
Passions	unrestrained				✓	
Perception	lack of			✓		
Practical	not	✓				
Presumptuous			✓			
Propensity to frown						Syco-psoric
Prostration of mind		✓				

Mental Symptoms	Rubric	Psora	Sycosis	Syphilis	Tubercular	Mixed Miasms
Quarrelsome			✓			
Rashness			✓			
Reactions	slow					Syphilo-psoric
Rejects	things when offered				✓	
Religion	deceitful in	✓				
Remembers	of distant past, events		✓			
Repeats			✓			
Responsibility	lack of				✓	
Restless	drives from bed, mental					Syphilo-psoric
Restless	frequently, changes places				✓	
Restless	menses, before					Psora-sycotic
Restless	mental	✓				
Restless	new moon, before	✓				
Restless	not why, knows					Psora-sycotic
Restless	objects, to gain					Syco-psoric
Restless	physical		✓			
Restless	posture, changing		✓			
Retain	cannot, information				✓	
Ridiculous			✓			
Rude and malicious						Syphilo-psoric
Rudeness			✓			
Sadness		✓				
Secretiveness						Psora-sycotic
Self-confidence	lack of					Syphilo-sycotic
Selfish			✓			
Solitude	prefers			✓		
Speech	rapid					Syco-psoric
Speech	slow					Syphilo-psoric
Spell	cannot		✓			
Stubborn						Syco-tubercular
Stupefaction						Psora-sycotic
Suicidal	disposition			✓		
Suicide				✓		
Suicide	planning					Syco-syphilitic
Sulky		✓				
Sullen					✓	
Suspicious			✓			
Sympathetic	not at all				✓	
Talks	himself, to					Syco-psoric
Things	new, wants				✓	
Things	rejects, in children, when offered				✓	
Things	unnecessary, desires					Tuberculo-psoric
Things	which make them sick, crave				✓	
Thoughtful		✓				
Thoughts	fast					Syco-psoric
Thoughts	fictitious	✓				
Thoughts	inconsistent	✓				
Thoughts	vanish	✓				
Timid		✓				
Timid	to school, on going	✓				
Tolerance	lack of				✓	
Torture	others, mentally		✓			
Torture	others, physically			✓		
Torture	siblings				✓	
Trust	cannot					Syco-syphilitic
Untidy		✓				
Violent	tendency					Syphilo-sycotic
Weakness	memory, of	✓				
Worry	does not				✓	

MIASMATIC DIAGNOSIS: MIASMATIC REPERTORY OF VERTIGO SYMPTOMS

Vertigo Symptoms	Rubric	Psora	Sycosis	Syphilis	Tubercular	Mixed Miasms
Vertigo	anaemia, from	✓				
Vertigo	base of brain, beginning at					Syphilo-tubercular
Vertigo	by rest, ameliorated					Psora-tubercular
Vertigo	consciousness, with momentary loss of	✓				
Vertigo	digestive disturbances, with	✓				
Vertigo	emotional disturbances, from	✓				
Vertigo	falling, with sensation of	✓				
Vertigo	feeling of intoxication, with	✓				
Vertigo	floating feeling, with	✓				
Vertigo	floating on air, as if	✓				
Vertigo	flushing of the face, with				✓	
Vertigo	forgetfulness, with total			✓		
Vertigo	formication, with sensation of		✓			
Vertigo	indigestion, from	✓				
Vertigo	in ears, with roaring	✓				
Vertigo	insects crawling, with feeling of		✓			
Vertigo	movement, aggravated by	✓				
Vertigo	night, aggravated at			✓		
Vertigo	opening eyes, returning on					Psora-sycotic
Vertigo	quiet, ameliorated by being				✓	
Vertigo	reading and writing, aggravated by	✓				
Vertigo	reading, on	✓				
Vertigo	restlessness, with		✓			
Vertigo	riding in a boat or car, on	✓				
Vertigo	sleep, ameliorated by				✓	
Vertigo	sun rising, aggravated by the	✓				
Vertigo	sun setting, ameliorated by the	✓				
Vertigo	vision, with temporary loss of	✓				
Vertigo	warmth, aggravated by	✓				
Vertigo	with dissatisfaction				✓	
Vertigo	with impatience				✓	
Vertigo	writing, on	✓				

MIASMATIC DIAGNOSIS: MIASMATIC REPERTORY OF HEAD SYMPTOMS

Head Symptoms	Rubric	Psora	Sycosis	Syphilis	Tubercular	Mixed Miasms
Discharge	behind ears, from, aggravated by working in water				✓	
Eruptions	in scalp, with pus, aggravated by washing			✓		
Eruptions	in scalp, aggravated by heat of bed					Psora-syphilitic
Eruptions	in scalp, aggravated in open air	✓				
Eruptions	in scalp, burn	✓				
Eruptions	in scalp, burn, aggravated in open air and evening	✓				
Eruptions	in scalp, do not suppurate	✓				
Eruptions	in scalp, dry	✓				
Eruptions	in scalp, dry, brown and become dead scales	✓				
Eruptions	in scalp, moist			✓		
Eruptions	in scalp, ulcerative			✓		
Eruptions	in scalp, warts		✓			
Eruptions	pus, in scalp, oozing			✓		
Fontanelles	open			✓		
Hair	a thick heavy crust					Syphilo-tubercular
Hair	after an illness, falls out	✓				
Hair	after childbirth, falls out				✓	
Hair	alopecia in circular spots		✓			
Hair	alopecia, after acute illness	✓				
Hair	breaks and splits, rough, harsh and sticks together				✓	
Hair	dandruff, bran-like	✓				
Hair	dandruff with thick yellow crust					Syphilo-tubercular
Hair	difficult to comb	✓				
Hair	dry, dead like hemp	✓				
Hair	eyebrows, eyelashes and beard, falling from			✓		
Hair	fishy odour		✓			
Hair	from beard, falls out			✓		
Hair	immature greyish hair		✓			
Hair	in bunches, tendency to fall			✓		
Hair	in-growing			✓		
Hair	in-growing eyelash, causing much irritation in conjunctiva			✓		
Hair	lustreless, dry	✓				
Hair	matted	✓				
Hair	moist, gluey			✓		
Hair	odour, sour					Syco-syphilitic
Hair	of beard, often in-growing and suppurating			✓		
Hair	of elderly people, eyelashes break and turn inward			✓		
Hair	oily					Syphilo-tubercular
Hair	on midline of head, grey	✓				
Hair	over scapula					Psora-sycotic
Hair	premature grey hair, too much		✓			
Hair	split at ends, breaks	✓				
Hair	spotty, baldness		✓			
Hair	thin	✓				
Hair	too early, becomes grey					Psora-sycotic
Hair	white in spots, becomes	✓				
Hair	with offensive odour, greasy			✓		

Head Symptoms	Rubric	Psora	Sycosis	Syphilis	Tubercular	Mixed Miasms
Head	devoid of perspiration	✓				
Head	long in comparison to body			✓		
Head	odour like old hay, sweat				✓	
Head	of fishy odour, sweats		✓			
Head	of musty odour, sweats					Syco-tubercular
Head	of offensive odour, sweats				✓	
Head	sour, odour		✓			
Head	uncovered, cannot bear				✓	
Headache	after midnight, aggravated			✓		
Headache	after sleep, ameliorated	✓				
Headache	aggravated at night, occipital			✓		
Headache	aggravated by rest, occipital			✓		
Headache	aggravated by rest, temporal			✓		
Headache	at night, aggravated by lying down			✓		
Headache	lying down and rest, aggravated by			✓		
Headache	night, aggravated at			✓		
Headache	sleep, ameliorated before			✓		
Headache	base of brain, at			✓		
Headache	before and during, hunger					Psora-tubercular
Headache	being quiet and sleep, ameliorated by					Psora-tubercular
Headache	bilious attacks, with	✓				
Headache	changing place, ameliorated by					Syphilo-sycotic
Headache	cold, ameliorated by			✓		
Headache	cold application, ameliorated by			✓		
Headache	despondency, with				✓	
Headache	dull, heavy					Syphilo-sycotic
Headache	during, child knocks or pounds head					Syphilo-tubercular
Headache	during, hungry				✓	
Headache	during new or full moon				✓	
Headache	during sleep, aggravated			✓		
Headache	during, strikes head				✓	
Headache	eating, ameliorated by				✓	
Headache	especially after midnight, aggravated early morning		✓			
Headache	especially on holidays, extremely painful				✓	
Headache	examinations, aggravated by preparing for				✓	
Headache	exertion, aggravated by			✓		
Headache	for days, lasts			✓		
Headache	from hunger	✓				
Headache	from meeting strangers				✓	
Headache	from sun	✓				
Headache	frontal		✓			
Headache	gentle motion, ameliorated by		✓			
Headache	head, bands around				✓	
Headache	heat, aggravated by				✓	
Headache	in vertex		✓			
Headache	into the pillow, with boring the head				✓	
Headache	lying down, aggravated by			✓		
Headache	long standing				✓	
Headache	meeting and entertaining strangers, aggravated by				✓	
Headache	morning, aggravated in	✓				
Headache	morning, ameliorated in			✓		
Headache	motion, ameliorated by			✓		
Headache	movement, aggravated by				✓	
Headache	movement, ameliorated by			✓		
Headache	new and full moon, during				✓	
Headache	nose bleed, ameliorated by				✓	
Headache	not amenable to treatment				✓	
Headache	of extremities, with coldness				✓	
Headache	in morning, persistent	✓				

Head Symptoms	Rubric	Psora	Sycosis	Syphilis	Tubercular	Mixed Miasms
Headache	in morning, returning	✓				
Headache	on head, during, cannot bear heat	✓				
Headache	on head, with offensive sweat			✓		
Headache	one-sided	✓				
Headache	one-sided, at base of brain			✓		
Headache	paroxysmal	✓				
Headache	periodical				✓	
Headache	persistent					Psora-tubercular
Headache	preparing for examinations, aggravated by				✓	
Headache	profuse offensive sweat, on head, associated with			✓		
Headache	red face, with	✓				
Headache	rest, aggravated by			✓		
Headache	rest, ameliorated by					Psora-tubercular
Headache	rest and warmth, ameliorated by	✓				
Headache	riding, aggravated by			✓		
Headache	riding in a carriage, aggravated by				✓	
Headache	rolling of head, with					Syco-tubercular
Headache	rush of blood, with				✓	
Headache	sleep, aggravated by			✓		
Headache	sensation of heat and flushing, with					Psora-tubercular
Headache	sensation of heaviness, with		✓			
Headache	severe	✓				
Headache	severe, with sensation of band					Tuberculo-syphilitic
Headache	sharp	✓				
Headache	suppressed eruptions, from				✓	
Headache	temporal			✓		
Headache	throbbing	✓				
Headache	warmth of bed, aggravated by			✓		
Headache	with cold and cough				✓	
Headache	with coldness of body					Psora-sycotic
Headache	with crying		✓			
Headache	with extreme weakness				✓	
Headache	with fever		✓			
Headache	with hot extremities				✓	
Headache	with involvement of gastric tract		✓			
Headache	with restlessness		✓			
Headache	with sadness					Psora-sycotic
Headache	with very cold extremities				✓	
Headache	with weakness					Psora-sycotic
Headache	with worrying					Psora-sycotic

MIASMATIC DIAGNOSIS: MIASMATIC REPERTORY OF EYE SYMPTOMS

Eye Symptoms	Rubric	Psora	Sycosis	Syphilis	Tubercular	Mixed Miasms
Aching	dull		✓			
Blurred	vision	✓				
Burning						Psora-syphilitic
Cataract			✓			
Coldness	sensation of	✓				
Colours	different, visualising	✓				
Conjunctivitis		✓				
Cornea	inflammation of	✓				
Cornea	ulceration of			✓		
Corneal	incoordination and inflammation		✓			
Daylight	intolerance of	✓				
Dryness	eye, of	✓				
Eye	agg. at night, complaints			✓		
Eye	agg. by rain and change of weather, disorders		✓			
Eye	agg. by warmth of bed, complaints			✓		
Eye	sunken				✓	
Glandular	structure change				✓	
Glaucoma			✓			
Haematoma					✓	
Iritis						Psora-sycotic
Itching	not amel. by rubbing, in canthi	✓				
Itching	rub, desire to	✓	.			
Itching	rub lids, desire to	✓				
Lachrymal	disturbed, functioning					Syphilo-tubercular
Lens	changes in, refractory				✓	
Lens	deformities			✓		
Lids	granulation of					Syco-tubercular
Lids	in pain, closed				✓	
Lids	together in morning, matted	✓				
Neuralgia	agg. by warmth			✓		
Neuralgia	amel. by cold			✓		
Neuralgia	amel. by warmth				✓	
Neuralgia	change of weather, agg. by rain		✓			
Neuralgia	in eye				✓	
Opacity	lens, of		✓			
Opacity	with degenerative changes, to lens					Syco-syphilitic
Pain	amel. by closing eyes				✓	
Photophobia	due to condylomata		✓			
Photophobic	artificial lights, in				✓	
Photophobic	of artificial light, with intolerance			✓		
Ptosis						Syco-syphilitic
Pupil	dilatation, chronic				✓	
Red	appearance					Psora-tubercular
Red	scaly, lids				✓	
Redness	heat, with sensation of				✓	
Retinal	detachment				✓	
Retinoblastoma			✓			
Sand	sensation of	✓				
Sensation	raw			✓		
Spots	eyes, before	✓				
Styes						Syco-tubercular
Sunlight	agg. by	✓				
Tarsal	tumours		✓			

197

Eye Symptoms	Rubric	Psora	Sycosis	Syphilis	Tubercular	Mixed Miasms
Vision	blurred, letters run together	✓				
Weakness	paralytic			✓		
Zigzag	objects	✓				

MIASMATIC DIAGNOSIS: MIASMATIC REPERTORY OF EAR SYMPTOMS

Ear Symptoms	Rubric	Psora	Sycosis	Syphilis	Tubercular	Mixed Miasms
Abscesses	in ear					Tuberculo-syphilitic
Anxiety	ear problems	✓				
Appearance	dirty	✓				
Canal	dry	✓				
Cold	brings earache, exposure to				✓	
Crawling	in ear	✓				
Discharge	cheesy				✓	
Discharge	curdled				✓	
Discharge	no complaints about, copious				✓	
Discharges	carrion-like, odour				✓	
Dryness	in ear	✓				
Earache	at night, appears				✓	
Eruptions	around ear				✓	
Eruptions	around ear, pimples				✓	
Eruptions	around ear, with pus			✓		
Eruptions	fissures					Syphilo-tubercular
Eruptions	humid				✓	
Eruptions	incrustations				✓	
Eruptions	moist, around ear				✓	
Flushed	appearance				✓	
Hear	cannot			✓		
Hearing	with curdled discharge, loss				✓	
Itching	in ear	✓				
Long	appearance			✓		
Mastoiditis					✓	
Noise	better in, hears		✓			
Noise	pain, causes	✓				
Noise	startled from	✓				
Noise	tolerate, cannot	✓				
Noises	in ear	✓				
Ossicles	destroyed					Syphilo-tubercular
Otitis Media	agg. at night			✓		
Otitis Media	agg. by warmth			✓		
Otitis Media	daytime, no pain, agg. at night				✓	
Otitis Media	offensive pus, with			✓		
Otitis Media	other complaints, accompanies			✓		
Otitis Media	when appears with other diseases, prognosis good, in children				✓	
Otitis Media	with exudation					Syco-tubercular
Otitis Media	with ulceration			✓		
Pain	agg. by change of weather		✓			
Pain	agg. in the day		✓			
Pain	agg. at night					Syphilo-tubercular
Pain	amel. during day				✓	
Pain	burning			✓		
Pain	bursting			✓		
Pain	pulsating		✓			
Pain	recurrent				✓	
Pain	restless, makes her		✓			
Pain	stitching		✓			
Pain	tearing				✓	
Pain	wandering					Syco-tubercular
Pulsation	in ear, sensation of					Psora-tubercular
Scales	dry	✓				

Ear Symptoms	Rubric	Psora	Sycosis	Syphilis	Tubercular	Mixed Miasms
Structural	changes			✓		
Suppuration	sore throat, following				✓	
Swollen	thick appearance		✓			
Tonsillitis	ear pain, with				✓	

MIASMATIC DIAGNOSIS: MIASMATIC REPERTORY OF NOSE SYMPTOMS

Nose Symptoms	Rubric	Psora	Sycosis	Syphilis	Tubercular	Mixed Miasms
Adenoids	swollen		✓			
Air	amel., open				✓	
Anosmia				✓		
Blocked	due to thickened membranes, sensation		✓			
Boils	in nose	✓				
Boils	in septum					Psora-syphilitic
Burning	of septum		✓			
Clinkers	brown			✓		
Clinkers	dark green			✓		
Clinkers	offensive			✓		
Clinkers	with offensive breath, offensive			✓		
Closed	room agg				✓	
Cold	amel. by natural discharges, symptoms	✓				
Cold	easily, catch					Psora-tubercular
Cold	heat, begins with	✓				
Cold	in morning, agg	✓				
Cold	nasal symptoms, agg.	✓				
Cold	recurrent catching				✓	
Cold	redness, begins with	✓				
Coryza	greenish		✓			
Crust	dark, thick, green			✓		
Crust	formation of		✓			
Discharge	stopped feeling, amel. slightly		✓			
Discharges	acrid			✓		
Discharges	amel., slightest		✓			
Discharges	fish brine, odour of		✓			
Discharges	in cold, thin		✓			
Discharges	old cheese, like				✓	
Discharges	purulent		✓			
Discharges	sulphur, like				✓	
Discharges	thin	✓				
Discharges	watery	✓				
Discharges	yellow					Syco-tubercular
Dryness	sensation of	✓				
Epistaxis	bright red				✓	
Epistaxis	by, amel				✓	
Epistaxis	cold application, amel. by				✓	
Epistaxis	from fever				✓	
Epistaxis	from overexertion				✓	
Epistaxis	from trivial cause				✓	
Flat	appearance			✓		
Flushing	face, in				✓	
Growths	nostrils, in		✓			
Hay Fever	discharges, acrid			✓		
Hay Fever	discharges, blood-streaked				✓	
Hay Fever	discharges, watery	✓				
Hay Fever	hourly, stuffed alternating with clear nostrils				✓	
Hay Fever	periodical				✓	
Hay Fever	sneezing, with					Psora-tubercular
Hyposensitivity	to smell	✓				
Mucus Membrane	red	✓				
Nasal	agg. at night, symptoms			✓		
Nasal	agg. by warmth of bed, symptoms			✓		

Nose Symptoms	Rubric	Psora	Sycosis	Syphilis	Tubercular	Mixed Miasms
Nasal	agg. by damp, symptoms		✓			
Nasal	amel. by abnormal discharges, symptoms					Syco-syphilitic
Nasal	leading to mouth breathing, openings narrow				✓	
Nasal	narrow, openings				✓	
Nasal Septum	deviated		✓			
Nasal Turbinate	swelling of		✓			
Nose	agg. by damp, complaints		✓			
Nose	agg. by cold, complaints	✓				
Nose	agg. by sleep, complaints	✓				
Nose	agg. in closed room, complaints				✓	
Nose	agg. in morning, complaints	✓				
Nose	amel. by abnormal discharges, complaints		✓			
Nose	amel. by nose bleed, complaints				✓	
Nose	amel. by open air, complaints				✓	
Nose	amel. by warmth, complaints	✓				
Nose	amel. by natural discharges, complaints	✓				
Nose	during fever, bleeding				✓	
Nose	from destruction of nasal septum, flat appearance			✓		
Nose	slightest cause, bleeding from				✓	
Nostril	in, growths		✓			
Nostril	leads to mouth breathing, stoppage of one	✓				
Nostril	small				✓	
Nostril	ulceration of			✓		
Odour	disturb sleep	✓				
Odour	fainting, cause	✓				
Odour	headaches, cause	✓				
Odour	nausea, cause	✓				
Odour	tolerate, cannot	✓				
Polyps						Mixed miasmatic
Post Nasal	drip				✓	
Recurrent	cold, catching of				✓	
Redness	mucus membrane, of	✓				
Rhinitis			✓			
Septum	burning	✓				
Septum	destroyed			✓		
Septum	dirty appearance	✓				
Septum	dry	✓				
Septum	dry, hot	✓				
Sinusitis			✓			
Sleep	cold symptoms, agg. by	✓				
Smell	diminished, sense of			✓		
Smell	due to increased sensitivity, heightened sense of	✓				
Smell	lost, sense of					Psora-syco-syphilitic
Smell	weak, sense of	✓				
Sneezing			✓			
Sneezing	cold, with	✓				
Snuffles	haemorrhage, with				✓	
Snuffles	moist		✓			
Snuffles	periodical				✓	
Ulcerated	nose			✓		
Warmth	nasal symptoms, amel. by	✓				
Watery	coryza		✓			

MIASMATIC DIAGNOSIS: MIASMATIC REPERTORY OF MOUTH SYMPTOMS

Mouth Symptoms	Rubric	Psora	Sycosis	Syphilis	Tubercular	Mixed Miasms
Aromatic Food	aversion to	✓				
Burnt	taste	✓				
Calculi	salivary ducts, in		✓			
Caries	teeth, in			✓		
Decayed	teeth			✓		
Dental	imperfect, arch				✓	
Eat	strong tasting food, does not like to	✓				
Eructation	of fat	✓				
Eructation	recently, of food eaten	✓				
Foetor Oris						Psora-syphilo-tubercular
Gum	with pus, boils					Syco-syphilitic
Gums	oozing blood					Syphilo-tubercular
Gums	soft					Syphilo-tubercular
Haematemesis					✓	
Leucoplakia			✓			
Leucoplakia	fungal infection, with			✓		
Lips	burning	✓				
Odour	mouth, from			✓		
Saliva	offensive			✓		
Saliva Duct	stones of		✓			
Salivation	hawking with				✓	
Salivation	increased					Psora–sycotic
Salivation	into long threads, can be drawn			✓		
Salivation	ropy			✓		
Stomatitis		✓				
Tartar	easily lodged	✓				
Taste	bitter	✓				
Taste	blood, of				✓	
Taste	burnt, of food as if	✓				
Taste	coppery, metallic			✓		
Taste	eggs, of rotten				✓	
Taste	fishy		✓			
Taste	food rejected due to abnormal	✓				
Taste	in morning, of blood				✓	
Taste	in open air, bitter	✓				
Taste	lost, sense of					Mixed miasmatic
Taste	of pus				✓	
Taste	perverted			✓		
Taste	salty				✓	
Taste	sour	✓				
Taste	sweetish				✓	
Taste	unpleasant			✓		
Teeth	bleeding				✓	
Teeth	cresentric, crowns			✓		
Teeth	deformed			✓		
Teeth	irregular					Syphilo-tubercular
Teeth	loose			✓		
Teeth	painful				✓	
Teething	with catching cold, painful					Syphilo-tubercular
Teething	with convulsions, painful					Syphilo-tubercular
Teething	with diarrhoea, painful					Syphilo-sycotic
Thrush						Psora-syphilitic
Tongue	burning	✓				
Tongue	dry	✓				

Mouth Symptoms	Rubric	Psora	Sycosis	Syphilis	Tubercular	Mixed Miasms
Tongue	moist			✓		
Tongue	teeth on, imprints of	✓				
Tongue	white coating				✓	
Tongue	yellowish coating		✓			
Tumours			✓			
Ulcers	mouth, in					Syphilo-tubercular
Warts			✓			

MIASMATIC DIAGNOSIS: MIASMATIC REPERTORY OF FACIAL SYMPTOMS

Facial Symptoms	Rubric	Psora	Sycosis	Syphilis	Tubercular	Mixed Miasms
Acne	hard			✓		
Acne	recurrent				✓	
Acne	simple	✓				
Anaemic	appearance	✓				
Appearance	dull			✓		
Beard	broken, hair			✓		
Beard	stubby			✓		
Bloated	appearance				✓	
Bloated	after sleep, appearance				✓	
Cheek	during dentition, red spots				✓	
Cheek	flushed				✓	
Cheek	high, bones			✓		
Cheek	with worms, red spots				✓	
Cheeks	on, red spots				✓	
Cheeks	one cold, one hot				✓	
Chin	during evening, flushed				✓	
Complexion	smooth				✓	
Congestion	venous					Psora-sycotic
Cool	to touch			✓		
Cyanotic	blue appearance	✓				
Cyst	dermoid		✓			
Dry		✓				
Dry	unwashed appearance	✓				
Erysipelas						Mixed miasmatic
Eyelashes	broken			✓		
Eyelashes	glossy				✓	
Eyelashes	irregularly curved			✓		
Eyelashes	soft				✓	
Eyelashes	stubby			✓		
Eyelids	crusty			✓		
Eyelids	inflamed, red					Psora–tubercular
Eyelids	scaly					Syphilo-sycotic
Eyes	around, blue ring					Tuberculo-psoric
Eyes	bright				✓	
Eyes	sunken					Psora–tubercular
Face	after rising, pale					Psora–tubercular
Face	bloated, after sleep					Syco-tubercular
Face	bluish					Syco-tubercular
Face	dropsical		✓			
Face	dull, morose			✓		
Face	greasy			✓		
Face	greyish			✓		
Face	inverted inwards, shape	✓				
Face	old looking			✓		
Face	pale	✓				
Face	puffy		✓			
Face	pyramidal, inverted appearance				✓	
Face	round				✓	
Face	shallow		✓			
Face	swollen		✓			
Face	yellowish		✓			
Features	sharp				✓	
Flushes	to head and chest, of heat				✓	
Greasy	appearance			✓		

Facial Symptoms	Rubric	Psora	Sycosis	Syphilis	Tubercular	Mixed Miasms
Hot flush	before menses, in face					Psora-sycotic
Hot flush	during climacteric, in face					Psora-sycotic
Hot flush	periodical					Psora–tubercular
Lips	burning, itching				✓	
Lips	fissured					Syphilo-tubercular
Lips	flushed				✓	
Lips	red				✓	
Lips	swollen		✓			
Lips	thick					Syco-syphilitic
Lips	vesicles, itching					Syco-psoric
Nose	flat			✓		
Pale	appearance	✓				
Perspiration	droplets of water, with			✓		
Perspiration	excessive		✓			
Perspiration	fishy odour, with		✓			
Perspiration	none	✓				
Pyramid	shape, inverted				✓	
Rough	skin					Psora-syphilitic
Smooth	of skin, appearance				✓	
Sunken	with blue rings, eyes					Psora-tubercular
Swollen	appearance		✓			
Unwashed	appearance	✓				
Voice	coarse			✓		
Voice	deep			✓		
Voice	hollow			✓		
Warts	on face		✓			

MIASMATIC DIAGNOSIS: MIASMATIC REPERTORY OF RESPIRATORY SYMPTOMS

Respiratory Symptoms	Rubric	Psora	Sycosis	Syphilis	Tubercular	Mixed Miasms
Abscess	lung, in			✓		
Anoxaemia		✓				
Anoxia		✓				
Anxiety	all respiratory complaints, with	✓				
Asthma	abdomen, amel. lying on		✓			
Asthma	agg. early morning		✓			
Asthma	expectoration, with profuse		✓			
Asthma	move, compelled to		✓			
Band	round the chest, sensation	✓				
Bronchioles	dilated		✓			
Bronchitis						Psora-tubercular
Burning	in chest	✓				
Chest	alternate with headache, complaints				✓	
Chest	barrel like				✓	
Chest	complaints, depressions with			✓		
Chest	expand fully, cannot				✓	
Chest	hopeful during, complaints				✓	
Chest	narrow				✓	
Chest	pigeon-like				✓	
Chilled	being, fear of				✓	
Cold	agg.				✓	
Colds	from cold, agg.	✓				
Colds	from warmth, amel.	✓				
Colds	in winter, agg.	✓				
Colds	natural discharges, amel. by	✓				
Cough	barking		✓			
Cough	deep, prolonged				✓	
Cough	expectoration, without				✓	
Cough	hollow				✓	
Cough	in evening, agg. by lying down				✓	
Cough	in morning, agg.				✓	
Cough	paroxysmal			✓		
Cough	teasing				✓	
Cough	teasing, dry					Psora-tubercular
Cough	tight				✓	
Covering Up	warmth amel.				✓	
Depressions	in chest, irregular			✓		
Discharges	natural, amel. by	✓				
Dry	cough, spasmodic	✓				
Dryness	throat, of	✓				
Dyspnoea	bed, before going		✓			
Dyspnoea	down, on lying		✓			
Dyspnoea	painful		✓			
Dyspnoea	passing stool, amel. by	✓				
Dyspnoea	stairs, on ascending		✓			
Emphysema			✓			
Exhaustion					✓	
Expansion	cannot be fully achieved, of lung				✓	
Expectoration	bloody				✓	
Expectoration	clear	✓				
Expectoration	difficult				✓	
Expectoration	float, does not				✓	
Expectoration	musty				✓	
Expectoration	offensive			✓		

Respiratory Symptoms	Rubric	Psora	Sycosis	Syphilis	Tubercular	Mixed Miasms
Expectoration	pus-like				✓	
Expectoration	salty				✓	
Expectoration	scanty	✓				
Expectoration	sticky				✓	
Expectoration	sweet				✓	
Expectoration	tasteless					Psora-syphilitic
Expectoration	thread-like			✓		
Expectoration	yellow-greenish			✓		
Fear	cold, of catching				✓	
Fear	in cold air, of breathing	✓				
Fibrosis	lung, of		✓			
Haemoptysis					✓	
Headache	chest complaints, alternates with				✓	
Headache	cough, induced by				✓	
Hoarseness	before menses, agg.			✓		
Hopeful	advanced condition, in				✓	
Humidity	all respiratory symptoms, agg.		✓			
Hypertrophy	nasal turbinate, of		✓			
Hypoxia	birth, at	✓				
Inhalation	incomplete				✓	
Lung	abscess			✓		
Lung	fibrosis		✓			
Lung	than the other, one larger				✓	
Milk	agg.				✓	
Mucus	in throat, tickling				✓	
Nasal	blockage		✓			
Night	respiratory symptoms, agg.					Syphilo-tubercular
Nodules	vocal chords, on		✓			
Oedematous	nose		✓			
Oedematous	tonsils		✓			
Oedematous	uvula		✓			
Pains	pressure, amel. by		✓			
Pharyngitis						Psora-tubercular
Phlegm	of, accumulation	✓				
Pleurisy					✓	
Pneumonia	consolidation of lung, with		✓			
Pulmonary Tuberculosis					✓	
Quinsy						Syphilo-tubercular
Rain	all respiratory symptoms, agg.		✓			
Rawness	throat, in			✓		
Recurrent	cough and cold				✓	
Respiration	accelerated		✓			
Respiration	laboured				✓	
Respiration	painful				✓	
Respiration	poor				✓	
Respiration	weakness, with				✓	
Respiratory	by cold and in winter, complaints agg.	✓				
Respiratory	by warmth, complaints amel	✓				
Respiratory	in morning, symptoms agg.	✓				
Restless	to move, compelled		✓			
Season	agg., changes in		✓			
Sensation	amel. by pressure, stitching		✓			
Sensation	band-like	✓				
Sensation	stitching			✓		
Sensitive	to catch cold, nose and throat	✓				
Shallow	respiration	✓				
Shoulders	rounded				✓	
Slow	respiration	✓				
Soreness	throat, in			✓		
Stitching	pain		✓			

Respiratory Symptoms	Rubric	Psora	Sycosis	Syphilis	Tubercular	Mixed Miasms
Swelling	with cough and cold, of glands				✓	
Swelling	with cough and cold, of tonsils				✓	
Tonsillitis	recurrent				✓	
Ulceration	respiratory system, in			✓		
Ulcerative	sore throat			✓		
Upper Respiratory	chest infections	✓				
Vocal Chord	nodules		✓			
Voice	husky					Psora-tubercular
Warm	amel., covering up				✓	
Winter	all respiratory symptoms, agg.	✓				

MIASMATIC DIAGNOSIS: MIASMATIC REPERTORY OF CARDIAC SYMPTOMS

Cardiac Symptoms	Rubric	Psora	Sycosis	Syphilis	Tubercular	Mixed Miasms
Anxiety	heart, felt in	✓				
Anxiety	in morning, agg.	✓				
Aortic	regurgitation		✓			
Band	sensation of	✓				
Blood	with weakness, rushes to chest					Psora-tubercular
Bradycardia		✓				
Breathing	at intervals, difficult and oppressed					Syco-tubercular
Breathing	on climbing stairs, difficult				✓	
Cardiac	change of position, symptoms amel. by			✓		
Cardiac	change of weather, symptoms agg. by		✓			
Cardiac	cold, symptoms amel. by			✓		
Cardiac	coughing, symptoms agg. by	✓				
Cardiac	daytime, symptoms amel. in			✓		
Cardiac	eating, symptoms agg. by	✓				
Cardiac	eructation, symptoms amel. by	✓				
Cardiac	evening, symptoms agg. in	✓				
Cardiac	extremes of temperature, symptoms agg. by			✓		
Cardiac	fainting, symptoms				✓	
Cardiac	from disappointment, symptoms	✓				
Cardiac	from excitement, symptoms	✓				
Cardiac	from fear, symptoms	✓				
Cardiac	from loss of friends, symptoms	✓				
Cardiac	heat, symptoms agg. by		✓			
Cardiac	high altitudes, symptoms agg. in				✓	
Cardiac	laughing, symptoms agg. by	✓				
Cardiac	lying down, symptoms amel. by					Psora-tubercular
Cardiac	movement, symptoms agg. by	✓				
Cardiac	night, symptoms agg. at					Syphilo-tubercular
Cardiac	of rheumatic complaints, symptoms from suppression	✓				
Cardiac	of rheumatic origin, agg. by motion, symptoms		✓			
Cardiac	open air, symptoms amel. in				✓	
Cardiac	perspiration, symptoms agg. by			✓		
Cardiac	pressure on chest, symptoms agg. by				✓	
Cardiac	rest, symptoms amel. by	✓				
Cardiac	sitting up, symptoms agg. on				✓	
Cardiac	sudden, failure			✓		
Cardiac	walking gentle, symptoms amel. by	✓				
Cardiac	warmth of bed, symptoms agg. by			✓		
Cardiac	with anxiety, symptoms	✓				
Cardiac	with depression, symptoms					Syphilo-psoric
Cardiac	with emotional, symptoms alternate				✓	
Cardiac	with fear of incurable disease, symptoms	✓				
Cardiac	with ringing in ears, symptoms				✓	
Cardiac	with sadness, symptoms	✓				
Cardiac	with weakness, symptoms				✓	
Circulation	of increased, sensation	✓				
Congenital	abnormalities, anomaly			✓		
Congenital	abnormalities, developmental					Syphilo-sycotic
Congenital	abnormalities, structural			✓		
Discharges	good prognosis, amel.		✓			
Dizzy	sitting up, on				✓	
Dropsical						Syco-psoric

Cardiac Symptoms	Rubric	Psora	Sycosis	Syphilis	Tubercular	Mixed Miasms
Dyspnoea	obesity, caused by		✓			
Dyspnoea	with blueness, painful					Psora-tubercular
Dyspnoea	with pain		✓			
Emaciation	persistent				✓	
Emotional	with cardiac symptoms, symptoms alternate				✓	
Empty	heart in, sensation	✓				
Endocarditis	bacterial, ulcerative			✓		
Faint	sitting up, on				✓	
Flabbiness	with prolonged cardiac problems		✓			
Flesh	falling away				✓	
Fluttering	in heart, sensation		✓			
Gout	of heart		✓			
Hammering	in heart, sensation	✓				
Heart	felt in, anxiety	✓				
Heart	so takes pulse, thinks, will stop	✓				
Heaviness	cannot explain, felt in heart				✓	
Heaviness	heart, felt in	✓				
Hypertrophy	heart, of		✓			
Mitral	regurgitation		✓			
Myocardial Infarctions			✓			
Obesity	causes dyspnoea		✓			
Oppression	morning, agg. in	✓				
Pain	agg. by arm movement, soreness in precordium		✓			
Pain	altitude, agg. at				✓	
Pain	at night, agg. by pressure on chest				✓	
Pain	coughing, agg. from	✓				
Pain	cutting	✓				
Pain	eating, agg. from	✓				
Pain	electric shock, like		✓			
Pain	eructation, amel. by	✓				
Pain	evening, agg. in	✓				
Pain	in precordium, agg. by movement, stitching					Syco-psoric
Pain	in precordium, stitching			✓		
Pain	laughing, agg. by	✓				
Pain	lying down, amel. by	✓				
Pain	movement, agg. by	✓				
Pain	neuralgic	✓				
Pain	open air, amel. in				✓	
Pain	piercing	✓				
Pain	precordium, soreness in		✓			
Pain	precordium to scapula		✓			
Pain	precordium to shoulder		✓			
Pain	rare, unless rheumatic		✓			
Pain	rest, amel. by	✓				
Pain	scapula to precordium		✓			
Pain	sharp	✓				
Pain	shoulder to precordium		✓			
Pain	sitting up, agg. by				✓	
Pain	comes suddenly, goes suddenly	✓				
Palpitations	of body, with violent shaking					Syco-tubercular
Palpitations	to head, rush of blood					Tuberculo-syphilitic
Palpitations	with red face, rush blood				✓	
Preoccupation	heart's condition, with	✓				
Pulse	bounding, full	✓				
Pulse	but feeble, rapid				✓	
Pulse	but rapid, feeble				✓	
Pulse	irregular			✓		
Pulse	soft	✓				
Pulse	tension, lacks		✓			

Cardiac Symptoms	Rubric	Psora	Sycosis	Syphilis	Tubercular	Mixed Miasms
Pulse	thread-like				✓	
Rheumatic	heart		✓			
Rush	to chest, of blood				✓	
Sensation	band, of	✓				
Sensation	fullness, of	✓				
Sensation	goneness, of	✓				
Sensation	in precordium, of heaviness				✓	
Sensation	soreness, of	✓				
Sensation	weakness, of	✓				
Tachycardia			✓			
Thrombosis						Syco-tubercular
Ulcerative	bacterial endocarditis			✓		
Uncomfortable	sensations	✓				
Valves	dilatation of		✓			
Valvular	degeneration			✓		
Valvular	disturbance		✓			

MIASMATIC DIAGNOSIS: MIASMATIC REPERTORY OF STOMACH SYMPTOMS

Stomach Symptoms	Rubric	Psora	Sycosis	Syphilis	Tubercular	Mixed Miasms
Acidity		✓				
Aggravation	eating, after	✓				
Aggravation	fat, from		✓			
Aggravation	green leafy vegetables, from		✓			
Aggravation	juicy fruit, from		✓			
Aggravation	meat, from		✓			
Aggravation	onion, from		✓			
Aggravation	protein, after eating	✓				
Alcohol	abuse of			✓		
Allergy	foods, to various				✓	
Amelioration	abdomen, lying on		✓			
Amelioration	belching, from	✓				
Amelioration	gentle motion, by	✓				
Amelioration	hot drinks, from					Psora–sycotic
Amelioration	violent motion, by		✓			
Amelioration	walking, by		✓			
Appetite	poor	✓				
Aversion	animal food, to				✓	
Aversion	boiled food, to	✓				
Aversion	cold food, to	✓				
Aversion	during fevers, to sweets	✓				
Aversion	green leafy vegetables, to		✓			
Aversion	juicy fruits, to		✓			
Aversion	meat, to					Syco-syphilitic
Aversion	meat and milk, to		✓			
Aversion	milk, to					Psora-sycotic
Aversion	onion, to		✓			
Bilious		✓				
Bilious	gentle motion, amel. by	✓				
Bilious	hot food and drinks, amel. from	✓				
Bilious	rest, amel. by	✓				
Bilious	sleep, amel. by	✓				
Burning		✓				
Colic	of three months, in baby		✓			
Colic	restlessness, with		✓			
Colic	twist, with		✓			
Colic	vaccination, from		✓			
Colic	with knees drawn up, three month's baby		✓			
Constriction	eating, especially after	✓				
Crampy	pain		✓			
Craving	beer		✓			
Craving	but refuses when offered esp. in children, for certain foods	✓				
Craving	coffee	✓				
Craving	cold food			✓		
Craving	cold or hot food		✓			
Craving	in fever, for acid	✓				
Craving	meat				✓	
Craving	meats and greasy food, but these do not suit them, highly seasoned foods	✓				
Craving	peculiar things				✓	
Craving	potatoes				✓	
Craving	pungent and salty foods, for alcohol, table salt		✓			

Stomach Symptoms	Rubric	Psora	Sycosis	Syphilis	Tubercular	Mixed Miasms
Craving	refuses, then					Psora-tubercular
Craving	salt				✓	
Craving	stimulants	✓				
Craving	tea	✓				
Craving	then vomits bile, sweet	✓				
Craving	to supply the nerve force, for tea, coffee, tobacco	✓				
Craving	tobacco				✓	
Craving	which makes them sick, for food				✓	
Degenerative	ulcers			✓		
Depression	stomach problems, with			✓		
Desire	acid	✓				
Desire	alcohol					Syco-syphilo-tubercular
Desire	and greasy foods, for salty				✓	
Desire	and hot foods, for sweet	✓				
Desire	and tobacco, for tea, coffee			✓		
Desire	and wine, for sour, sweet, chalk, lime, pencil				✓	
Desire	aromatic food				✓	
Desire	beer		✓			
Desire	betel-nut etc., for coconut		✓			
Desire	but cannot assimilate, for milk				✓	
Desire	coconut		✓			
Desire	coffee					Psora-syphilitic
Desire	cold, drinks			✓		
Desire	cold, food					Syco-tubercular or syphilitic
Desire	fat					Psora-tubercular
Desire	food, icy cold				✓	
Desire	gravy		✓			
Desire	hot food, piping				✓	
Desire	indigestible things, for				✓	
Desire	meat				✓	
Desire	meat, fat, seasoned	✓				
Desire	meat, for very spicy			✓		
Desire	meat, ghee, oily and fried foods, for spicy foods	✓				
Desire	oily things					Psora-tubercular
Desire	pastry	✓				
Desire	pickles	✓				
Desire	potatoes				✓	
Desire	pungent		✓			
Desire	salt/salty					Syco-tubercular
Desire	seasoned food		✓			
Desire	sour					Psora-syphilitic
Desire	spicy	✓				
Desire	spicy things, hot					Psora-tubercular
Desire	stimulants			✓		
Desire	sweet	✓				
Desire	tea					Syphilo-tubercular
Desire	tobacco					Syphilo-tubercular
Desire	warm food		✓			
Desire	which agg. the condition, for food				✓	
Desire	which disagrees, food				✓	
Desire	wine			✓		
Discomfort	eating, after		✓			
Distention		✓				
Distention	gas, from	✓				
Dullness	with, stomach complaints			✓		
Dyspepsia		✓				
Eating	few hours after, agg	✓				

Stomach Symptoms	Rubric	Psora	Sycosis	Syphilis	Tubercular	Mixed Miasms
Eating	follows, headache	✓				
Eating	follows, sleepiness	✓				
Eating	follows, weariness	✓				
Empty	feeling	✓				
Empty	in morning, feeling	✓				
Eructation	bitter	✓				
Eructation	colic, with		✓			
Eructation	loud		✓			
Eructation	sour	✓				
Faint	hunger, with					Psora-tubercular
Fat	by, agg.					Syco-tubercular
Fat	thrives on				✓	
Flatulent		✓				
Flushed	face				✓	
Fullness		✓				
Gastric	agg. at night, symptoms			✓		
Gastric	agg. from extremes of temperature, symptoms			✓		
Gastric	agg. from warmth, symptoms			✓		
Gastric	amel. by hot drinks, symptoms		✓			
Gastric	amel. by violent motion, symptoms		✓			
Gastric	amel. by walking, symptoms		✓			
Gastric	amel. dry weather, symptoms				✓	
Gastric	amel. from lying on abdomen, symptoms		✓			
Gastric	amel. in open air, symptoms				✓	
Gastric	with anxiety, symptoms	✓				
Gastric	with flushed face, symptoms				✓	
Gastric	with giddiness, symptoms	✓				
Gastric	with sweat, symptoms	✓				
Gastric	with vertigo, symptoms	✓				
Gastritis		✓				
Glands	mesenteric, intestinal, swelling				✓	
Gnawing	sensation of	✓				
Green Leafy	vegetables, agg. by		✓			
Haematemesis					✓	
Headache	eating, after	✓				
Heartburn		✓				
Hunger	10-11 a.m.	✓				
Hunger	after full meal, morbid	✓				
Hunger	capacity, eat beyond		✓			
Hunger	constant				✓	
Hunger	diarrhoea follows, eat beyond capacity	✓				
Hunger	in pregnancy, for unnatural things	✓				
Hunger	indigestible things, for	✓				
Hunger	night, at					Psora-syphilitic
Hunger	satisfied, easily	✓				
Hunger	unnatural things, for, such as chalk	✓				
Intestinal	swollen, glands				✓	
Intolerant	spices, to		✓			
Liver	pain	✓				
Melaena					✓	
Meat	but agg. from, desires		✓			
Mesenteric	swollen, glands				✓	
Milk	allergy				✓	
Milk	disagrees				✓	
Nausea	with, faint feeling	✓				
Oesophagitis		✓				
Oily	agg.				✓	
Onion	agg.		✓			
Pain	burning			✓		
Pain	bursting			✓		

Stomach Symptoms	Rubric	Psora	Sycosis	Syphilis	Tubercular	Mixed Miasms
Pain	colic		✓			
Pain	liver, in	✓				
Pain	tearing			✓		
Pain	throbbing	✓				
Pain	ulcerative			✓		
Polyps	gastric tract, of the		✓			
Pressure	endured, cannot be	✓				
Protein	by, agg.	✓				
Salt	thrives on				✓	
Sensation	after eating, beating	✓				
Sensation	after eating, of oppression	✓				
Sensation	after eating, of throbbing	✓				
Sensation	beating	✓				
Sensation	cold	✓				
Sensation	constriction	✓				
Sensation	distension	✓				
Sensation	eating after, of constriction	✓				
Sensation	fullness	✓				
Sensation	gnawing	✓				
Sensation	heaviness	✓				
Sensation	hot	✓				
Sensation	oppression	✓				
Sensation	stone-like	✓				
Sensation	throbbing	✓				
Sensation	weight	✓				
Sleepiness	after eating	✓				
Spinach	by, agg.		✓			
Starch	difficult, assimilation					Syphilo-tubercular
Stone	in stomach, like feeling	✓				
Touch	from, agg.	✓				
Tumours	gastric tract, of		✓			
Ulcers				✓		
Vomiting		✓				
Weariness	eating, after	✓				

MIASMATIC DIAGNOSIS: MIASMATIC REPERTORY OF ABDOMINAL SYMPTOMS

Abdominal Symptoms	Rubric	Psora	Sycosis	Syphilis	Tubercular	Mixed Miasms
Abdomen	at night, symptoms agg.			✓		
Abdomen	by cold, symptoms amel.			✓		
Abdomen	by warmth, symptoms agg.			✓		
Abdomen	felt through the abdominal wall, beating of aorta				✓	
Abdomen	in open air, symptoms amel.				✓	
Abdomen	involvement of, lymphatic				✓	
Abdomen	or as a large plate turned bottom side up, saucer shaped, inverted,				✓	
Acidity		✓				
Aggravation	fruit				✓	
Aggravation	greasy food				✓	
Aggravation	milk				✓	
Aggravation	oily food				✓	
Alcoholism	tendency to			✓		
Amelioration	in general, in open air				✓	
Appendicitis			✓			
Appendicular Colic			✓			
Ascites						Syco-psora-tubercular
Assimilate	starch, inability to				✓	
Assimilate	the nutritious substances of food, inability to	✓				
Bleeding	per rectum				✓	
Bloating	eating, after	✓				
Burning	sensation			✓		
Bursting	sensation			✓		
Cholecystitis		✓				
Cholelithiasis			✓			
Cirrhosis	liver, of					Syphilo-sycotic
Colic	appendicular		✓			
Colic	birth, from			✓		
Colic	food, from simple			✓		
Colic	in lower abdomen, abdominal					Syco-tubercular
Colitis		✓				
Constipation		✓				
Constriction	abdomen, felt in	✓				
Cramps	beans, from	✓				
Cramps	potatoes, from	✓				
Diarrhoea	brain symptoms, appear or disappear during				✓	
Diarrhoea	breakfast, after				✓	
Diarrhoea	due to taking food beyond capacity of digestion, of various types	✓				
Diarrhoea	during dentition, child frequently suffers				✓	
Diarrhoea	in general		✓			
Diarrhoea	or breakfast, after food				✓	
Diarrhoea	with crampy pain in lower abdomen, stools expelled in jet			✓		
Digest	starches, cannot easily				✓	
Discomfort	after eating			✓		
Discomfort	lying on abdomen, amel. by			✓		
Distention		✓				
Drunkard						Syphilo-sycotic
Duodenitis		✓				

Abdominal Symptoms	Rubric	Psora	Sycosis	Syphilis	Tubercular	Mixed Miasms
Dysentery				✓		
Dysentery	at night, agg.			✓		
Dysentery	perspiration, with			✓		
Dyspepsia		✓				
Eating	after agg.	✓				
Eating	bloating, agg. after	✓				
Empty	sensation	✓				
Extremists	or really cold things, likes hot				✓	
Feeling	and waterbrash, heartburn	✓				
Feeling	in the morning, empty	✓				
Flatulence	in abdomen, causes rumbling and gurgling				✓	
Flatulence	in lower abdomen				✓	
Flatulence	in lower abdomen, causes pain				✓	
Full	sensation	✓				
Glands	swollen, intestinal				✓	
Glands	swollen, mesenteric				✓	
Gurgling	abdomen, in	✓				
Gurgling	after eating, in abdomen	✓				
Heartburn		✓				
Heaviness	with distension of abdomen, occasional	✓				
Hernia						Psora-syco-tubercular
Hunger	esp. during fever and pregnancy, for indigestible things	✓				
Hunger	for unnatural things such as. chalk and clay, excessive	✓				
Hungry	a full meal, even after	✓				
Hungry	for a meal, cannot wait	✓				
Hungry	of digestion, they eat beyond their capacity	✓				
Intolerance	of spices		✓			
Liver	degeneration			✓		
Liver	fatty, degeneration			✓		
Liver Cells	degeneration of			✓		
Milk	agg. from				✓	
Muscles	laxation of				✓	
Nausea & Vomiting		✓				
Nausea	quiet and sleep, amel. by rest	✓				
Nausea	weakness after, before stool				✓	
Nausea	with vomiting at regular intervals, bilious	✓				
Pain	amel. by hard pressure, paroxysmal		✓			
Pain	and stomach, in liver	✓				
Pain	bends forwards, patient		✓			
Pain	bruised	✓				
Pain	compels to bend forward, abdominal		✓			
Pain	crampy		✓			
Pain	gentle pressure, amel. by	✓				
Pain	hard pressure, amel. by		✓			
Pain	hard pressure, crampy amel. by		✓			
Pain	heat, amel. by	✓				
Pain	on bending, stitching		✓			
Pain	paroxysms		✓			
Pain	pressive	✓				
Pain	pulsating		✓			
Pain	sore	✓				
Pain	stitching		✓			
Pain	wandering		✓			
Pain	which comes in paroxysms, crampy, colicky and spasmodic		✓			
Papilloma				✓		
Peristalsis	accelerated			✓		
Peristalsis	arrhythmic			✓		
Peristalsis	causing dysentery, arrhythmic			✓		

Abdominal Symptoms	Rubric	Psora	Sycosis	Syphilis	Tubercular	Mixed Miasms
Peristalsis	slow	✓				
Piles			✓			
Piles & Fistulas	alternate with heart disease				✓	
Prefers	with salt and pepper, fat meats, well-seasoned foods		✓			
Pressure	on abdomen, agg. from				✓	
Rumbling	abdomen, in	✓				
Rumbling	after eating, in abdomen	✓				
Sensation	burning			✓		
Sensation	bursting			✓		
Sensation	tearing			✓		
Spasm	dysenteric, perverted intestinal peristalsis leading to			✓		
Spasm	with profuse perspiration, in dysentery			✓		
Stool	blood, with :				✓	
Stool	of changeable character				✓	
Stool	with jelly-like mucus			✓		
Stool	with odour of rotten eggs, greasy and bloody					Tuberculo-syphilitic
Stool	with scrapings of mucus membrane			✓		
Swelling	of intestinal and mesenteric glands				✓	
Taste	musty or fishy		✓			
Tearing	sensation			✓		
Thrive	also require much salt, better on fats and fat foods				✓	
Touch	agg., on abdomen	✓				
Touch	cannot endure	✓				
Ulcer	duodenal				✓	
Umbilicus	fish brine odour, thin yellow/green discharge with		✓			
Umbilicus	protruding		✓			
Umbilicus	swollen		✓			
Umbilicus	with yellow discharge, ulceration				✓	
Worm	complaints				✓	

MIASMATIC DIAGNOSIS: MIASMATIC REPERTORY OF SEXUAL SYMPTOMS

Sexual Symptoms	Rubric	Psora	Sycosis	Syphilis	Tubercular	Mixed Miasms
Abortion	spontaneous			✓		
Abortion	spontaneous, recurrent					Syphilo-tubercular
Air	amel., open				✓	
Amenorrhoea		✓				
Anorexia	during menses, loss of appetite				✓	
Anxiety	menses, with	✓				
Auditory	during menses, hallucinations				✓	
Azoospermia				✓		
Backache	menses, during					Syco-tubercular
Bleeding	uterus, from				✓	
Burning	in womb, sensation			✓		
Cervical	dysplasia			✓		
Cervical	erosion			✓		
Climacteric	flushing					Syco-tubercular
Coition	due to polyps, painful				✓	
Coition	due to weakness, impossible			✓		
Cold	with menses, extremities				✓	
Conception	difficult					Psora-sycotic
Depression	leucorrhoea, with				✓	
Desire	lack of	✓				
Desire	unrestrained				✓	
Diarrhoea	menses, with					Syco-tubercular
Discharges	bland	✓				
Discharges	natural, amel.	✓				
Discharges	scanty	✓				
Dwells	in males, on sexual thoughts					Syco-psoric
Dwindling	testes	✓				
Dysfunctional	uterine bleeding				✓	
Dysmenorrhoea	colic		✓			
Dysmenorrhoea	exhaustive				✓	
Dysmenorrhoea	paroxysmal		✓			
Dysmenorrhoea	puberty, begins at	✓				
Dysmenorrhoea	sharp	✓				
Ectopic	pregnancy		✓			
Ejaculation	easy	✓				
Ejaculation	premature	✓				
Endometriosis			✓			
Endometrium	mottled appearance		✓			
Epistaxis	menses, with				✓	
Erection	but strong desire, absent			✓		
Erection	even with voluptuous dreams, weak	✓				
Erection	frequent					Syco-tubercular
Erection	insufficient	✓				
Erection	painful					Syphilo-tubercular
Erection	strong					Syco-tubercular
Erection	weak	✓				
Erosion	cervical			✓		
Erosion	vulva			✓		
Fainting	menses, with					Syphilo-tubercular
Fears	menses, with					Psora-tubercular
Fever	menses, with				✓	
Fibroids	uterus, of		✓			
Fibroma			✓			
Foetus	stillborn				✓	

Sexual Symptoms	Rubric	Psora	Sycosis	Syphilis	Tubercular	Mixed Miasms
Gloomy	menses, during			✓		
Haemospermia					✓	
Headache	menses, during				✓	
Hysterical	menses, after				✓	
Imbalance	hormones, of		✓			
Impotency	lack of desire, from	✓				
Infertility	failure to release ovum, from			✓		
Infertility	hormonal imbalance, from		✓			
Infertility	long lasting menses, from				✓	
Itching	pudenda	✓				
Itching	voluptuously, pudenda					Psora-sycotic
Labour	cannot nurse the child, exhausting				✓	
Labour	exhausting				✓	
Labour	long		✓			
Labour	painful		✓			
Leucorrhoea	acrid			✓		
Leucorrhoea	after menses, yellow				✓	
Leucorrhoea	amel.					Syco-syphilitic
Leucorrhoea	before and after menses, thick				✓	
Leucorrhoea	before menses, yellow				✓	
Leucorrhoea	bland	✓				
Leucorrhoea	depression, with			✓		
Leucorrhoea	dry cough, with				✓	
Leucorrhoea	faintness, with				✓	
Leucorrhoea	fish-brine, odour of		✓			
Leucorrhoea	greenish-yellow		✓			
Leucorrhoea	mental weakness, during		✓			
Leucorrhoea	mental weakness, from		✓			
Leucorrhoea	musty, odour				✓	
Leucorrhoea	offensive			✓		
Leucorrhoea	palpitation, with				✓	
Leucorrhoea	purulent				✓	
Leucorrhoea	putrid			✓		
Leucorrhoea	resulting vesicles, acrid and itching					Syco-syphilitic
Leucorrhoea	scanty	✓				
Leucorrhoea	starchy				✓	
Leucorrhoea	stringy			✓		
Leucorrhoea	thin		✓			
Leucorrhoea	vitality poor, with				✓	
Leucorrhoea	watery				✓	
Leucorrhoea	weakness excessive, with				✓	
Leucorrhoea	weakness, from				✓	
Libido	increased		✓			
Libido	lack of	✓				
Lochia	acrid			✓		
Lochia	biting		✓			
Lochia	burning			✓		
Lochia	clots					Psora-sycotic
Lochia	excoriating			✓		
Lochia	foetid					Psora-syphilitic
Lochia	offensive					Psora-syphilitic
Lochia	stains			✓		
Lochia	stringy			✓		
Lochia	yellowish		✓			
Mastodynia			✓			
Masturbation	excessive				✓	
Melancholia	menses, with			✓		
Menses	abundant				✓	
Menses	acrid			✓		
Menses	after, hysterical				✓	
Menses	anxiety, with					Psora-tubercular

221

Sexual Symptoms	Rubric	Psora	Sycosis	Syphilis	Tubercular	Mixed Miasms
Menses	backache, with					Syco-tubercular
Menses	before, feels unwell				✓	
Menses	bright red				✓	
Menses	burning			✓		
Menses	clots, many				✓	
Menses	copious				✓	
Menses	diarrhoea, with					Syco-tubercular
Menses	during puberty, slow and intermittent onset	✓				
Menses	during, depression			✓		
Menses	during, eyes sunken				✓	
Menses	during, fainting			✓		
Menses	during, fears					Psora-tubercular
Menses	during, gloomy			✓		
Menses	during, hallucinations				✓	
Menses	during, headache				✓	
Menses	during, nausea				✓	
Menses	during, bitter vomiting				✓	
Menses	during, weakness				✓	
Menses	epistaxis, with				✓	
Menses	exhaustive				✓	
Menses	fever, with				✓	
Menses	fish brine, odour of		✓			
Menses	foetid blood	✓				
Menses	frequent, too				✓	
Menses	from anaemia, scanty	✓				
Menses	in extremities, cold				✓	
Menses	irregular			✓		
Menses	long duration, infertility from				✓	
Menses	mental restlessness, with	✓				
Menses	pain, warmth amel.		✓			
Menses	painful		✓			
Menses	painful, colicky		✓			
Menses	painful, spasmodic		✓			
Menses	pale, appearance during	✓				
Menses	prolonged				✓	
Menses	sad, during	✓				
Menses	scanty	✓				
Menses	short	✓				
Menses	with flow, pain		✓			
Metastatic	of uterus, cancers				✓	
Mottled	of endometrium, appearance		✓			
Nausea	menses, during				✓	
Necrosis				✓		
Oligospermia		✓				
Ovarian	tumours		✓			
Ovary	polycystic		✓			
Ovum	ripen, failing to					Syco-syphilitic
Pallor	with menses, of face	✓				
Pelvis	inflammation, of		✓			
Polyps	bleeding, uterine				✓	
Polyps	bleeding, vaginal				✓	
Polyps	uterine					Psora-syco-tubercular
Polyps	vaginal					Psora-tubercular
Polyuria	menses, during		✓			
Pregnancy	during, craving for peculiar things	✓				
Pregnancy	ectopic		✓			
Prostatic	on urination, fluid	✓				
Prostatic	with straining at stool, fluid	✓				
Pruritus		✓				
Pruritus	meat, agg. by		✓			
Pruritus	sexual organs, in		✓			

Sexual Symptoms	Rubric	Psora	Sycosis	Syphilis	Tubercular	Mixed Miasms
Pruritus	vulvae		✓			
Restlessness	with menses, mental	✓				
Sad	menses, during	✓				
Scrotum	swelling of		✓			
Scrotum	with swelling, pain in		✓			
Semen	during micturition, discharge				✓	
Semen	during stool, discharge				✓	
Semen	nightly, discharge				✓	
Semen	without erection, discharge	✓				
Semen	without excitement, discharge	✓				
Sexual	at night, symptoms agg.					Syphilo-tubercular
Sexual	by change of weather, symptoms agg.		✓			
Sexual	by cold, symptoms agg.	✓				
Sexual	by humidity, symptoms agg.		✓			
Sexual	by menstrual discharges, symptoms amel.	✓				
Sexual	by rain, symptoms agg.		✓			
Sexual	by rest, symptoms agg.		✓			
Sexual	by unnatural discharges, symptoms amel.					Syco-syphilitic
Sexual	by warmth, symptoms agg.			✓		
Sexual	by warmth, symptoms amel.	✓				
Sexual	during summer, symptoms agg.			✓		
Sexual	in open air, symptoms amel.				✓	
Sterility						Psora-sycotic
Stillbirth					✓	
Testes	dwindling	✓				
Testes	of, disappearance	✓				
Testes	painful		✓			
Testes	swollen		✓			
Ulcerated	tumours			✓		
Uterine	dysfunctional, bleeding				✓	
Uterus	haemorrhage, profuse				✓	
Uterus	retroflexed		✓			
Uterus	retroverted		✓			
Uterus	with bleeding, retroflexed				✓	
Uterus	with bleeding, retroverted				✓	
Uterus	with infection, bleeding				✓	
Vagina	hypersensitive		✓			
Vagina	sore			✓		
Vertigo	menses, with				✓	
Violence	sexual			✓		
Visual	with menses, disturbances				✓	
Voluptuous	with prostatic fluid discharge, dreams	✓				
Vomiting	menses, during				✓	
Vulvae	ulceration			✓		
Warts	genital		✓			
Weakness	menses, during				✓	
Womb	burning sensation			✓		

MIASMATIC DIAGNOSIS: MIASMATIC REPERTORY OF URINARY SYMPTOMS

Urinary Symptoms	Rubric	Psora	Sycosis	Syphilis	Tubercular	Mixed Miasms
Acidic	urine	✓				
Air	amel., open				✓	
Albuminuria						Syco-tubercular
Anuria		✓				
Bladder	burning			✓		
Bladder	bursting			✓		
Bladder	constriction, sense of	✓				
Bladder	full, sense of	✓				
Bladder	in old people, sense of full	✓				
Bladder	papillomas of		✓			
Burning	urinary meatus, in	✓				
Burning	urine has contacted, of parts				✓	
Calculi	complications of		✓			
Calculi	renal			✓		
Cold	agg.	✓				
Colourless	urine				✓	
Constriction	sense of	✓				
Contraction	urethra, in		✓			
Cramps	micturition, during		✓			
Cystitis		✓				
Depression	kidney problems, with			✓		
Depression	prostrate problems, with			✓		
Diabetes Insipidus						Syco-tubercular
Diabetes Mellitus						Mixed miasmatic
Discharge	amel., natural	✓				
Dropsy	renal		✓			
Enuresis						Psora-tubercular
Enuresis	fear of school, with	✓				
Enuresis	from discomfort, wakes		✓			
Enuresis	habitual		✓			
Enuresis	in children, nocturnal					Psora-tubercular
Enuresis	in first sleep					Syco-tubercular
Flow	diminished					Syco-syphilitic
Full	in old people, sensation	✓				
Haematuria					✓	
Haematuria	in sleep				✓	
Involuntary	nocturnal				✓	
Irritation	where urine has contacted, in parts			✓		
Kidney	fibrous changes in					Psora-syphilitic
Melancholia	kidney problems, with			✓		
Melancholia	prostrate problems, with			✓		
Micturition	after fright, stops	✓				
Micturition	after tension, stops	✓				
Micturition	amel.	✓				
Micturition	anxiety, with				✓	
Micturition	becoming chilled, stops after	✓				
Micturition	before thunderstorm, frequent desire		✓			
Micturition	burning, with					Psora-syco-syphilitic
Micturition	frequent					Psora-sycotic
Micturition	infrequent		✓			
Micturition	involuntary	✓				
Micturition	irritation			✓		
Micturition	painful		✓			
Micturition	restlessness, with					Syco-tubercular

224

Urinary Symptoms	Rubric	Psora	Sycosis	Syphilis	Tubercular	Mixed Miasms
Micturition	smarting	✓				
Micturition	weakness follows				✓	
Nephroblastoma			✓			
Nephritis		✓				
Night	agg., symptoms				✓	
Oedema	nephrotic syndrome, with		✓			
Oliguria		✓				
Oliguria	from chill	✓				
Oliguria	from fright	✓				
Oliguria	from tension	✓				
Pain	pulsating			✓		
Pain	stitching			✓		
Pain	wandering			✓		
Phosphaturia	fever, after	✓				
Polyps	with bleeding, of bladder				✓	
Polyps	of bladder					Syco-tubercular
Polyuria	during rain		✓			
Polyuria	nocturnal				✓	
Profuse	urine					Syco-tubercular
Prostate	enlargement		✓			
Prostate	with bleeding, enlargement					Syco-tubercular
Prostatitis	fluid, with oozing of					Psora-sycotic
Prostatitis	from sexual over-indulgence		✓			
Pyaemia				✓		
Pyelitis		✓				
Renal	calculi		✓			
Renal	full moon, spasm agg.				✓	
Renal	new moon, spasm agg.				✓	
Renal	recurrent, spasm				✓	
Spasms	bladder, in		✓			
Spasms	urethra, in		✓			
Stress	from coughing, incontinence	✓				
Stress	from laughing, incontinence	✓				
Stress	from sneezing, incontinence	✓				
Stress	incontinence	✓				
Thunderstorm	before, desire to urinate increases		✓			
Tickling	in urethra, sensation				✓	
Tumours	malignant, of kidney					Syco-syphilitic
Urethra	stricture of			✓		
Urethritis		✓				
Urinary	agg. damp weather, symptoms		✓			
Urinary	anxiety, symptoms with	✓				
Urinary	apprehension, symptoms with	✓				
Urinary	at night, symptoms agg.				✓	
Urinary	cramps		✓			
Urinary	fear of incurable disease, symptoms with	✓				
Urinary	by change of weather, symptoms agg.		✓			
Urinary	by cold, symptoms agg.	✓				
Urinary	by damp, symptoms agg.		✓			
Urinary	by rain, symptoms agg.		✓			
Urinary	by warmth, symptoms agg.			✓		
Urinary	in open air, symptoms amel.				✓	
Urinary	in summer, symptoms agg.			✓		
Urine	acid	✓				
Urine	brownish	✓				
Urine	colourless				✓	
Urine	copious				✓	
Urine	dark	✓				
Urine	deposits, white	✓				
Urine	deposits, yellow/white	✓				
Urine	in, pus			✓		

Urinary Symptoms	Rubric	Psora	Sycosis	Syphilis	Tubercular	Mixed Miasms
Urine	odour, carrion-like				✓	
Urine	odour, fish brine		✓			
Urine	odour, fishy		✓			
Urine	odour, musty				✓	
Urine	odour, putrid				✓	
Urine	pale				✓	
Urine	passes, frequently					Psora-sycotic
Urine	phosphates, with				✓	
Urine	profuse				✓	
Urine	protein, with				✓	
Urine	pus, with			✓		
Urine	red					Syphilo-tubercular
Urine	scanty	✓				
Urine	sugar, with				✓	
Urine	yellowish					Psora-sycotic
White	after fever, deposit in urine	✓				
White/yellow	after fever, deposit in urine	✓				

MIASMATIC DIAGNOSIS: MIASMATIC REPERTORY OF RECTAL SYMPTOMS

Rectal Symptoms	Rubric	Psora	Sycosis	Syphilis	Tubercular	Mixed Miasms
Black	stool		✓			
Bleeding	rectum, from				✓	
Bruised	sensation	✓				
Burning	in rectum, sensation			✓		
Bursting	in rectum, sensation			✓		
Cancer	of rectum					Syco-tubercular
Colic	restlessness, with		✓			
Congestion	heat and flushing, with				✓	
Congestion	portal area, of				✓	
Constipation		✓				
Constipation	coated tongue, with	✓				
Constipation	diarrhoea, alternates with				✓	
Constipation	drowsiness, with	✓				
Constipation	fetor oris, with	✓				
Constipation	headache, with				✓	
Constipation	heaviness, with	✓				
Constipation	loss of appetite, with	✓				
Constipation	nausea, with	✓				
Constipation	no desire to work, with	✓				
Constipation	obstinate					Psora-tubercular
Constipation	pain in other areas, with	✓				
Constipation	prolonged			✓		
Constipation	prolonged, headache, with			✓		
Constipation	sleepiness, with	✓				
Crampy	pain		✓			
Diarrhoea			✓			
Diarrhoea	acrid		✓			
Diarrhoea	after taking cold things, painless offensive	✓				
Diarrhoea	agg. night			✓		
Diarrhoea	alternates with, constipation				✓	
Diarrhoea	amel. by rocking, with colic		✓			
Diarrhoea	anticipatory tension, from	✓				
Diarrhoea	bad news, from	✓				
Diarrhoea	by change of weather, agg.		✓			
Diarrhoea	by cold, agg.					Syco-tubercular
Diarrhoea	by eating fruit, agg.					Syco-tubercular
Diarrhoea	by getting wet, agg.		✓			
Diarrhoea	by hot food, amel.	✓				
Diarrhoea	by meat, agg.				✓	
Diarrhoea	by milk, agg.				✓	
Diarrhoea	by oily food, agg.				✓	
Diarrhoea	by potatoes, agg.				✓	
Diarrhoea	by pressure, amel.					Psora-sycotic
Diarrhoea	by teething, agg.				✓	
Diarrhoea	by warm drinks, amel.	✓				
Diarrhoea	by warmth in abdomen, amel.					Psora-sycotic
Diarrhoea	by warmth, amel.					Psora-sycotic
Diarrhoea	cold debilitating perspiration, with				✓	
Diarrhoea	cold, from				✓	
Diarrhoea	cold food, from	✓				
Diarrhoea	corrosive		✓			
Diarrhoea	dentition, during					Syphilo-tubercular
Diarrhoea	desires to be carried, with colic in children		✓			
Diarrhoea	expulsive		✓			

Rectal Symptoms	Rubric	Psora	Sycosis	Syphilis	Tubercular	Mixed Miasms
Diarrhoea	fish brine odour, of		✓			
Diarrhoea	fright, from	✓				
Diarrhoea	getting wet, from		✓			
Diarrhoea	gluttony, from	✓				
Diarrhoea	green		✓			
Diarrhoea	gushes		✓			
Diarrhoea	insecure feeling in rectum, with		✓			
Diarrhoea	milk, from				✓	
Diarrhoea	morning, in					Psora-tubercular
Diarrhoea	painful		✓			
Diarrhoea	painless, from fright	✓				
Diarrhoea	restlessness, with		✓			
Diarrhoea	seaside, at				✓	
Diarrhoea	sour		✓			
Diarrhoea	warm perspiration, with				✓	
Diarrhoea	weakness, follows	✓				
Diarrhoea	with colic, agg. at night					Syco-syphilitic
Diarrhoea	with crying, painful		✓			
Dysentery				✓		
Fissures	foetid discharge, with			✓		
Fissures	putridity, with			✓		
Fistulas	anal					Syphilo-tubercular
Gurgling	abdomen, in	✓				
Haemorrhoids	bleeding				✓	
Haemorrhoids	blind		✓			
Haemorrhoids	itching, with					Psora-sycotic
Haemorrhoids	leads to asthma, suppression				✓	
Haemorrhoids	leads to heart problems, suppression				✓	
Haemorrhoids	painful		✓			
Haemorrhoids	sensitive					Psora-sycotic
Ineffectual	for several days, desire for stool	✓				
Ineffectual	for stool, desire	✓				
Insecurity	feeling of		✓			
Intestine	of, scrapings				✓	
Irritable Bowel Syndrome	with abundance of blood				✓	
Irritable Bowel Syndrome	with abundance of pus			✓		
Itching	haemorrhoids					Psora-sycotic
Lienteria				✓		
Mucus	jelly-like				✓	
Obstipation						Psora-tubercular
Odour	coming from anus, fish-like		✓			
Pain	bruised	✓				
Pain	crampy		✓			
Pain	pressive	✓				
Pain	pulsating		✓			
Pain	sore	✓				
Pain	stitching		✓			
Pain	throbbing in abdomen, with	✓				
Pain	with pulsation of rectum, stitching		✓			
Polyps	bleeding				✓	
Prolapse	rectum, of					Psora-sycotic
Pruritis	from diarrhoea, in rectum					Psora-sycotic
Pyogenic	inflammation				✓	
Rectal	amel. by warm drinks, symptoms	✓				
Rectal	amel. by warm food, symptoms	✓				
Rectal	amel. by warmth, symptoms	✓				
Rectal	amel. pressure by, symptoms	✓				
Rectal	asthma, diseases alternating with				✓	
Rectal	chest diseases, symptoms alternating with				✓	

Rectal Symptoms	Rubric	Psora	Sycosis	Syphilis	Tubercular	Mixed Miasms
Rectal	heart diseases, symptoms alternating with				✓	
Rectal	lung diseases, symptoms alternating with				✓	
Rectal	with depression, symptoms			✓		
Rectal	with melancholy, symptoms			✓		
Rumbling	abdomen, in	✓				
Sore	rectum, in	✓				
Stitching	with pulsation of rectum, pains		✓			
Stool	absent, desire	✓				
Stool	acrid			✓		
Stool	afterwards, likes to be alone					Syphilo-tubercular
Stool	ash colour				✓	
Stool	before, nausea				✓	
Stool	black			✓		
Stool	bloody				✓	
Stool	by eating cold food, agg.					Psora-tubercular
Stool	by excessive eating, agg.					Syco-tubercular
Stool	by exposure to cold, agg.				✓	
Stool	changeable				✓	
Stool	colic, with		✓			
Stool	curd, like				✓	
Stool	desire, ineffectual	✓				
Stool	ejects forcefully		✓			
Stool	green		✓			
Stool	green, bloody				✓	
Stool	gushes		✓			
Stool	hard	✓				
Stool	mucus, with		✓			
Stool	odour, mouldy				✓	
Stool	odour, musty				✓	
Stool	offensive					Psora-syphilo-tubercular
Stool	painless				✓	
Stool	polychromatic					Syco-tubercular
Stool	rotten eggs, odour of				✓	
Stool	scrapings of intestine, with			✓		
Stool	slimy					Syco-syphilitic
Stool	sour		✓			
Stool	sticky		✓			
Stool	undigested food, contains	✓				
Stool	watery					Psora-sycotic
Stool	weakness after				✓	
Stool	yellowish			✓		
Weakness	diarrhoea, from					Psora-syphilitic
Worms						Psora-tubercular
Worms	irritation, with					Psora-tubercular
Worms	nose and rectum, with itching in					Psora-tubercular
Worms	pin				✓	
Worms	recurrent infestation				✓	
Worms	thread					Psora-tubercular
Worms	various types				✓	

MIASMATIC DIAGNOSIS: MIASMATIC REPERTORY OF SKIN SYMPTOMS

Skin Symptoms	Rubric	Psora	Sycosis	Syphilis	Tubercular	Mixed Miasms
Abscess	surgery line, in			✓		
Acne	menses, with		✓			
Acne	painful		✓			
Allergy	skin, manifested on				✓	
Angry	of skin eruptions, appearance				✓	
Angry	with oozing of blood, appearance of skin eruptions					Syphilo-tubercular
Anxiety	suppressed skin eruptions, from	✓				
Apprehension	suppressed skin eruptions, from	✓				
Beard	skin eruptions, falls from			✓		
Bedsores				✓		
Boils					✓	
Boils	heal slowly			✓		
Boils	in healing, difficulty				✓	
Boils	offensive discharge, with			✓		
Boils	painful	✓				
Boils	pus, with profuse					Syphilo-tubercular
Boils	recurrent				✓	
Boils	scurfy scales, shedding	✓				
Boils	sensitive	✓				
Boils	small	✓				
Boils	spread, which			✓		
Broken	beard		✓			
Burning	sensation				✓	
Capillaries	web-like, spider		✓			
Cauliflower	warts, like		✓			
Condylomatas			✓			
Copper	colour of eruption			✓		
Corns			✓			
Cracks						Psora-syphilitic
Cracks	feet, of					Psora-syphilitic
Cracks	hands, of					Psora-syphilitic
Crusts	fine	✓				
Crusts	heavy			✓		
Crusts	light	✓				
Crusts	small	✓				
Crusts	thick		✓			
Cysts			✓			
Dandruff		✓				
Depigmentation				✓		
Dirty	of skin, appearance	✓				
Discharges	bland	✓				
Discharges	offensive			✓		
Discharges	scanty	✓				
Dry	of skin, appearance	✓				
Dry	scales	✓				
Ecchymosis					✓	
Eczema		✓				
Eczema	exfoliating			✓		
Eczema	pus, with			✓		
Eruption	flat			✓		
Eruption	pale				✓	
Eruption	to heal, slow			✓		
Eruption	vesicular			✓		

Skin Symptoms	Rubric	Psora	Sycosis	Syphilis	Tubercular	Mixed Miasms
Eruptions	circumscribed, spots in		✓			
Eruptions	coloured copper			✓		
Eruptions	dry	✓				
Eruptions	fingers, around				✓	
Eruptions	flexures, in			✓		
Eruptions	groupings, in circular		✓			
Eruptions	hair falls out of beard, due to		✓			
Eruptions	heal, slow to					Psora-syphilitic
Eruptions	mouth, around				✓	
Eruptions	patchy		✓			
Eruptions	raw ham, like			✓		
Eruptions	rings, in		✓			
Eruptions	Scaly, thick scales		✓			
Eruptions	spots, in circumscribed		✓			
Eruptions	vesicular		✓			
Erysipelas			✓			
Fear	from suppressed skin eruptions, of incurable diseases	✓				
Fibroma			✓			
Fine	skin				✓	
Fissures				✓		
Freckles					✓	
Gangrene				✓		
Glandular	with skin eruptions, swellings				✓	
Growths	clearness of skin, abnormal				✓	
Haemangiomas					✓	
Harsh	appearance	✓				
Herpes						Syco-tubercular
Herpes Genitalis			✓			
Herpes Zoster			✓			
Herpes	recurrent					Syco-tubercular
Hives					✓	
Hyper-pigmentation			✓			
Itching	burning, with					Psora-syphilitic
Itching	by cold, agg.	✓				
Itching	exudation, without	✓				
Itching	in late evening, agg.	✓				
Itching	in winter, agg.	✓				
Itching	like sweat, amel. by natural discharges	✓				
Itching	pudenda	✓				
Itching	undressing, agg. by	✓				
Itching	voluptuous					Psora-sycotic
Itching	without pus	✓				
Keloids			✓			
Leprosy						Syphilo-tubercular
Lipoma			✓			
Localised	in rash, spots		✓			
Melanomas			✓			
Moles			✓			
Moles	hairy tufts, with			✓		
Moles	pinhead		✓			
Molluscum Contagiosum			✓			
Necrosis				✓		
Nettle Rash					✓	
Nose	red, tip				✓	
Offensive	discharges			✓		
Oily	skin		✓			
Painless	ulcerations				✓	
Papule		✓				
Parasites	itching, with	✓				

Skin Symptoms	Rubric	Psora	Sycosis	Syphilis	Tubercular	Mixed Miasms
Parasites	thickening of skin, with		✓			
Parasites	tickling, with	✓				
Parasites	ulceration, with			✓		
Parasites	with oozing of blood, with tickling				✓	
Patches	urine coloured				✓	
Patches	wine coloured		✓			
Perspiration	as a whole, agg.				✓	
Perspiration	offensive				✓	
Perspiration	results in lung symptoms, suppressed				✓	
Perspiration	sleep, during		✓			
Perspiration	thickly oozing		✓			
Petechial	haemorrhage				✓	
Pigment	disturbed, metabolism		✓			
Pigmentation	altered		✓			
Pigmentation	circles in		✓			
Pimples	dry	✓				
Pruritus		✓				
Pruritus	anus, in		✓			
Pruritus	by meat, agg.		✓			
Pruritus	nose, in		✓			
Pruritus	sexual organs, in		✓			
Pruritus	vulvae, in		✓			
Psoriasis						Mixed miasmatic
Purpura					✓	
Rawness				✓		
Red	capillaries					Tuberculo-sycotic
Red	skin, angry looking		✓			
Relief	of suppressed eruptions, from reappearance	✓				
Ringworm						Syco-tubercular
Ringworm	follows chronic bronchitis, suppression					Syco-tubercular
Ringworm	follows chronic headache, suppression		✓			
Ringworm	follows rheumatic disease, suppression		✓			
Ringworm	follows stomach disorders, suppression		✓			
Ringworm	suppression of				✓	
Rough	skin	✓				
Rough	to touch, skin	✓				
Scar	tumours		✓			
Scratching	temporarily relieves	✓				
Skin	agg. after itching, symptoms				✓	
Skin	agg. by meat, symptoms		✓			
Skin	agg. by milk, symptoms				✓	
Skin	agg. by oily foods, symptoms				✓	
Skin	agg. by touch, symptoms				✓	
Skin	agg. by undressing, symptoms				✓	
Skin	agg. by warmth, symptoms			✓		
Skin	agg. by warmth of bed, symptoms					Syphilo-tubercular
Skin	agg. by wet weather, symptoms		✓			
Skin	agg. in humid weather, symptoms		✓			
Skin	agg. in summer, symptoms			✓		
Skin	amel. by abnormal discharges, symptoms			✓		
Skin	amel. by pressure, symptoms		✓			
Skin	amel. in dry weather, symptoms					Syco-tubercular
Skin	amel. in open air, symptoms				✓	
Skin	angry appearance, symptoms				✓	
Skin	Barber's shop, symptoms contracted at		✓			
Skin	bluish				✓	
Skin	dry, symptoms	✓				
Skin	in localised spots, symptoms		✓			
Skin	look haemorrhagic, symptoms				✓	
Skin	obstinate, symptoms				✓	
Skin	pale, appearance				✓	

Skin Symptoms	Rubric	Psora	Sycosis	Syphilis	Tubercular	Mixed Miasms
Skin	recurrent, symptoms				✓	
Skin	smooth				✓	
Skin	tags		✓			
Skin	thickened		✓			
Skin	ulceration			✓		
Skin	with exhaustion, symptoms				✓	
Soreness				✓		
Spider's Web	of veins, appearance		✓			
Squamous				✓		
Stubby	beard		✓			
Suppression	results in depression, of skin disease			✓		
Suppression	results in a lack of enthusiasm, of skin disease					Syphilo-tubercular
Suppression	results in diseases of the nerve centres, of skin disease		✓			
Suppression	results in heart disease, of skin disease		✓			
Suppression	results in impaired intellect, of skin disease			✓		
Suppression	results in liver disease, of skin disease		✓			
Suppression	results in reproductive disorders, of skin disease		✓			
Suppression	results in ulcerative states, of skin disease				✓	
Suppuration	marked					Syphilo-tubercular
Sweat	forehead, on	✓				
Sweat	scanty	✓				
Sweat	sour odour, of	✓				
Thickened	skin		✓			
Thrombosis	venous				✓	
Tinea Barbae			✓			
Tinea Favosa					✓	
Tinea Vesicular			✓			
Ulceration				✓		
Ulceration	blood, with			✓		or Syphilo-tubercular
Ulceration	burns after			✓		
Ulceration	haemorrhage, with				✓	
Ulceration	night, agg. at			✓		
Ulceration	open			✓		
Ulceration	painless			✓		
Ulceration	pus, with			✓		
Ulceration	scalds after			✓		
Ulceration	warmth of bed, agg. by			✓		
Ulcers					✓	
Unhealthy	appearance	✓				
Unwashed	appearance	✓				
Urticaria					✓	
Vaccination	consequence of, skin disorders as a:		✓			
Vaccination	warts follow		✓			
Varicose Veins			✓		✓	
Varicose Veins	flushed, red				✓	
Verrucae			✓			
Vesicular	during menses, eruptions isolated		✓			
Vesicular	eruptions			✓		
Vesicular	flat and red, eruptions			✓		
Vesicular	recurs in menstrual period, eruptions slow to heal					Syco-tubercular
Vesicular	slow to heal, eruptions					Syco-syphilitic
Vulvae	ulceration			✓		
Warts			✓			
Warts	dryness, with					Syco-psoric
Warts	face on		✓			
Warts	genitals, on		✓			
Warts	hands, on		✓			

Skin Symptoms	Rubric	Psora	Sycosis	Syphilis	Tubercular	Mixed Miasms
Warts	relieves, reappearance of		✓			
Warts	vaccination, after		✓			
Water	tolerate, cannot	✓				
Wine	coloured moles		✓			
Wine	coloured patches		✓			

MIASMATIC DIAGNOSIS: MIASMATIC REPERTORY OF NAIL SYMPTOMS

Nail Symptoms	Rubric	Psora	Sycosis	Syphilis	Tubercular	Mixed Miasms
Asymmetrical						Syphilo-tubercular
Bends				✓		
Bends	easily			✓		
Break	easily				✓	
Brittle						Syphilo-tubercular
Bumps			✓			
Concave	shaped					Syphilo-tubercular
Convex			✓			
Corrugated			✓			
Dome	shaped		✓			
Dry		✓				
Flush	nails, on pressing				✓	
Glossy					✓	
Grooves	longitudinal			✓		
Hang Nails					✓	
Harsh		✓				
Irregular	shape of nail					Syco-syphilitic
Irregular	with thick edges	✓				
Longitudinal	grooves			✓		
Nails	easily lost				✓	
Panaritiums	pus, with			✓		
Pitted				✓		
Protuberances			✓			
Pus	at cuticle points			✓		
Pus	cuticle and nail, at junction of				✓	
Ridged			✓			
Ridges	horizontal		✓			
Ridges	longitudinal		✓			
Scalloped	edges				✓	
Split	easily					Syphilo-tubercular
Spoon	shaped			✓		
Stained	dark				✓	
Stained	spots				✓	
Stained	white				✓	
Stitching	in nail bed, pain		✓			
Tear	easily				✓	
Thick			✓			
Thin					✓	
Whitlow					✓	

MIASMATIC DIAGNOSIS: MIASMATIC REPERTORY OF EXTREMITY SYMPTOMS

Extremity Symptoms	Rubric	Psora	Sycosis	Syphilis	Tubercular	Mixed Miasms
Abnormalities	six fingers, such as		✓			
Anasarca	localised		✓			
Ankle	stumbles, joint			✓		
Ankle	weak, joint				✓	
Ankles	weak				✓	
Arthritis Deformans			✓			
Bone	in long bones, pain			✓		
Bone	metastasis			✓		
Bone	pains			✓		
Bone	sarcoma			✓		
Bones	curved				✓	
Bones	fragile			✓		
Bones	soft				✓	
Bones	weak				✓	
Bruised	pains	✓				
Burning	hands	✓				
Burning	pains			✓		
Burning	sweating soles with, feet	✓				
Burning	with sweating palms, hands	✓				
Bursting	pains			✓		
Caries	bones, of			✓		
Circulation	poor	✓				
Clumsy	easily, drop things				✓	
Cold	agg.		✓			
Cold	amel.				✓	
Cramps		✓				
Cramps	extremities, in lower				✓	
Deformities	limbs, of			✓		
Delayed	in children, walking				✓	
Dry	hands	✓				
Energy	lacking				✓	
Exertion	fatigues, physical		✓			
Exhausted	easily				✓	
Exhausted	night, at				✓	
Extremities	cold					Psora-tubercular
Extremities	unnoticed, cold				✓	
Falls	easily			✓		
Fatigue	exertion, from physical		✓			
Feet	damp				✓	
Feet	perspiring				✓	
Fingers	blunt, appearance				✓	
Fingers	equal, appearance				✓	
Fingers	long, appearance				✓	
Flabbiness	exercise, from lack of				✓	
Fragile	bones			✓		
Gangrene	inflamed			✓		
Gout			✓			
Hands	compressed, easily				✓	
Hands	flabby					Syco-tubercular
Hands	moist				✓	
Hands	perspiring				✓	
Hands	soft				✓	
Hands	thin				✓	
Humidity	agg.		✓			

Extremity Symptoms	Rubric	Psora	Sycosis	Syphilis	Tubercular	Mixed Miasms
Inflammation		✓				
Inflammation	chronic		✓			
Inflammatory	in joints, deposits		✓			
Joint	pains	✓				
Joints	diminished, strength				✓	
Keyboard	causes swelling, typing					Syco-tubercular
Keyboard	fatigues, typing				✓	
Lameness			✓			
Lancinating	pains			✓		
Meat	agg.		✓			
Motion	agg., beginning of			✓		
Muscle	wasting				✓	
Muscles	during sleep, twitch	✓				
Necrosis	bones, of				✓	
Neuralgia						Psora-tubercular
Neuralgia	by quiet, amel.				✓	
Neuralgia	by rest, amel.				✓	
Neuralgia	by motion, amel.				✓	
Neuralgia	by warmth, amel.				✓	
Night	agg.				✓	
Nodular	growths				✓	
Nodular	of glandular origin, growths				✓	
Numbness			✓			
Numbness	tingling, with	✓				
Numbness	with tingling, when sitting agg. by pressure	✓				
Oedema	localised		✓			
Oedematous	swelling		✓			
Onset	slow					Syphilo-sycotic
Osteoarthritis			✓			
Osteomyelitis						Psora-syphilitic
Osteoporosis						Syco-syphilitic
Ostitis		✓				
Pain	aching, in bones				✓	
Pain	amel. by motion, neuralgic				✓	
Pain	amel. by quiet, neuralgic				✓	
Pain	amel. by rest, neuralgic				✓	
Pain	amel. by warmth, neuralgic				✓	
Pain	at seaside, agg.			✓		
Pain	burning			✓		
Pain	bursting			✓		
Pain	by abnormal discharges, amel.			✓		
Pain	by appearance of fibrous growths, amel.		✓			
Pain	by appearance of old ulcers, amel.		✓			
Pain	by appearance of warts, amel.		✓			
Pain	by approach of thunderstorm, agg.					Syphilo-tubercular
Pain	by change of position, amel.			✓		
Pain	by discharge of pus, amel.			✓		
Pain	by fruit, agg.				✓	
Pain	by lying on abdomen, amel.		✓			
Pain	by milk, agg.				✓	
Pain	by nose bleeding, amel.				✓	
Pain	by offensive sweat, amel. temporarily				✓	
Pain	by oily food, agg.				✓	
Pain	by pressure, amel.		✓			
Pain	by pressure in the chest, agg.				✓	
Pain	by rain, agg.		✓			
Pain	by return of suppressed normal discharges, amel.		✓			
Pain	by sea-voyage, agg.			✓		
Pain	by slow motion, amel.		✓			
Pain	by stretching, amel.		✓			

Extremity Symptoms	Rubric	Psora	Sycosis	Syphilis	Tubercular	Mixed Miasms
Pain	by sweat, agg.			✓		
Pain	by thunderstorm, agg.					Syphilo-tubercular
Pain	during daytime, amel.				✓	
Pain	in closed room, agg.				✓	
Pain	in cold of winter, amel.			✓		
Pain	in dry weather, amel.					Syco-tubercular
Pain	in extremes of temperature, agg.			✓		
Pain	in lukewarm climate, amel.			✓		
Pain	in open air, amel.				✓	
Pain	in summer, agg.			✓		
Pain	long bones, in			✓		
Pain	neuralgic	✓				
Pain	night, agg. at approach of				✓	
Pain	night, at agg.					Syphilo-tubercular
Pain	tearing			✓		
Pain	temporarily by sweat, amel.				✓	
Pain	winter, amel.			✓		
Pains	by approach of night, agg.			✓		
Pains	at night, agg.			✓		
Pains	bones, in			✓		
Pains	by scratching, amel.	✓				
Pains	by standing, agg.	✓				
Pains	by approach of storm, agg.					Syphilo-tubercular
Pains	by beginning to move, agg.		✓			
Pains	by bending, agg.		✓			
Pains	by change of weather, agg.		✓			
Pains	by crying, amel.	✓				
Pains	by damp, agg.		✓			
Pains	by eating, amel.	✓				
Pains	by heat, amel.	✓				
Pains	by hot application, amel.	✓				
Pains	by humidity agg.		✓			
Pains	by meat, agg.		✓			
Pains	by movements, agg.			✓		
Pains	by moving, amel.		✓			
Pains	by natural discharges, amel.					Psora
Pains	by perspiration, agg.				✓	
Pains	by reappearance of suppressed skin eruptions, amel.	✓				
Pains	by rest, agg.		✓			
Pains	by rubbing, amel.		✓			
Pains	by stooping, agg.		✓			
Pains	by unnatural discharges, amel.		✓			
Pains	by warmth of bed, agg.				✓	
Pains	during daytime, agg.	✓				
Pains	during thunderstorm, agg.					Syphilo-tubercular
Pains	in extremes of temperature, agg.				✓	
Pains	in summer, amel.	✓				
Pains	on stretching, amel.			✓		
Pains	through mucus membranes, amel. unnatural discharges			✓		
Pains	unnatural discharges, amel. from greenish-yellow			✓		
Pallid				✓		
Paralysis	incoordination, with					Syco-syphilitic
Paralysis	muscle wasting, with				✓	
Periosteum	with deposits, inflamed			✓		
Periostitis		✓				
Perspiration	cold				✓	
Perspiration	offensive, of palms				✓	
Perspiration	offensive, soles of				✓	

238

Extremity Symptoms	Rubric	Psora	Sycosis	Syphilis	Tubercular	Mixed Miasms
Perspiration	palms, of				✓	
Perspiration	soles, of				✓	
Physical	fatigues, exertion		✓			
Physical	fatigues, slight exertion		✓			
Piano	causes swelling, playing					Syco-tubercular
Piano	fatigues, playing				✓	
Power	in joints, lost				✓	
Pressive	pains		✓			
Puffy			✓			
Pulsating	in bones, pain					Syco-syphilitic
Pulsating	in muscles, pain		✓			
Rested	never, seems				✓	
Rheumatism			✓			
Rickets						Syphilo-tubercular
Seaside	at, agg.				✓	
Sea Voyage	agg.				✓	
Shooting	in bones, pain					Syco-syphilitic
Shooting	pain, muscles in		✓			
Shooting	pains			✓		
Sore	pains		✓			
Soreness			✓			
Sprain	of joints, easy		✓			
Stamina	lacking					Psora-sycotic
Standing	agg.	✓				
Standing	difficult	✓				
Stiffness			✓			
Stitching	in bones, pain					Syphilo-sycotic
Stitching	in muscles, pain		✓			
Stitching	pains		✓			
Stooping	agg.		✓			
Strength	lacking				✓	
Strength	with the sun, comes and goes				✓	
Stretching	agg.		✓			
Stumbles	easily				✓	
Summer	agg.			✓		
Sweat				✓		
Sweat	of palms, offensive				✓	
Sweat	of soles, offensive				✓	
Tearing	in bones, pain					Syco-syphilitic
Tearing	in muscles, pain		✓			
Tearing	pains			✓		
Thin	appearance				✓	
Thunderstorm	agg.					Mixed miasmatic
Tired	little exertion, from		✓			
Tophi	in joints, deposits		✓			
Ulceration	bone marrow, of			✓		
Ulcers				✓		
Varicose Veins	lower extremities, in	✓				
Wandering	in bones, pain		✓			
Wandering	in muscles, pain		✓			
Warmth	desires	✓				
Weakness	joints, in				✓	
Weakness	paralytic					Syco-syphilitic
Winter	in, agg.	✓				
Wrists	drop				✓	
Wrists	weak				✓	

MIASMATIC DIAGNOSIS: MIASMATIC REPERTORY OF SLEEP SYMPTOMS

Sleep Symptoms	Rubric	Psora	Sycosis	Syphilis	Tubercular	Mixed Miasms
Awakening	weariness, with				✓	
Dreams	anxiety, of	✓				
Dreams	anxious	✓				
Dreams	dead bodies, of			✓		
Dreams	death, of			✓		
Dreams	destruction, of			✓		
Dreams	fanciful		✓			
Dreams	fear, of	✓				
Dreams	fearful faces, of	✓				
Dreams	fearful images, of	✓				
Dreams	frightening	✓				
Dreams	gloomy foreboding, of				✓	
Dreams	lascivious					Psora-sycotic
Dreams	sad	✓				
Dreams	sex, of perverted				✓	
Dreams	sexual		✓			
Dreams	suicidal				✓	
Dreams	vivid	✓				
Exhausted	sleep, after				✓	
Grinding	during sleep, of teeth	✓				
Head	during sleep, rolls			✓		
Muscles	during sleep, twitch					
Restless	sleep		✓			
Salivation	sleep, during	✓				
Screams	sleep, during			✓		
Short	sleeps		✓			
Sleep	at night, disturbed			✓		
Sleep	at the seaside, disturbed			✓		
Sleep	by change of position, amel.			✓		
Sleep	by sweat, disturbed			✓		
Sleep	during summer, disturbed			✓		
Sleep	in closed room, disturbed				✓	
Sleep	in damp weather, restless		✓			
Sleep	in stuffy room, disturbed				✓	
Sleep	restless		✓			
Sleep Walking		✓				
Sleepless	day, during	✓				
Snoring		✓				
Somnambulism		✓				
Stool	during sleep, passes	✓				
Sweat	during sleep, on head	✓				
Talking	sleep, during	✓				
Teeth	during sleep, gnashing of	✓				
Unrefreshing	sleep				✓	
Unrefreshing	sleep, depression with				✓	
Unrefreshing	sleep, exhaustion with				✓	
Unrefreshing	sleep melancholia with				✓	
Urine	during sleep, passes	✓				
Wakes	sleep, then returns		✓			
Weariness	awakening, on				✓	
Worms	expelled during sleep, round like	✓				

MIASMATIC DIAGNOSIS: MIASMATIC REPERTORY OF MODALITY SYMPTOMS

Modality Symptoms	Rubric	Psora	Sycosis	Syphilis	Tubercular	Mixed Miasms
Aggravation	and moist cold, in damp cold		✓			
Aggravation	closed room, in				✓	
Aggravation	cold, from	✓				
Aggravation	during damp cold weather, of joint pains		✓			
Aggravation	extremes of temperature, from			✓		
Aggravation	from warmth, during summer			✓		
Aggravation	fruits, greasy and oily food, from milk				✓	
Aggravation	heat, from		✓			
Aggravation	humid atmospheres, in		✓			
Aggravation	movements, from			✓		
Aggravation	natural discharges, from			✓		
Aggravation	night, at			✓		
Aggravation	perspiration, from			✓		
Aggravation	pressure, from				✓	
Aggravation	rainy season, during		✓			
Aggravation	rest, from		✓			
Aggravation	sea voyage, from			✓		
Aggravation	seaside, at			✓		
Aggravation	sleep, during	✓				
Aggravation	standing, from	✓				
Aggravation	sunset to sunrise, from				✓	
Aggravation	thunderstorm, during					Mixed miasmatic
Aggravation	warmth of bed, from				✓	
Aggravation	winter, during	✓				
Amelioration	any natural discharge, from		✓			
Amelioration	as fibrous growths appear, of mental condition		✓			
Amelioration	as warts appear, of mental condition		✓			
Amelioration	by offensive foot or axillary sweat, temporary				✓	
Amelioration	by return of acute gonorrhoeal manifestation, markedly		✓			
Amelioration	change of position, from			✓		
Amelioration	cold, from			✓		
Amelioration	diarrhoea, perspiration etc., from	✓				
Amelioration	discharge of pus, through			✓		
Amelioration	dry atmosphere, in		✓			
Amelioration	dry weather, in		✓			
Amelioration	eliminative processes, by		✓			
Amelioration	from breaking open of old sores, in general		✓			
Amelioration	heat, from	✓				
Amelioration	in dry weather, by stretching		✓			
Amelioration	in open air, during daytime				✓	
Amelioration	like leucorrhoea, from any abnormal discharge					Syco-syphilitic
Amelioration	like menses, by return of suppressed normal discharges		✓			
Amelioration	like urine, sweat, menses etc., by natural discharges	✓				
Amelioration	lukewarm climate, in			✓		
Amelioration	lying down, by	✓				
Amelioration	morning, in		✓			
Amelioration	motion, from		✓			
Amelioration	nasal discharge, from		✓			

Modality Symptoms	Rubric	Psora	Sycosis	Syphilis	Tubercular	Mixed Miasms
Amelioration	nose bleeding, by				✓	
Amelioration	or pressure, from lying on stomach		✓			
Amelioration	slow motion, by		✓			
Amelioration	stretching, by		✓			
Amelioration	summer, during	✓				
Amelioration	sunrise to sunset, from			✓		
Amelioration	winter, during			✓		

PART — VI
MIASMATIC PRESCRIBING :
MIASMATIC WEIGHTAGE OF MEDICINES

Medicine	Psoric	Sycotic	Syphilitic	Tubercular	Chilly or Hot
ABIES CANADENSIS	++	+	+	++	C++
ABIES NIGRA	++	+	+	+	
ABROTANUM	++	+++	++	++	C+
ABSINTHIUM	++	+	++	+	
ACALYPHA INDICA	++	+	+	+++	
ACETANILIDUM	++	++	+	+	C++
ACETIC ACID	++	+	+	+++	C++
ACONITUM NAPELLUS	++	+	+	++	C+
ACONITUM NAPELLUS	+++	++	+	+++	C+
ACTAEA RACEMOSA	+	+++	+	+	C+
ACTEA SPICATA	++	+++	++	+	C+
ADONIS VERNALIS	++	++	+	++	
ADRENALIN	++	++	+	+	
AESCULUS HIPPOCASTANUM	++	++	+	+	H++
AETHIOPS MERCURIALIS-MINERALIS	++	+	+++	++	
AETHUSA CYNAPIUM	++	+	+	+	H+
AGARICUS MUSCARIUS	+	++	+	+++	C+++
AGAVE AMERICANA	++	+++	++	++	
AGNUS CASTUS	+	+++	+	+	C+
AGRAPHIS NUTANS	++	++	+	++	C+
AILANTHUS GLANDULOSA	+	++	++	+++	
ALETRIS FARINOSA	++	+	+	+	C++
ALFALFA	++	++		+	
ALLIUM CEPA	++	++	+	++	H++
ALLIUM SATIVUM	++	+	+	+++	C+
ALNUS	++	+	+	++	
ALOE SOCOTRINA	++	++	+	++	H++
ALSTONIA SCHOLARIS	++	+	+		
ALUMEN	++	++	+	++	C++
ALUMINA	++	+	+	+	C+++
ALUMINA SILICATA	++	+	++	+	C++
AMBRA GRISEA	+	+			C+
AMBROSIA	++	+	+	++	
AMMONIACUM-DOREMA	++	++	+	+	C+
AMMONIUM BENZOICUM	++	+++			
AMMONIUM BROMATUM	++	++			C+
AMMONIUM CARBONICUM	++	+		+++	C++
AMMONIUM CAUSTICUM	++	+	++	+++	
AMMONIUM IODATUM	++	++			
AMMONIUM MURIATICUM	++	++			H+
AMMONIUM PHOSPHORICUM	++	+++			
AMMONIUM PICRATUM	++	+	+	++	
AMMONIUM VALERIANICUM	++	+		+	
AMPELOPSIS	++	++	+	++	
AMYGDALUS PERSICA	++	++	+	++	C+
AMYLENUM NITROSUM	++		+	+	H++
ANACARDIUM	++	++	++	+	H+
ANAGALLIS	++	+++	+	+	
ANATHERUM	++	++	++	+	
ANEMOPSIS CALIFORNICA	++	++	+	++	
ANGUSTURA VERA	++	+++	+++	+	
ANHALONIUM	++	+++	++	+	
ANILINUM	++	++		+	
ANTHEMIS NOBILIS	++	++	+	+	H+
ANTHRACINUM	++	+	+++	++	C+

L denotes leading remedies within each miasm.

Medicine	Psoric	Sycotic	Syphilitic	Tubercular	Chilly or Hot
ANTHRAKOKALI	++	++	+	+	
ANTIMONIUM ARSENICOSUM	++	++	+	++	
ANTIMONIUM CRUDUM	++	++	+	+	C+
ANTIMONIUM SULPHURATUM ARUATUM	++	++	+	++	
ANTIMONIUM TARTARICUM	++	++		+	C+
ANTIPYRINE	++	++	++	++	C+
APIS MELLIFICA	++	++	+	+	H++
APIUM GRAVEOLENS	++	+++	+	++	
APOCYNUM CANNABINUM	+	+++	+	+	C+
APOCYUM ANDROSAEMIFOLIUM	++	+++	+	+	
APOMORPHIA	++	+	++		
AQUILEGIA	++	++	+	+	
ARAGALLUS LAMBERTI	+	++	+	+	
ARALIA RACEMOSA	++	++	+	++	
ARANEA DIADEMA	++	+++	+	++	C+++
ARBUTUS ANDRACHNE	++	+++			
ARECA	+	++		+	
ARGEMONE MEXICANA	++	++			
ARGENTICUM METALLICUM	+	++	++	+	H+
ARGENTICUM NITRICUM	+++	+++	+++	+++	H++
ARISTOLOCHIA MILHOMENS	++	++	++	++	
ARNICA MONTANA	++	++	++	+++	C+
ARSENICUM ALBUM	+++	+++	+	++	C+++
ARSENICUM BROMATUM	++	+	+++	+	
ARSENICUM HYDROGENISATUM	++	++	++	+++	C++
ARSENICUM IODATUM	+++	++	+	+++ L	H+
ARSENICUM METALLICUM	++	+	+++	++	
ARSENICUM SULF. FLAVUM	++	+	++		
ARTEMISIA VULGARIS	++		+++	++	
ARUM DRACONTIUM	++	++	+++	+	
ARUM TRIPHYLLUM	++		++	++	C+
ARUNDO	++	+	++	++	
ASAFOETIDA	++	+	+++	+	H++
ASARUM EUROPUM	++	+	+		C++
ASCLEPIAS SYRIACA	++	+++			
ASCLEPIAS TUBEROSA	++	++	+	+	
ASIMINA TRILOBA	++	+	++	+	
ASPARAGUS OFFICINALIS	+	++	++	++	
ASPIDOSPERMA	++	++			
ASTACUS FLUVIATILIS	++	+		+	C++
ASTERIAS RUBENS	+	+++	+	+	C+
ASTRAGALUS MOLLISSIMUS	++	+	++	+	
AURUM METALLICUM	++	+	+++ L	++	C++
AURUM MUR. NATRONATUM	++	+++	++	+	
AVENA SATIVA	+++	+	+	+	
AZADIRACHTA INDICA	++	++	+		C+
BACILLINUM	++	+++	++	+++ L	H+
BADIAGA	++	++	+	++	C++
BALSAMUM PERUVIANUM	++	+	+	++	
BAPTISIA TINCTORIA	++		++	+	H+
BAROSMA CRENATA	++	++			
BARYTA ACETICA	++	++	++	+	C+
BARYTA CARBONICUM	++	++	+	+++	C+++
BARYTA IODATA	++	+++	++	+++	H+++
BARYTA MURIATICA	++	++	+++	++	
BELLADONNA	+++		+	+++	C++
BELLIS PERENNIS	+++	+++	+	+	C+
BENZENUM COAL NAPHTHA	++	+	+++	+	
BENZOICUM ACIDUM	+	+++		+	C+
BERBERIS AQUIFOLIUM – MAHONIA	+	++	+++	+	
BERBERIS VULGARIS	+	+++		+	C+
BETA VULGARIS	++	+	+	+++	
BETONICA	+	++			

L *denotes leading remedies within each miasm.*

Medicine	Psoric	Sycotic	Syphilitic	Tubercular	Chilly or Hot
BISMUTHUM	++	++	+	++	H+
BLATTA AMERICANA	++	+++			
BLATTA ORIENTALIS	++	+++	+	++	
BOLETUS LARICIS – POLYPORUS OFFICINALE	++	+	++	+++	C+
BORAX	++	++	+		H++
BORICUM ACIDUM	++	++	++	++	C++
BOTHROPS LANCIOLATUS – LACHESIS LANCIOLATUS	++	++	+++	+++	
BOTULINUM	++	++	+		
BOVISTA	++	+		++	H+
BRACHYGLOTTIS	++	++	+	+	C+
BROMIUM	+	++		++	H++
BRYONIA ALBA	++	+++	+	++	H++
BUFO	++	++	+++	++	H+
BUTYRIC ACID	++	++	+++	+	
CACTUS GRANDIFLORUS	++	+		+++	H+
CADIMUM SULPH	++	++	+++	++	C+
CAHINCA	++	++	+	++	
CAJUPUTUM	+++	++	+	+	
CALADIUM	+	++		+	C+
CALC FLUORICA	++	++	+++	++	C++
CALC SILICATA	++	+++	+	+	C++
CALCAREA ACETICA	++	++	++	+	
CALCAREA ARSENICA	++	+	+	++	C++
CALCAREA CARBONICA	+++ L	+++	++	+++ L	C++
CALCAREA IODATA	++	+++	+	+++	H++
CALCAREA PHOSPHORICA	++	+	++	+++	C++
CALCAREA SULPHURICA	++	+	++	++	H++
CALENDULA	++	+	+++	+	C+
CALOTROPIS	++	+	+++	++	
CALTHA PALUSTRIS	++	++	+		
CAMPHORA	++	+		++	C++
CAMPHORA MONO-BROMATA	++	+	++	+	
CANCHALAGUA	++	+	++	++	
CANNABIS INDICA	++	+	+		H++
CANNABIS SATIVA	++	+++	+++	+	C+
CANTHARIDES	++	+	+++	++	C+
CAPSICUM	++	+	+	++	C+++
CARBO ANIMALIS	+	++	+++	+++	C++
CARBO VEGETABILIS	++	+	++	+++	C++
CARBOLIC ACID	++	+	++	+	C++
CARBONEUM HYDROGENISATUM	++	+	+++	+	
CARBONEUM OXYGENISATUM	++	++	++	++	C+
CARBONEUM SULPHURATUM	+++	+	++	++	C+
CARDUUS MARIANUS	++	+++	+	++	C++
CARLSBAD	++	++	+	++	C++
CASCARA SAGRADA –RHAMNUS PURSHIANA	+++	++	+		
CASCARILLA	++	++	+	++	
CASTANEA VESCA	++	++	++	+	
CASTOR EQUI	++	+++	++	+	
CASTOREUM	++	+	+	++	
CATARIA NEPETA	++	++			
CAULOPHYLLUM	++	+++	+	++	C+
CAUSTICUM	+++	+++	++	+++	C++
CEANOTHUS	++	+++	+	+	C+
CEDRON- SIMARUBA FERROGINEA	++	++	+	+++	
CENCHRIS CONTORTRIX	++	++	++	+++	
CEREUS BONPLANDII	+	++	+	++	
CERIUM OXALICUM	++	++	+	++	
CHAMOMILLA	++	++	++	+	H++
CHAPARRO AMARGOSO	++	++	+	++	
CHELIDONIUM MAJUS	++	+	++		C+
CHELONE	++	++	+	++	
CHENOPODI GLAUCI APHIS	++	++	+	+	

L *denotes leading remedies within each miasm.*

Medicine	Psoric	Sycotic	Syphilitic	Tubercular	Chilly or Hot
CHENOPODIUM ANTHELMINTICUM	++	++	+	++	C+
CHIMAPHILA UMBELLATA	++	+++	+	++	C+
CHININUM SULPHURICUM	++	++	+	++	H+
CHINUNUM ARSENICOSUM	+++	++	+	+++	C+
CHIONANTHUS	++	++		++	
CHLOLESTERINUM	++	+++	+	++	
CHLORALUM	++	++	+	++	
CHLOROFORMUM	++	++	++	++	
CHLORUM	++	++	++	+	
CHROMICUM ACIDUM	++	++	++	++	
CHRYSAROBINUM	++	++	++	+	
CICUTA VIROSA	++		++		C++
CIMEX – ACANTHIA	++	+	+	+	
CINA	++	++	+	++	H+
CINCHONA OFFICINALIS	++	++	+	+++	C++
CINERARIA	++	++		+	
CINNABARIS	++	+	++		C+
CINNAMONUM	++	++	++	+++	
CISTUS CANADENSIS	++	++	+	+++	C++
CITRUS VULGARIS	++	+			
CLEMATIS	+	++	+++	+	C++
COBALTUM	++	++	+	++	
COCA	++	+	++	++	C+
COCAINA	++	++	++	++	
COCCINELLA SEPTEMPUNCTATA	++	+·	+	+	
COCCULUS	++	+	+	++	C++
COCCUS CACTI	+	+	++	+	C++
COCHELEARIA ARMORACIA - ARMORACIA SATIVA	++	+	++	++	
CODEINUM	++	+	+	++	
COFFEA	++	++		+	C++
COLCHICUM	++	++	+		C+
COLLINSONIA CANADENSIS	++	++		++	C+
COLOCYNTHIS	++	++	+		C+
COMOCLADIA DENTATA	++	++	++	+	H+
CONDURANGO	++	++	+++	+	
CONIUM MACULATUM	++	++	+	+	C++
CONVALLARIA MAJALIS	++	++	+	++	H+
COPAIVA	++	++	+	+	
CORALLIUM	++	+++	+	++	C+
CORALLORHIZA	++	+	+	++	
CORNUS CIRCINATA	++	++	+	+	
CORYDALIS	++	+	+++	+	
COTYLEDON	++	++			
CRATAEGUS	++	++	+	+	H+
CROCUS SATIVA	++			++	H+
CROCUS SATIVA	++	+	+	+++	H++
CROTALUS HORRIDUS	++	++	+	+++	H+
CROTON TIGLIUM	++	+	+	+	H+
CUBEBA	++	++	+	+	
CUCURBITA CITRULLUS	++	++			
CUCURBITA PEPO	++	++		++	
CUPHEA	++	+			
CUPRUM ACETICUM	++	++	+	++	C+
CUPRUM ARSENITUM	++	++	++	+	C+
CUPRUM METALLICUM	++	++	++	+	C++
CURARE	++	+	+	++	C++
CYCLAMEN EUROPAEUM	++	++		++	C++
CYPRIPEDIUM	++	++			
DAPHNE INDICA	++	+++	+		C+
DIGITALIS PURPUREA	++	++		+	C++
DIOSCOREA VILLOSA	++	++	+		H+
DIOSMA LINCARIS	++	++	++	++	
DIPHTHERINUM	++	+	+	++	C++

L *denotes leading remedies within each miasm.*

Medicine	Psoric	Sycotic	Syphilitic	Tubercular	Chilly or Hot
DOLICHOS PURIENS	++	++	+	+	
DORYPHORA	+	+++	+		
DROSERA ROTUNDIFOLIA	++	+	+	++	C++
DUBOISIA	++	++	+	++	C+
DULCAMARA	++	++	+	+	C++
ECHINACEA – RUDBECKIA	++	++	+++L	++	C+
ELAPS CORALLINUS	++	++	++	+++	C++
ELATERIUM – ECBALIUM	++	+++			C+
EOSIN	++	++	++	++	
EPIGEA REPENS	++	+++	+	+	
EPIPEGUS – OROBANCHE	++	++			C+
EQUISETUM HYEMALE	++	++		+	C+
ERECHTHITES	++	++	+	+++	
ERIGERON – LEPTILON CANDENSE	++	++	++	+++	
ERIODICTYON	++	++	+	+++	C+
ERYNGIUM AQUATICUM	++	++	+	+	
ESCHSCHOLTZIA CALIFORNICA	++	++	+	+	
EUCALYPTUS GLOBULUS	++	+++	++	++	
EUGENIA JAMBOS	++	+	++	+	H+
EUONYMUS ATROPURPUREA	++	++	++	++	H+
EUPATORIUM AROMATICUM	++	++	++	+	
EUPATORIUM PERFOLIATUM	++	+	+	++	C+
EUPATORIUM PURPUREUM	++	+++	+	++	C++
EUPHORBIA LATHYRIS	++	++	++	+	C++
EUPHORBIUM	++	++	++	+++L	H+
EUPHRASIA	++	+	+	+	H+
EUPION	++	+++	+	+	
FABIANA IMBRICATA	++	+++	+	+	
FAGOPYRUM	+++	++	+	++	H+
FEL TAURI	++	+++			
FERRRUM PICRICUM	++	+++	+	+	
FERRUM IODATUM	++	++	+	+++	H++
FERRUM MAGNETICUM	++	++	+	+	
FERRUM METALLICUM	++	++	+	++	C+
FERRUM PHOSPHORICUM	++		+	++	C++
FICUS RELIGOSA	++	+	+	++	
FILIX MAS	++	+	+	++	
FLUORICUM ACIDUM	++	+	+++	++	H++
FORMALIN	++	++	++	+	
FORMICA RUFA	++	++	++	++	C++
FRAGARIA	++	++	+	+	
FRANCISCEA	++	+++	++	++	
FRAXINUS AMERICANA	++	+++			
FUCHSINA – MAGENTA	++	++	+	++	
FUCUS VESICULOSUS	++	+++			H+
FULIGO LIGNI	++	++	++	++	
GALANTHUS NIVALIS	++	++	+	++	
GALIUM APARINE	++	++	++	++	
GALLICUM ACIDUM	++	++	++	+++	
GAMBOGIA	++	++	+	++	H+
GAULTHERIA	++	++		+	
GELSEMIUM	+	++	+	+	H++
GENTIANA LUTEA	++	++			
GERANIUM MACULATUM	++	+	++	+++	H+
GETTYSBURG WATER	++	++	+	+	
GINSENG	++	+++	+	++	C+
GLONOINE	++	+	+	++	H++
GLYCERINUM	++	++	+	+	
GNAPHALIUM	++	+++	+	+	
GOLONDRINA	++	++	+	+	
GOSSYPIUM	++	++	+	+	
GRANATUM	++	++	+	++	
GRAPHITES	+++	++	++	++	C+++
GRATIOLA	++	++	++	++	H+

L *denotes leading remedies within each miasm.*

Medicine	Psoric	Sycotic	Syphilitic	Tubercular	Chilly or Hot
GRINDELIA	++	+++	+	+	
GUACO	++	+	+++	++	
GUAIACUM	++	++	++	++	
GUAREA	++	++	+	+	C+
GUN POWDER	++	++	+++ L	++	C++
GYMNOCLADUS	++	++	+	++	C+
HAEMATOXYLON	++	++	+	++	C++
HAMAMELIS VIRGINICA	++	+	+	+++	H+
HEDEOMA	++	++	+	+	
HEKLA LAVA	++	+++	+++	++	
HELIANTHUS	++	++	+	+	
HELLEBORUS	++	+++	++	+++	C+
HELODERMA	++	++	+	+	C+++
HELONIAS	+++	+++	+	+	
HEPAR SULPHURIS	+++	++	+++	++	C+++
HEPATICA	++	+++	+	+	
HERACLEUM	++	++			
HIPPOMANES	++	++	+	+	
HIPPOZAENIUM	++	+++	+++	+++L	
HIPPURIC ACID	++	++	+	+	H+
HOANG NAN	++	++	+++	++	
HOMARUS	++	++	++	++	C+
HURA BRAZILIENSIS	++	++	++	+	
HYDRANGEA	++	+++	+	++	
HYDRASTIS	++	++	+++	++	C+
HYDROCOTYLE	++	+++	++	++	
HYDROCYANIC ACID	+++	++	+++	++	
HYDROPHOBINUM (LYSSINUM)	++	++	+++	+++	C++
HYOSCYAMUS	++	+++	+	++	C+
HYPERICUM	+++	++	++	++	C+
IBERIS	++	+	+	+++	C+
ICHTHYOLUM	++	+++	++	+++	
IDOFORMUM	++	++	+	+++L	
IGNATIA	+++	++	+	+++	C+
ILEX AQUIFOLIUM	++	+	+	++	C++
ILLICIUM	++	+++	+	+	
INDIGO	++	++	++	++	C+
INDIUM	++	+++	++	+	C+
INDOL	+++	++	+	+	
INSULIN	++	++	+	+	
INULA	++	++	+	+++	
IODUM	++	+	++	+++ L	H+++
IPECACUANHA	++	+	++	+++	C+
IRIDIUM	+++	++	+	+	H+
IRIS VERSICOLOR	++	+	++	++	H+
JACARANDA	++	+++	+++	++	
JATROPHA	++	++	+	++	
JEQUIRITY	++	++	+++	++	
JONOSIA ASOCA	++	+++	++	+++	
JUGLANS REGIA	++	++	+++	++	
JUGULANS CINEREA	++	++	+	++	C+
JUNCUS EFFUSES	++	+++			
JUNIPERUS COMMUNIS	++	+++	+	++	
JUSTICIA ADHATODA	++	+		++	C+
KALI IOD (HYDRIODICUM)	++	++	+++	+	H+
KALI ARSENICUM	++	++	+++	+	C+
KALI BICHROMICUM	++	++	+++	++	C++
KALI BROMATUM	++	++	+	++	
KALI CARBONICUM	++	++	+	+++	C+++
KALI CHLORICUM	++	++	+++	++	
KALI CYANATUM	+++	+	+++	+	
KALI MURIATICUM	++	+	+	++	C+
KALI NITRICUM	++	+++	++	+++	C+
KALI PERMANGANICUM	++	++	+++	++	

L *denotes leading remedies within each miasm.*

Medicine	Psoric	Sycotic	Syphilitic	Tubercular	Chilly or Hot
KALI PHOSPHORICUM	++	++	++	+	C+
KALI SILICATUM	++	++	+	++	C++
KALI SULPHURICUM	++	+++	+	++	C++
KALMIA LATIFOLIA	++	+++			C+
KAOLIN	++	+++	+	+	
KOUSSO	++		+	++	
KREOSOTUM	++	+	+++ L	++	C++
LABURNUM	++	++	++	+	
LAC CANINUM	++	++	+	++	H+
LAC DEFLORATUM	++	+			C+
LACHESIS	++	+++	++	+++	H++
LACHNANTHES	++	++	+	++	
LACTICUM ACIDUM	++	+	+	++	C+
LACTUCA VIROSA	+	++			H+
LACTUCA VIROSA	++	+++			
LAMIUM	+	++	+	+	
LAPIS ALBUS	++	+++	+	++	
LAPPA	++	++	+	+	
LATHYRUS	++	++	+		C+
LATRODECTUS MACTANS	++	+	+		
LAUROCERASUS	++	+		+	H+
LECITHIN	++	+	+	++	
LEDUM PAL	++	+++	+	+	H++
LEMNA MINOR	++	++		+	C+
LEPIDIUM BONARIENSE	++	++	+	+	
LEPTANDRA	+	++	+	+++	
LIATRIS SPICATA	++	+++	++	+	
LILIUM TIGRINUM	++	+++	+	+	H+
LIMULUS	++	++			
LINARIA	++	++	+	+	
LINUM USITATISSIMUM	+++	++	+	+	
LITHIUM CARBONICUM	++	+++	+	+	
LOBELIA INFLATA	++	++	+		C++
LOBILIA PURPURASCENS	+++	+	+	+	
LOLIUM TEMULENTUM	++	++	+		
LONICERA XYLOSTEUM	++	++	+++	++	
LUPULUS	++	++			H+
LYCOPODIUM	+++ L	+++	++	+++	C++
LYCOPUS VIRGINICUS	++	+++	+	++	C+
MAGNESIA MURIATICA	++	++	+	++	H+
MAGNESIA PHOSPHORICA	++	+++	+	++	C++
MAGNESIA SULPHURICA	++	++	+	+	H+
MAGNESIS CARBONICA	+++	++	+	++	C++
MAGNOLIA GRANDIFLORA	++	++	+	+	C+
MALANDRINUM	++	++	+	+	H+
MANCINELLA	++	+++	++	+	
MANGANUM ACETICUM	++	++	+++	++	C++
MANGIFERA INDICA	++	+	+	+++	
MECURIALIS PERENNIS	+++	++	++	+	
MEDORRHINUM	++	+++ L	++	++	H++
MEDUSA	++	+++	+	+	
MEL CUM SALE	++	+++			
MELILOTUS	+++	++	+	++	H+
MENISPERNUM	++	++			
MENTHA PIPERITA	++	++	+	+	
MENTHOL	+++	++	+	+	
MENYANTHES	++	++	+	+	
MEPHITIS	++	+++	+	+	
MERCURIUS CORROSIVUS	+++	+++	+++	++	C++
MERCURIUS CYANATUS	++	++	+++	+++	C++
MERCURIUS DULCIS	++	+++	++	+++	C++
MERCURIUS IODATUS FLAVUS	++	+++	+++	+++	C++
MERCURIUS IODATUS RUBER	++	+++	+++	++	C++
MERCURIUS SOLUBILIS	+++	++	+++ L	+++	C++

L *denotes leading remedies within each miasm.*

Medicine	Psoric	Sycotic	Syphilitic	Tubercular	Chilly or Hot
MERCURIUS SULPHURICUS	++	+++	++	+	
METHYLENE BLUE	++	+++	+++	++	
MEZEREUM	++	++	+++ L	++	C+++
MICROMERIA	++	++			
MILLEFOLIUM	++	++	++	+++ L	
MITCHELLA	++	+++	+	++	
MOMORDICA BALSAMINA	++	++	+	++	
MORPHINUM	++	++	+++	+	
MOSCHUS	++	++	+	++	C++
MUREX	++	+++	++	+	C+
MURIATIC ACID	++	++	+++	+++	C +
MYGALE LASIODARA	++	+++	+	+	
MYOSOTIS	++	+++	++	+++	
MYRICA	++	+++	+	+	
MYRISTICA SEIBIFERA	++	+	+++	+	
MYRTUS COMMUNIS	++	+++	++	+++	C+
NAJA TRIPUDIANS	++	+	++	+++	H++
NAPHTHALINE	+++	+++	++	+++	
NARCISSUS	++	++	+		
NATRUM ARSENICUM	++	++		+	C+
NATRUM CARBONICUM	++	++	+		H+
NATRUM CHLORATUM	++	+++	++	++	H+
NATRUM MURIATICUM	+++	+++	++	++	C++/H±
NATRUM NITRICUM	++	+++	+	+++	
NATRUM PHOSPHORICUM	++	++	+	++	H+
NATRUM SALICYLICUM	++	++	+	+++	
NATRUM SULPHURICUM	++	+++ L	+	+	C+
NICCOLUM	++	++		++	
NICCOLUM SULPHURICUM	++	++	+++	++	H+
NITRI SPIRITUS DULCIS	++	+++			C+
NITRI SPIRITUS DULCIS	+++	+++	+	++	C++
NITRIC ACID	++	+++ L	+++ L	+++	C++
NITRO-MURIATIC ACID	++	+++	++	++	
NUPHAR LUTEUM	+++	++		+	
NUX MOSCHATA	+++	++	+	++	C++
NUX VOMICA	+++	++	+	++	C+++
NYCTANTHES ARBOR-TRISTIS	+++	++			
OCIMUM CANUM	++	+++	+		
OENANTHE CROCATA	++	++	++		
OLEANDER	++	++		+	C++
OLEUM ANIMALE	++	+	+	+	H+
OLEUM JECORIS ASELLI	++	+	++	+++	C++
OLEUM SANTALI	++	+++		+	
ONISCUS ASELLUS	++	+++	+	+	
ONOSMODIUM	++	++	+	++	
OOPHORINUM	++	+++		++	
OPERCULINA TURPETHUM	++	+++	++	++	
OPIUM	+++	++	++	+	H++
OPUNTIA- FICUS INDICA	++	++			
OREODAPHNE	++	++			
ORIGANUM	++	+++		+	
ORNITHOGALUM UMBELLATUM	++	++	+++	+	C+
OSMIUM	++	++	+	++	
OSTRYA VIRGINICA	++	+++			
OVI GALLINAE PELLICULA	++	++		+	
OXALICUM ACIDUM	++	++	+	+++	C+
OXYDENDRON	++	+++			
OXYTROPIS	++	++	+		
PAEONIA	++	++	+++	++	C++
PALLADIUM	++	+++	+	+	
PARAFFINE	+++	++	++	++	
PAREIRA BRAVA	++	+++	+	+	
PARIS QUADRIFOLIA	++	++	+	+	
PARTHENIUM	++	++	+	++	

L *denotes leading remedies within each miasm.*

Medicine	Psoric	Sycotic	Syphilitic	Tubercular	Chilly or Hot
PASSIFLORA INCARNATA	++	+++	++	++	
PAULLINIA SORBILIS	++	++	+	++	
PENTHORUM	++	+++	+	+	
PERTUSSIN	++	++	+	+	
PETROLEUM	+++	++	++	++	C++
PETROSELINUM	++	+++			
PHASEOLUS	++	++		++	
PHELLANDRIUM	++	++	+	+++	C++
PHOSPHORICUM ACIDUM	++	++	+	+++ L	C++
PHOSPHORUS	+++	++	+++	+++ L	C+++
PHYSALIS	++	+++	+	++	C++
PHYSOSTIGMA	++	++	+++	++	H+
PHYTOLACCA	++	++	+++ L	++	C++
PICRIC ACID	++	++	+	+	H++
PILOCARPUS	++	++	+	+++	H+
PINUS SYLVESTRIS	++	++	+	++	
PIPER METHYSTICUM	++	+++	+	+	C+
PIPER NIGRUM	++	++	+	+	
PITUITRIN	++	+++		+	
PIX LIQUIDA	++	+		++	
PLANTAGO MAJOR	++	++	+	+	C+
PLATANUS OCCIDENTALIS	++	++			
PLATINA	++	+++	+	++	H+
PLUMBUM METALLICUM	++	+++	+	+	C+
PODOPHYLLUM	++	++			
POLYGONUM PUNCTATUM	++	++	++	+	C+
POLYPORUS PINICOLA	+++	+++			
POPULUS CANDICANS	++	++	+	+	
POPULUS TREMULOIDES	++	++	+	++	
POTHOS FOETIDUS	++	++		+	H+
PRIMULA VERIS	++	++			C+
PRIMULA OBCONICA	++	+++	++	++	
PROPYLAMIN	++	++		+	
PRUNUS SPINOSA	++	++			
PSORINUM	+++ L	++	++	+++	C+++
PTELEA	++	++			H+
PULEX IRRITANS	++	+	+++	+	
PULSATILLA	++	+++ L	+	++	H/C
PYROGENIUM	++	++	+++	++	C+
QUASSIA	++	++	++	+	
QUERCUS GLANDIUM SPIRITUS	++	++	++		
QUILLAYA SAPONARIA	+++	++	+	+	
RADIUM	++	+++ L	++	+	C+
RANUNCULUS BULBOSUS	++	++	+	+	C+++
RANUNCULUS SCELERATUS	++	++	++	+	C+
RAPHANUS	++	+++		+	
RATANHIA	++	++	+++	++	
RHAMNUS CALIFORNICA	++	+++	+		
RHEUM	+++	++			C+
RHODIUM	++	+++	+		
RHODODENDRON	++	+++		+	C+
RHUS AROMATICA	++	+++	+	++	
RHUS GLABRA	++	+++	+	+	
RHUS TOXICODENDRON	+++	+++	++	++	C++
RHUS VENENATA	++	++	+++	+	C+
RICINUS COMMUNIS	++	++	+	++	
ROBINIA	+++	++			
ROSA DAMASCENA	++	+	+	++	
RUMEX CRISPUS	++	+	+	++	C++
RUTA GRAVEOLENS	++	+++	+		C++
SABADILLA	++	++	+++	++	C+++
SABAL SERRULATA	+++	+++			
SABINA	++	++	+	+++	H++
SACCHARUM OFFICINALE	++	++	++	+	

L *denotes leading remedies within each miasm.*

Medicine	Psoric	Sycotic	Syphilitic	Tubercular	Chilly or Hot
SALICYLICUM ACIDUM	++	+	+	++	C+
SALIX NIGRA	++	++	+	++	
SALVIA OFFICINALIS	++	++		++	
SAMBUCUS NIGRA	++	++	+	++	C+
SANGUINARIA	++	+	++	+++	C+
SANGUINARIA NITRICA	++	+++	++	+	
SANICULA	++	+++	+	+	C+
SANTONINUM	++	++		+++	
SAPONARIA	++	++	+	+	
SAPONARIA	++	++	++	++	H+
SARCOLACTIC ACID	++	++	+	++	
SARRACENIA PURPUREA	++	+			C+
SARSAPARILLA	++	+++	++	+	C+
SCROPHULARIA NODOSA	++	+++	++	+++	C+
SCUTELLARIA	++	++	++	+	
SECALE CORNUTUM	++	++	++	+++	H++
SEDUM ACRE	++	++	+		
SELENIUM	++	+++	+	++	H++
SEMPERVIVUM TECTORUM	++	++	++	+++	
SENECIO AUREUS	++	++	++	++	C+
SENEGA	++	++	+	+	C++
SENNA	++	++			
SEPIA	++	+++ L	+	++	C+++
SERUM ANGUILLAR (EEL SERUM)	++	+++			
SILICEA	++	++	+++	+++ L	C+++
SILPHIUM	++	+++	++	+	
SINAPIS NIGRA	++	++		+++	
SKATOL	++	+	+++	+	
SKOOKUM CHUCK	+++	++	+	+++	
SOLANUM LYCOPERSICUM	++	+++		+	C++
SOLANUM NIGRUM	++	++	+++	+	
SOLIDAGO VIRGA	++	++	+	+++	
SPARTIUM SCOPARIUM	+++	++	+++	+	
SPIGELIA	++	++	+	+++	C++
SPIRAEA ULMARIA	++	+++	+	+	H+
SPIRANTHES	++	+++			
SPONGIA TOSTA	++	++		+++	H+
SQUILLA	++	++	+	++	
STANNUM	+++	++	++	+++ L	C++
STAPHYSAGRIA	++	+++ L	++	++	C++
STELLARIA MEDIA	+++	+++	+++ L	+	H++
STERCULIA	++	++	+		
STICTA	++	+++	+	++	C++
STIGMATA MAYDIS	++	+++			
STILLINGIA	++	+++	+++		C+
STRAMONIUM	++	+++	+	+	C++
STRONTIA	++	+++	+	+++	C+++
STROPHANTHUS HISPIDUS	++	+++		+	
STRYCHNIA PHOSPHORICA	++	+++	+	+	
STRYCHNINUM	++	++	++	+	
SUCCINUM	++	++		+	
SULFONAL	+++	+++		++	
SULPHUR	+++ L	++	+++	+++	H+++
SULPHUR IODATUM	++	+++	++	+	H+++
SULPHURICUM ACIDUM	++	++	+++	+++	C++
SULPHUROSUM ACIDUM	++	++	+++	++	
SUMBUL	+++	+++	+		C+
SYMPHORICARPUS RACEMOSA	++	++		+	
SYMPHYTUM	++	++	+	+	
SYPHILINUM	+++	++	+++ L	++	C++
SYZYGIUM JAMBOLANUM	+++	+	+++	++	
TABACUM	++	++	+		H+
TANACETUM VULGARE	+++	++	++		
TANNIC ACID	++	+++	+	++	

L *denotes leading remedies within each miasm.*

Medicine	Psoric	Sycotic	Syphilitic	Tubercular	Chilly or Hot
TARAXACUM	+++	+	+	+++	
TARENTULA CUBENSIS	++	+	+++L	++	
TARENTULA HISPANIA	++	+++	++	+++	H++
TARTARICUM ACIDUM	+++	++			H+
TAXUS BACCATA	++	+++	+	+++	
TELLURIUM	++	+++	++	++	C++
TEREBINTHINA	++	+++	++	+++ L	C+
TEUCRIUM MARUM VARUM	+++	+++	+	++	H+
THALLIUM	++	++	++	++	
THASPIUM AUREUM	++	++	+++		
THEA	++	+	+	++	C++
THERIDION	++	+++	++	+++	C+
THERIDION	+++	+++L	++	++	C++
THIOSINAMINUM	++	+++	+		
THLASPI BURSA PASTORIS	++	+++	+	+++ L	
THUJA OCCIDENTALIS	++	+++ L	++	++	C+++
THYMOL	++	+++		+	
THYMUS SERPYLLUM	++	++	+		
THYMUS SERPHYLLUM	+++	+++	+	+	
THYROIDINUM	++	+++ L	++	+++	C+++
TILIA EUROPA	++	++	++	+++	H++
TITANIUM	++	++	+	+++	
TONGO	++	++			
TORULA CEREVISIAE	++	+++	+		
TRIBULUS TERRESTRIS	++	+++		+	
TRIFOLIUM PRATENSE	++	++	+++	+	H+
TRILLIUM PENDULUM	++	++	++	+++ L	
TRINITROTOLUENE	+++	+	++	+++	
TRIOSTEUM PERFOLIATUM	++	+++	+	+	
TRITICUM – AGROPYRON REPENS	++	+++	+	+	
TROMBIDIUM	++	++	+++	+	
TUBERCULINUM	+++	+++	++	+++ L	C+++
TURNERA	++	+++			
TUSSILAGO PETASITES	++	+++			
UPAS TIENTE	++	++	+	+	
URANIUM NITRICUM	++	+++	++	++	
UREA	++	++	+	+++	
URTICA URENS	++	+++ L	+	+++	
USNEA BARBATA	+++	++		+	
USTILAGO MAYDIS	++	+++	+	++	
UVA URSI	++	+++	+	++	
VACCININUM	++	+++			
VALERIANA	++	++	+	+	C+
VANADIUM	++	++	++	++	
VANILLA	++	++		++	
VARIOLINUM	++	++	+	++	
VERATRUM ALBUM	+++	+++		++	C++
VERATRUM VIRIDE	++	+++	+	++	
VERBASCUM	+++	++	+	+++	
VERBENA	++	+	++	+	
VESPA CRABRO	++	++	+	++	
VIBURNUM OPULUS	++	+++	+	+	H++
VINCA MINOR	+++	+	+	+++	
VIOLA ODORATA	++	++	+	++	C++
VIOLA TRICOLOR	+++	+++	+		C++
VIPERA	++	+++	++	++	
VISCUM ALBUM	++	+++	++	++	C+++
WYETHIA	++	++	+	++	
XANTHOXYLUM	++	++	+	+	
XEROPHYLLUM	++	++	++	++	C+
X-RAY	++	+++ L	++	+	C+
YOHIMBINUM	++	++	+	++	
YUCCA FILAMENTOSA	++	+++		+	
ZINCUM METALLICUM	++	+++	++	++	

L *denotes leading remedies within each miasm.*

Medicine	Psoric	Sycotic	Syphilitic	Tubercular	Chilly or Hot
ZINCUM VALERIANUM	++	++	++	++	
ZINGIBER	++	+++		+	C+

MIASMATIC DIAGNOSIS:
LEADING ANTI-MIASMATIC MEDICINES

LEADING ANTI-PSORIC MEDICINES:

ALOES, *Alumina*, Ambra, Ammon.carb., Anacard, Ant.c., *Apis.mel.*, Arg.nit., *Ars. alb.*, Ars. iod., Avena sativa, Baryta.carb., *Bell*, Borax, Bryonia, Bufo.r., Calc.ars., **CALC.CARB.**, Caps, Carbo veg., Causticum, Cist.c., Coc.c., Conium.mac., Cup.m., Digit, *Dulcamara*, Ferr.met., Ferr.phos., *Graph*, **HEP.SULPH**, Hypericum, *Ignatia*, Kali phos., *Kali.carb.*, Lac.c., Lach., Led., **LYCO.**, *Mag.c.*, Mag.m., Mang.acet, Melilotus, Merc Cor, Merc Sol, Mur.ac. Nat.c., Natrum Mur, Nuphar Luteum, Nux Moschata, Nux Vomica, Nyctanthes, Opium, Paraffinum, Petrol, Phos, Platinum, Plumb.met., **PSORIN**, Pyrog., Rheum, Rhus tox, Robinia, Sabal ser, Sarsap., Secele cor, Selen., Silicea, Spartium Scoparium, Stan.met., Stellaria media, Sulfonal, **SULPH.**, Sulph.ac. Sumbul, Syphilinum, Syzigium Jambo, Tanacetum vulgare, Taraxacum. Tarent, Tartaric acid, Teucrium marum varum., Theridon, Usnea barbata, Veratrum album, Verbascun Vinca minor, Viola tricolor, **ZINC. MET.**

LEADING ANTI-SYCOTIC MEDICINES:

Abrotanum, Actaea racemosa, Agaricus mus., Agnus castus, Argentum met., Alumina, Ammonium benzoicum, Ammonium phosphoricum, Anacardium, Anagallis, Angustura vera, Ant.crudum, Antimonium tart., Apocynum cannabinium, **ARANEA.**, Arbutus andrachne, Arg.nit., Ars alb., Asterius, Aurum mur natronatum, *Bacillinum*, Baryta carb., *Benzoic acid*, Berb. vulg., *Bryonia*, Calc.carb., *Calc.iod.*, Cannabis sat, Carbo.sulph., Carbo.veg., Carbo an, Caulophyllum, **CAUSTICUM**, Chamomilla, **CONIUM.**, Dulcamara., Graphites, Helleborus, Hepar sulph., Hyoscyamus, *Kali.sulph.*, Kalmia latifolia, *Lachesis*, *Lapis albus*, Ledum pal, Lilium tigrinum, Lithium carb, *Lycopodium.*, Lycopus virginicus, Mag Phos, Mancinella, Mang.acet, **MEDORRHINUM**, Mephites, Merc.cor, Merc. dulcis, Merc. iod. flavus, Merc. iod. ruber, Merc. sulph, Murex, Mygale lasiodora, Myrica, **NAT.SULPH.**, *Natrum mur*, Natrum nitricum, **NIT. AC.**, Nitri spiritus dulcis, Ocimum can, Oleum santali, Oophorinum, Operculina turpethum, Origanum, Ostrya virginica, Oxydendron, Palladium, Pareira brava, Passiflora incar, Penthorum, Petroselinum, Phosphorus, Physalis, Piper methysticum, Pituitrin, Platina, Plumbum Met, **PULSATILLA, PYROGEN, RADIUM BROMIDE.**, Raphanus, Rhamnus cali., Rhodium, Rhododenron, Rhus tox, Rhus aromatica, Rhus glabra, Ruta grav., Sabal ser., Sabina., Sanguinaria nit, Sanicula, *Sarsap*, Scrophularia, Secal., Selen., **SEPIA**, Serum Anguillar, Sinnab., Solanum Lycopers, Spiranthes, **STAPHYSAG.**, Stellaria media, Sticta pulmonalis, Stigmata maydis, Stillingia, Stramo, Strontia, Strophanthus hisp, Strychnia, Sulfonal, Sulphur iod., Sumbul, Tannic ac., Tarantula hisp., Taxus baccata, Tellurium, Terebinth, Teucrium marum varum, Theridion, Thiosinaminum, Thlaspi bursa pastoris, **THUJA**, Thymol, **THYROIDINUM**, Torula cerevisiae, Tribulus terrestris, Triosteum perfoliatum, Tuberculinum, Turnera, Tussilago petasites, Uranium Nitricum, **URTICA URENS**, Ustilago maydis, Uva ursi, Vaccininum, **VARIOLINUM;** Veratrum album, Veratrum Vir, Viburnum Op, Viola Tricolor, Viscum Album, **X-Ray**, Yucca filamentosa, Zincum Met, Zingiber,

LEADING ANTI-SYPHILITIC MEDICINES:

Anthracinum, Arg nit., Arg.met., Ars. bromatum, Ars. metallicum, Ars.alb., Ars.iod., Artemisia vulgaris, Aurum.mur.nat., Asafoetida., Aurm.iod., **AURUM MET.**, Aurum.brom., Badiaga, Baptisia, Calc.ars., *Calc.fl.*, Calc.iod.; Calc.s., Calendula, *Cannabis sat*, Cantharides, Carbo.an., Carbo.veg., Carbo.an., **CARCINOSIN., CINAB.**, *Clematis.*, Conium., Corallium.rub., **FLUORIC ACID.**, Guaiacum, *Hep.sulph.*, Hydrastis, **HYDROPHOBINUM**, Iodum., Kali.ars., **KALI.BICH.**, Kali.carb., **KALI.IOD.**, Kali.mur., Kali.sulph., Kalmia., **KREOSOTE.**, Lach., Ledum pal., Lycopodium, Manganum aceticum, Merc. iod flavus, *Merc.bin.iod., Merc.bromatus., Merc.cor., Merc.cyan., Merc.dulcis, Merc.iod.fl., Merc.iod.rub., Merc.proto iod.*, **MERC.SOL., MEZEREUM.**, Morphinum, Muriatic acid, Myristica seibifera, **NITRIC ACID**, Ornithogalum, Osmium., Paeonia, Petroleum., *Phos*, Phos.ac., Physostigma,

L denotes leading remedies within each miasm.

PHYTOLACCA, Pyrogen, Ratanhia, Rhus Ven, Sabadilla, Sarsaparilla, Silicea, Solanum nigram, Spartium scoparium, **STELLARIA**., Stillingia, Sulphur, Sulphuric acid, Sulphurosum acidum, **SYPHILINUM**., Syzigium jambo, **TARANTULA CUB**, Thaspium aureum, Trifolium pratese, Trombidium, Tuberculinum.

LEADING ANTI-TUBERCULAR MEDICINES:

Acalypha ind., *Acet.ac.*, Agaricus muscarius, Ailanthus glandulosa, Allium cepa, Allium sat., Ammonium carbonicum, Ammon causticum, Antim tart., Arg nit., *Arnica mont.*, **ARS. IOD., BACILLINUM,** Baptisia, Baryta carb, *Belladonna*, Bromium, Bufo, Cactus grandiflorus,**CALC.CARB.**, **CALC.IOD.**, *Calc.phos.*, *Calc.sulph.*, *Carbo.an.*, Carbo.veg., *Carcinosin,* Chin.ars., **CHINA**, Cistus can, Conium mac., Crotalus horridus, Dros., Dulc., Elaps., Ferr.ars., Ferr.i., *Ferr.phos.*, Galium.ap., *Hamamelis vir.*, Helleborus, Hep. sulph, **HYDRAS.,** Hydrophobinum, Iberis, Ignatia, **IOD**., *Ipecac, Kali.c.*, Kali.chl., Kali.iod., Kali.nit., Kali.p., Kali.s., Lac.def., Lach., Lachnanth., Laurocer., Leptandra, Lyco., Mangifera indica, Merc cyanatus, Merc dulcis, Merc iod. flavus, Merc sol, **MILLEFOLIUM**, Muriatic acid, Naja tripudians, Natrum salicyclicum, Natrum nitricum, *Nit.ac.,* Oleum jec., Oxalicum acidum, Phelland., **PHOS. ACID., PHOS.,** Pilocarpus, Plumbum met., Polygon.av., Psorinum, Sabina, Sang. Can., Santoninum, Scrophularia nodosa, Secale Cor, Sempervivum tectorum, Senecio.aureus, Seneg., Sepia, **SILICEA**., Sinapis nigra, Skookum chuck, Solidago virga, Spigelia, Spong. tosta, Stann. Met., Strontia, *Sulphur*, Sulphuric acid, Taraxacum, Tarent. cub., Taxus Buccata, **TEREBINTH**, Theridion, **THLASPI BURSA PASTORIS**, Thyroidinum, Tilia europa, Titanum, **TRILLIUM PENDULUM**, Tri nitro toluene, **TUBERCULINUM**, Urea, Urtica urens, Verbascum, Vinca minor.

LEADING TRI-MIASMATICS:

Arg.Nit., Calcarea.Carb., Carcinosin, Causticum, Hydrophobinum (Lyssin), Hep.sulph., Lycopodium., Merc sol, Nitric acid., Phosphorus, Stellaria media, Sulphur, Tuberculinum.

L denotes leading remedies within each miasm.

PART — VII
MIASMATIC PRESCRIBING :
MODERN CLASSICAL PRESCRIBING - PRACTICAL APPROACH - <u>CLASSICAL PRESCRIBING</u>

APPROACH- A

<u>NON-SUPPRESSED CASES: CASES WITH CLARITY OF SYMPTOMS</u>:

MTEK is an useful memory aid to arriving at a correct prescription.

- **M** = Miasmatic Totality
- **T** = Totality of Symptoms
- **E** = Essence (should include gestures, postures, behaviours etc)
- **K** = Keynotes (which should encompass PQRS symptoms, refer §153 and §209 of Hahnemann's Organon)

When the above criteria are considered and the steps below followed, a correct prescription can be made.

<u>Step-I</u>: Make the miasmatic diagnosis of the case i.e. ascertain the surface miasm.

<u>Step-II</u>: Assess the Totality of Symptoms + Essence + Keynotes and PQRS (if any) of the case and formulate the indicated remedy.

<u>Step-III</u>: Ensure that the indicated remedy covers the surface miasm, as diagnosed in Step I.

<u>Step-IV</u>: Administer the remedy, which encompasses the miasm as well as the Totality of Symptoms.

<u>Step-I</u>:

Make the miasmatic diagnosis of the case i.e. ascertain the surface miasm, this can be done by:

(a) **Head to foot assessment of symptoms** (please refer Miasmatic Prescribing by Subrata K. Banerjea);

(b) **Through clinical manifestation of disease**, e.g. hypo/scanty/less are psora (e.g. hypotension, atrophy, anaemia etc); hypers are sycotic (e.g. hypertension, hypertrophy, hyperplasia etc.); dyses are syphilitic (e.g. dystrophy, dysplasia etc.) and allergies and haemorrhages are tubercular (e.g. hay fever, menorrhagia etc).

(c) **Through psychic essence, nature and character of the individual case** (e.g. suspicious, jealous and exploiting in nature represents sycosis; destructive and cruel to animals represents syphilis; stubborn, changeable and impatient natures are tubercular etc.)

(d) We can diagnose the miasm from other, different aspects, e.g. reference to **hair falling**: alopecia with dry lustreless hair and bran-like dandruff is psora; circular or spotty baldness is sycotic; diffused hair falling is syphilitic, and thick yellow crusts in the hair are tubercular; in reference to **taste**: burnt is psoric; fishy is sycotic; metallic is syphilitic and taste of pus is tubercular; in reference to **pulse**: bradycardia is psoric; tachycardia is sycotic and irregular pulse is syphilitic; in reference to **bowels**: constipation is psoric; diarrhoea is sycotic; dysentery is syphilitic and malaena is tubercular; in reference to **pains**: neuralgic pains are psoric; joint pains are sycotic; bone pains are syphilitic and pains with exhaustion are tubercular.

(e) **Diathesis** (tendencies/pre-disposition) can also hint the miasm: eruptive diathesis is psoric; rheumatic-gouty, lithic-uric acid or proliferative diathesis is sycotic; suppurative-ulcerative is syphilitic and haemorrhagic diathesis is tubercular.

(f) Psoric secretions are watery, mucussy, serous; sycotics are purulent, yellowish; sticky, acrid, putrid and offensive are syphilitic and haemorrhagic secretions/discharges are tubercular.

(g) If you ask your patient what his hobbies are: 'hunting' reflects syphilitic taint; 'travelling' is tubercular, whereas 'gambling' is sycotic!

(h) Ask your patient: 'If you could take a week off and money would be no object, what would you do?' Mr. Psora is lazy and will do nothing; Mr. Tubercular will go on a round the world trip! Thereby you understand the innate dyscrasia and miasmatic nature of your patient.

(i) Miasmatic diagnosis can be made from nail appearance; e.g. dry harsh nails are psoric; thick, wavy, ribbed, corrugated, convex nails are sycotic; thin, spoon shaped concave nails are syphilitic and glossy and spotted nails are tubercular.

(j) Miasmatic observation of children: nervous, anxious, constipated children are psoric; restless, hyperactive (ADHD), colicky, diarrhoeic children are sycotic; withdrawn, dull, extremely forgetful, convulsive, dysenteric children are syphilitic and allergic, haemorrhagic, stubborn, impatient children are tubercular.

By such a prescription, which covers the miasmatic dyscrasia of the person, the chances of recurrence are eradicated and the axiom of 'rapid, gentle and permanent recovery' (Hahnemann's Organon §3) is encompassed. In cases of one-sided disease with a scarcity of symptoms, the action of the anti-miasmatic remedy is centrifugal, and by bringing the suppressed symptoms to the surface, allows a proper totality to be framed.

The miasmatic consideration is therefore of great importance as demonstrated in the following example:-

A person is suffering from features of gastric ulcer, which has been confirmed by radiography. As ulceration is syphilitic, the surface miasm is therefore syphilitic also. Let us say that the totality of symptoms (physical, emotional and essence) of the person reflects towards Kali Bichromicum, an anti-syphilitic remedy. The choice of remedy is therefore simple, as Kali Bich covers both the totality of symptoms and the surface miasm of this gastric ulcer case. Kali Bich will peel away the outer layer and reveal a second layer underneath. This second layer may perhaps manifest through the appearance of warts or moles on the face, an indication of suppressed sycosis and the next assessment of the case should include this new surface totality. Following Kentian ideology we now know that there needs to be a change in the plan of treatment, that is, the previous syphilitic plan needs to change to a current sycotic plan, and a new anti-sycotic medicine needs to be selected based on the presenting totality.

<u>**Step II**</u>:

Assess the Totality of Symptoms + Essence + Keynotes and PQRS (if any) of the case and formulate the indicated remedy.

Totality of symptoms:

(1) Each of the symptoms must be complete with regard to its location, sensation, modality and concomitant (Subrata's addition : Cause and onset, duration of the suffering and treatments he/she had in the past.)

(2) The symptoms should have a chronological order of development and progression.

(3) Environmental, occupational and other exogenous influences on the case must be evaluated.

(4) Then the background of the case from (a) the past history (with special reference to various forms of suppressions) and (b) the family history (inherited miasmatic influences), must be in the purview.

(5) The qualitative totality of all the symptoms (outwardly reflected picture of the internal essence of the disease) is the sole indication for the choice of the remedy.

Essence:

i) Acquaintance with the psychic essences and personification of 'Drug Pictures' [e.g. Mr. Lycopodiums are teachers, doctors, successful dictators, and politicians; and their personality characteristics reflect they are careful; cautious; conscientious; conservative; courteous; contained; avoid risk and commitments - Mr. Safe; Mr. Nux Vomicas are CEO, share brokers, salesman, and their personality characteristics reflect they are ambitious, impatient, arrogant, charismatic, aggressive, independent, confident, courteous, workaholics, perfectionists; Mrs. Pulsatillas are nursery nurses teachers, carers. and their personality characteristics reflect they are emotional-tearful, moody, changeable, pleasing, perceptive, affectionate, caring, forsaken, worriers; and Miss Phosphorus' can be artists, actors, receptionists, maitre d'hotel, politicians, and their personality characteristics reflect they are expressive, emotional, social, artistic, impressionable, gregarious, sympathetic and sensitive] with modern interpretations of old proving symptoms;

ii) To ascertain a clearer picture for the constitutional medicine e.g. ask about the **innate nature** of the person, for example 'Give ten words to describe yourself'. and when patient says I am **COMPASSIONATE**: - e.g. Arg-nit, Bell, Calc, Calc.Phos, Carcin, Caust, Coccul, Graph., Ign, Lach, Nat-c. Nat-m, Nit-ac, Nux-v, Phos, Puls., Sulph; **DUTIFUL** :- Calc, Calc-I, Carcin.,Cocculus, Ignatia, Kali-ars., Kali-c, Kali iod., Lyco, Nat-m, Puls; **EASY GOING** :- Ars, Calc, Carc, Lil.Tig., Lyco, Mag Mur., Nat-m, Nux-v, Phos-ac, Phos, Puls, Rhus Tox, Sepia, Sil., Sulph, Thuja; **FAMILY ORIENTED** :- Acet-ac, Anac., Ars, Baryta C., Calc, Calc-I, Calc-sil, Carc., Graph., Hep, Ign., Iod., Kali Br., Kali Nit., Kali Phos., Lyco.,Mag Carb., Nat Carb.,Nat Mur., Petr, Phos, Phos.Ac., Puls, Psor., Rhus-t, Sulph. etc. *These are modern extensions/ interpretations of old proving symptoms and not found in the Repertory books and Subrata has developed an extensive Repertory of Personality Characters.*

APPROACH- B

CONTAMINATED DRUG DEPENDENT CASES: CASES WITHOUT CLARITY OF SYMPTOMS:

i) In drug dependent cases placing emphasis on Lesser Known Medicines (e.g. Franciscea, Ginseng, Pimpenella, Stellaria, Viola etc. to open the *steroid dependant arthritic cases* with few uncontaminated symptoms and absence of clear modalities can prove beneficial; such lesser known organopathic medicines have capability to alleviate symptoms to certain extent, thereby giving the chance to wean off the conventional medication, and experience shows that after 40-50% weaning off; uncontaminated symptoms of the natural disease surface and give scope for constitutional prescribing) can succeed when well selected remedies fail;

ii) For example, in drug dependent asthma cases, when the patient is on an inhaler and/or steroids; in such cases it is very difficult to get a clear picture of the case. The artificial chronic disease is superimposed on the original natural disease, therefore symptoms are contaminated or suppressed and the patient cannot give a clear picture e.g., modalities, etc. In such cases, homoeopathic bronchodilators e.g., Aralia Racemosa, Blatta Orientalis, Aspidosperma, Cassia Sophera, Eriodictyon, Pothos Foetidus etc., can be prescribed on the basis of few available symptoms (according to §173--§178, Ref. Organon of Medicine) and gradually the conventional allopathic bronchodilator is withdrawn [Subrata asks the patient to sip the homoeopathic bronchodilator, medicine prescribed on the basis of symptomatic similarity, when the patient is out of breath and in need of conventional bronchodilator. Patient takes the homoeopathic medicine and tries to defer the conventional medicine as much as s/he can. In this way, a steroid dependent patient who used to take steroid/inhaler 8 hourly; can, with the help of homoeopathic medicine now defer the steroids to 12 hourly. This is the way conventional medication is gradually weaned off].

In the same way, for pain killer dependent Migraine cases, the artificial chronic disease is superimposed on the original natural disease, therefore symptoms are contaminated or suppressed and the patient cannot give a clear picture for a constitutional medicine as well as the modalities of the pain are masked. Therefore, the following medicines can be selected on the basis of few available symptoms, e.g., Acetanilidum, Anagyris, Bromium, Chionanthus Virginica, Epiphegus, Ferrum Pyro-Phosphoricum, Indium, Iris Versicolor, Kalmia Latifolia, Lac Defloratum, Melilotus, Menispernum, Menynanthes, Oleum Animale, Onosmodium, Saponin, Usnea Barbata, Yucca Filamentosa. Accordingly the conventional allopathic pain killer is gradually withdrawn and after approximately 50% weaning off of the conventional medicine, suppressed symptoms surface and now the patient can give much clearer modalities. This will lead to making a change in the plan of treatment and on the basis of 'MTEK' a constitutional prescription can now be made.

Similar example for Drug Dependent Hypertensive cases where the following medicines (Allium Sativa, Crataegus Oxyacantha, Eel Serum, Ergotinum, Lycopus Virginicus, Rauwolfia Serpentina, Spartium Scoparium, Strophanthus Hispidus) are capable of gradually weaning off the conventional medication.

iii) Generally experience shows after approximately 50% weaning off of the conventional medicine, suppressed symptoms surface and now the patient can give much clearer modalities. This will lead to making a change in the plan of treatment and on the basis of 'MTEK' a constitutional prescription can now be made. Through this approach, not only does the patient gain immediate confidence that homoeopathy works, but can also wean off the conventional medication to certain extent.

PART — VIII
MIASMATIC PRESCRIBING: MIASMATIC INTERPRETATION IN PRESCRIBING – CASE ILLUSTRATIONS

CASE-1

AN OBSTINATE LONG STANDING CASE OF PSORIASIS, COMPLETELY CURED

PRESENTING COMPLAINTS:

Mr. A.L. 52 yrs. old, came to me first on 11th April, 1987, complaining as follows:

(1) Eruptions all over the body, skin dries and peels off, no discharge of blood, fluid or pus. No itching, no pain.
(2) Scaly in character with profuse bran like scaling.
(3) The skin disease started in 1970, at the seaside in Goa and since then the patient has consulted various dermatologists without any appreciable change.
(4) It started on the trunk, chest and back, and slowly spread over almost all parts of the body covered by clothes.
(5) The face and scalp were clear from the beginning.
(6) Previously there was nothing on the palms but around 1978, one circular spot appeared near the wrist. The patient tried to conceal that during his office hours, so he put on gloves and subsequently it broke virulently in the palm and dorsum of both the hands.
(7) The patient also tried various Ayurvedic and Homoeopathic medicines and ointments without any permanent improvement.
(8) Occasional cough during winter.
(9) Appetite - Normal.
(10) Sweat - Profuse.
(11) Stool and urine - Normal.
(12) Sexual organs - Nothing abnormal is noted.
(13) Skin heals in normal time; does not suppurate.
(14) Temperament - Mild, quiet and non communicative, sympathetic, depressed, occasionally weepy.
(15) Memory - Normal.
(16) Fears - Nothing particular.
(17) Past History (i) Typhoid in 1964. (ii) Asthma in 1985. (iii) Psoriasis since 1970.
Patient had allopathic treatment for typhoid and asthma, including steroids for asthma.
(18) Vaccinations - No adverse reaction.
(19) Chilly patient who also catches cold easily.
(20) Likes spicy food, salt ++, salty +, cold food ++. Likes meat, but after eating red meat there is unusual irritation and discomfort in the skin.
(21) Though chilly, likes winter, which is better for skin. Dislikes rainy weather and damp. Easily affected by changes in weather.
(22) Thirst - Normal.
(23) Perspiration- Heavy and oily.
(24) Sleep and dreams - Nothing abnormal noted.
(25) Married with four children.

(26) Family History
- (i) Father died at the age of 45 with asthma.
- (ii) Mother died of hepatitis at the age of 48.

A. **PROVISIONAL DIAGNOSIS:** Psoriasis.

B. **MIASMATIC DIAGNOSIS:** Mixed miasmatic (preponderance of psora-sycosis).

MIASMATIC INTERPRETATION OF THE PSORIASIS CASE

PSORA	SYCOSIS	SYPHILIS	TUBERCULAR
• Skin dry and harsh • Mild, silent temperament	• Skin peels off • Skin scaly in character • Circular spots appeared near the wrist • Oily skin with thickly oozing perspiration • Psoriasis • Tendency to conceal the symptoms • H/O Asthma is Psora-sycotic • Desire for salt & salty foods • Meat causes uneasiness • Hates rainy weather & damp • F/H of asthma with father • Fish scale eruptions are tri-miasmatic	• Depressed	• Chilly • Catches cold easily • Desires salt

Psora 2   Sycosis 12   Syphilis 1   Tubercular 3

In this case there is a clear Sycotic preponderance in the history and the presenting symptoms reflect Sycosis as a surface miasm. On the basis of the totality of symptoms Thuja was chosen, which covered the surface miasm and the family history. Thuja also covers the surface symptoms as well as the surface miasm and therefore it is capable of peeling off this presenting layer. In this case there was no need to compare remedies miasmatically as the case was clearly Thuja (presenting symptoms and the surface miasm supports the prescription), however in few other cases below you will see how the miasmatic analysis helped to differentiate the remedy choice as the case was confused by excessive suppression.

This is a wonderful example of how miasmatic interpretation of a case helps the certainty of chronic prescribing as Thuja covers the miasmatic totality as well as the totality of symptoms therefore one can be confident to watch and wait for the movement of symptoms. In this case, you can see from the illustrations that after 50% improvement of the case, the appearances of the skin lesions were circular which confirmed that the patient still required a Sycotic medicine, therefore no change in the miasmatic plan of treatment was required. This reflects that miasmatic understanding helps in management and prognosis of the case and confirms any need for a change in the plan of treatment.

Note: Generally in psoriasis, one may find the dryness of Psora, squamous character of Syphilis and thickened skin with fish scale eruptions of Sycosis.

PRESCRIPTION CHART

Dates	Points in favour of the Prescription	Prescribed Medicine
11th Apr'87	(i) Eruptions are only in the covered areas; (ii) Oily & shiny appearance of the face; (iii) Change of weather affects the patient; (iv) Chilly patient but desires cold food; (v) Averse to rainy season (hydrogenoid); (vi) Sycotic coverage.	Thuja 30 1 dose followed (48 hours later) by Thuja LM 3 1 globule in a bottle of water to be sipped --- top up – sip --- top up continue like this for 1 week.
12th May'87	Severe <aggravation.	Thuja LM 5 1 globule in a bottle of water to be sipped --- top up – sip --- top up continue like this for 1 week.
11th Jun'87	Entire layer of skin from the sole came off, patient feeling better on the whole.	Thuja LM 7 1 globule in a bottle of water to be sipped --- top up – sip --- top up continue like this for 1 week.
10th Jul'87	Patient complaining of nocturnal fever, night sweats, hot flushes. No change in skin. Change in the plan of treatment. Anti-tubercular coverage.	Ars. Iod. 30 2 doses (1 globule in water to be divided into two doses) (alternate mornings)
25th Jul'87	Feeling better of the nocturnal fever. Wait and watch before any change.	Wait and watch.
31st Jul'87	Patient came back with severe dyspnoea (a return of an old symptom suppressed by allopathic medicine). Patient is having attacks at midnight and better in orthopnoea (bending forward with piled up pillows to lay on).	Ars. Alb. 30 2 doses (daily morning).
10th Aug'87	Dyspnoea is much better. Change of plan of treatment. Complementary of Arsenicum album, i.e. Thuja being prescribed again.	Thuja LM 9 1 globule in a bottle of water to be sipped --- top up – sip --- top up continue like this for 1 week.

Dates	Points in favour of the Prescription	Prescribed Medicine
8th Sep'87	As a whole psoriasis is better again and the patient feels well.	Thuja LM 11 1 globule in a bottle of water to be sipped --- top up – sip --- top up continue like this for 1 week.
26th Sep'87	Feeling better. Psoriasis disappearing from above downwards. Upper part of the trunk, palms, soles and the back are 50% better.	Thuja LM 13 1 globule in a bottle of water to be sipped --- top up – sip --- top up continue like this for 1 week.
29th Oct'87	Entire layer from the shin-bone came off. As a whole feeling better. Appetite increased. Depression is much less.	Thuja LM 15 1 globule in a bottle of water to be sipped --- top up – sip --- top up continue like this for 1 week.
3rd Dec'87	The eruptions are slowly disappearing. No new scales or patches have appeared.	Thuja LM 17 1 globule in a bottle of water to be sipped --- top up – sip --- top up continue like this for 1 week.
4th Jan'88	The eruptions are slowly disappearing. No new patches have appeared.	Thuja LM 19 1 globule in a bottle of water to be sipped --- top up – sip --- top up continue like this for week.
4th Feb'88	The eruptions are slowly disappearing. No new patches have appeared	Thuja LM 21 1 globule in a bottle of water to be sipped --- top up – sip --- top up continue like this for 1 week
7th Mar'88	Patient is much better. I have changed the scale and potency, to finish the case.	Thuja 10M 1 globule in a bottle of water to be sipped --- top up – sip --- top up continue like this for 10 days.
5th Apr'88	Much better. Wait and watch.	Wait and watch.
19th May'88	Much better. Wait and watch.	Wait and watch.

Dates	Points in favour of the Prescription	Prescribed Medicine
13th Jul'88	Much better. To finish the case and to observe if there is any residue to resolve and see if anything new appears.	Thuja 50M 1 globule in a bottle of water to be sipped --- top up – sip --- top up continue like this for 10 days.
5th Sep'88	Much better. To finish the case and to observe if there is any residue to resolve and see if anything new appears.	Thuja CM 1 globule in a bottle of water to be sipped --- top up – sip --- top up continue like this for 10 days.
21st Nov'88	Nothing noted to complain about. Overall very well. Still I asked him to visit, so that he can be prescribed a deep acting anti-tubercular to close.	Wait and watch.
30th Jan'89	Total cure. To finish the case deep acting Syco-tubercular remedy.	Bacillinum 200 1 globule in a bottle of water to be sipped --- top up – sip --- top up continue like this for 10 days.
	Instruction to the patient - only visit if any symptoms re occur.	

MIASMATIC APPROACH IN PSORIASIS TREATMENT

(1) Dr. H. Roberts says, Psoriasis is the marriage of all miasms, but its characteristics are predominantly Psoric and Sycotic.

(2) My approach for the treatment of chronic cases is always from the miasmatic point of view, the heritage that I have descended from, my three generations of homoeopaths. I do take up the whole case and from the totality of symptoms, I make a miasmatic totality and thereby arrive at a miasmatic diagnosis of the case. Then, I like to ensure that the remedy which is indicated by the totality of the symptoms, should cover the miasmatic totality too. Or in other words, the remedy should also cover the miasmatic background of the patient. In this way I am confident my prescribed remedy always covers both the totality of symptoms and the miasmatic dyscrasia of the patient and the cure becomes permanent as discussed in §3 of Hahnemann's Organon of Medicine

(3) In this case of Psoriasis, I started with a deep acting anti-sycotic remedy, as there was sycotic preponderance, but one should also remember, that polychrests like Thuja, do cover most of the miasms in greater or lesser degrees. So in this tri-miasmatic case of Psoriasis, Thuja not only covered the sycotic preponderance but also touched the other miasms.

(4) I've learnt from the collective experience of 106 years of my ancestral homoeopaths, who passed their gems of wisdom from one generation to the next, that in Psoriasis cases at any stage or at the end, you will find the tubercular miasmatic state will surface and a deep acting anti-tubercular remedy will be needed on the basis of the presenting totality of symptoms. This will ensure the cure is permanent. The `Medicine of Experience'! **I never prescribe for miasm but prescribe for miasmatic state and their presenting symptoms**. It is the ability of the physician to skilfully elicit the symptoms from the patient, in order to assess the surface and the latent miasms.

(5) In Case 1 above, Bacillinum was prescribed as a completing remedy which is a Syco (++) Tubercular (+++) remedy; and also, Bacillinum has the capacity to throw out to the surface the eruptions, which were suppressed previously by the use of allopathic steroid medicines. This property of Bacillinum has also been recognised by Dr. Burnett in terms of ringworm - repercussion.

CONCLUSION

This was a very interesting case of long-standing Psoriasis and through my miasmatic approach of prescribing, the patient has not only found relief from his problem but still over twenty years later enjoys permanent good health.

*Readers may view the pictures of the case (before and after treatment) in our website under Dermatological Diseases (**Case No. D001**- A case of Psoriasis in a middle aged man, completely cured by Thuja).*

CASE-2

A DIAGNOSED CASE OF ATOPIC DERMATITIS

Name of the Patient Mast. S.K.S, boy born in 1983

PRESENTING COMPLAINTS

(1)   Skin eruption especially on the face, since six months of age.
(2)   Multiple small, red eruptions; pustular and vesicular in type, for last five and half years Oozing fluid and pus. Cycle of pustules → oozes → pus and blood → becomes crusty → child picks and scratches → bleeds → pus → dries → crust again.
(3)   Itching (+++), better by gentle rubbing confirmed by observation and also confirmed by the parents. Hard scratching made the eruption bleed, feels a little better from gentle rubbing. (i) Itching of the skin aggravates at night, from warmth. (ii) Itching aggravates in summer, from heat of the sun. (iii) Itching aggravates by washing; hot or cold. (iv) Skin discomfort aggravation from sour foods and fruit. (v) Skin discomfort aggravation from sweat.
(4)   Stinging and cutting pains (++) with occasional burning in the affected areas of skin. The boy weeps and cries due to the tremendous discomfort which results from itching → bleeding and pus formation with a sensation of rawness of the affected areas and from picking the crusts.
(5)   Had alot of allopathic treatment, including cortisone ointments; and Ayurvedic (naturopathic) treatment without any appreciable or permanent change.
(6)   Chronic loose stool 4-5 times per day with froth and mucus (++) for last two years. This diarrhoea aggravates from motion, eating. Urging initiated after meals or any light food.
(7)   Occasional right sided abdominal pain.
(8)   Extremely painful (+++). Lymph glands around neck swollen for last 3 years (?Cervical lymphadenopathy as diagnosed by medical doctor). Aggravation from cold, touch, pressure; better from warm application.
(9)   HEAD - Occasional pain in forehead; aggravated in the sun and better by rest.
(10) EAR - Otorrhoea (discharge from ear) with itching.
(11) THROAT - Occasional throat pain, sore throat from cold, better by warm gargling.
(12) LUNGS - Occasional dry cough; aggravates at night.
(13) ABDOMEN – (i) Gas and distension in abdomen. (ii) Gurgling sound in stomach aggravation after full meals. (iii) Occasional right sided abdominal colic, which is aggravated by warm milk.
(14) STOMACH - Appetite decreased.
(15) URINE - Nothing abnormal.

(16) STOOL- (i) Ineffectual urging, aggravated after eating, with heavy feeling in abdomen. (ii) Profuse, yellowish stool with mucus (++), watery (++), frothy (++), less faecal matter. (iii) Loose, 4-5 times a day; aggravates after meals. (iv) Cramps in right side of abdomen, with urging, before evacuation; better after passing stool. (v) Due to profuse expulsion of stool, child exhausted after each evacuation.

(17) Mental Symptoms - angry, irritable temper (+), quarrelsome (+), fault-finding (+), obstinate and stubborn. Suspicious (+). Jealous of his friends as they can enjoy normal life whilst he can't. Silent, absent-minded (+), gloomy, timid, broods in silence. Likes to be alone (+). Fear of death (+). Disgusted with life as if the enjoyment of the entire childhood has been lost. Memory weak. Gradual loss of memory (+). This is mainly due to his absent-mindedness. Gloomy and morose (perturbed by the discomfort of the skin). Weeping mood (+). Involuntary sighing. He cries when reprimanded (+). The child is intensely sympathetic (++). He does everything slowly (+). He has a fear of ghosts (+), darkness (+), incurable diseases (+) and accidents (+).

(18) Has applied a profuse quantity of allopathic creams and lotions, and also tried herbal oils. Feels relieved for some period of time; thereafter it comes back again and generally returns worse than the previous state so he is afraid of trying anything, any more. Totally frustrated. Gonorrhoea of father.

(19) Past History - Skin disease from the age of 6 months, measles at the age of 3.

(20) First cause of breakdown of health (N.B.W.S. Never Been Well Since) - Skin disease. Cervical glands.

(21) Homoeopathic Generalities:

(22) Heat and cold reaction - Hot patient; likes open air; catches cold easily.

(23) Desires and aversions for food - Sweet +, pungent and hot +, salty +. Potato, meat and chicken +, rich, spicy and fatty food +, warm food +, cold drinks +, ice cream +. Thirsty.

(24) Sleep and dreams - Sleeps well during the later part of night. Disturbed sleep and difficulty in falling asleep due to skin discomfort. No recurrent dreams.

(25) Perspiration - Profuse sweat on face and axillae. Sour smelling. Stains the clothes yellow.

(26) Family History - Father had asthma, bronchitis; Mother had eczema during pregnancy with this child; cured by ointment.

(27) Previous Treatment - Allopathic or Pharmaceutical prescriptions. Ayurvedic or Naturopathy, including herbal oils. Homoeopathic medicines prescribed by colleagues. Bacillinum, Graphites and Sulphur in LM and different Centesimal scales all without any appreciable change.

(28) Provisional diagnosis- Exfoliative dermatitis with cervical lymphadenopathy, Atopic dermatitis.

CASE ANALYSIS, MIASMATIC DIAGNOSIS AND FINAL PRESCRIPTION

Miasmatic Analysis

PSORA	SYCOSIS	SYPHILIS	TUBERCULAR
- Itching+++ - Itching << washing - Itching << by eating sour fruit or food - Sun headache - Headache better by rest - Dry cough - Gas and distension in abdomen - Silent, timid - Unhealthy skin represents Psora. Also Psora creates irritation in general → physical itching → over the skin - Desires sweet, pungent and hot foods - Various fears - darkness, ghosts, accidents, incurable diseases	- Multiple vesicular eruptions - Skin stinging - Chronic loose stool - Yellowish stool - Cramp in right side of abdomen - Quarrelsome - Suspicious - Sympathetic - Profuse sweat - Stains the clothes yellow	- All sorts of boils, ulcers, which do not heal fast. - Discharge of pus, which is offensive. - Itching < at night, from warmth - Itching < summer - Skin discomfort < by sweat - Skin burning - Sensation of rawness - Stool with mucus - Discharge from ear - Sore throat from cold - Disgusted with life - Chronic loose motion dysentery (Recurrent problem Tubercular - Syphilitic) - Desires spicy ++ - Desires to be alone	- Oozing of blood - Swollen lymph glands around neck - Exhaustion after evacuation - Fault finding, critical - Stubborn - Recurrent and obstinate boils and pimples with profuse pus - Skin problem < at night, warmth < after itching and cold washing - Cervical lymph-adenopathy - As a result of suffering from severe diseases suppurative otitis media appears

Psora   11   Sycosis   10   Syphilis   13   Tubercular   9

This is a mixed miasmatic case with Psora-Syphilo-Tubercular preponderance. As the young boy had such a long history of suppression and therefore the symptoms were quite complicated, Croton Tig was indicated on the basis of the totality with special emphasis on a very peculiar modality, *itching better by gentle rubbing*. It covers the multi-miasmatic background with Psoric preponderance so once again it was a wonderful example of prescribing a medicine which covers the surface symptoms, as well as the surface miasm. By including the miasm in the prescription one can become more confident about the correct selection of the medicine and stay with the medicine with confidence. *The same principle will apply when, by virtue of repertorisation, you have finally ended with four or five top ranking medicines and are now feeling confused about the final selection. In such a case, evaluate the miasmatic background of the case and make sure your final indicated medicine not only covers the symptoms but the miasmatic expression of the case as well.*

FINAL PRESCRIPTION AND REMEDY REACTION

I started the case with Cortisone in homoeopathic potency with an idea to use tautopathy and remove the prolonged bad effect caused by Cortisone (pharmaceutical preparation). I think Cortisone had initially removed the bad effect and thereafter I switched on to Sulphur which I will confess was a mistake and there was no appreciable change. Also it was a case with Syphilo-psoric preponderance. Finally, I realised the presence of Croton Tig symptoms and re-visited the miasmatic analysis. The reasons for the prescription of Croton Tig has been given below in the chart.

Date	Report After Last Medication	Prescription done On the Basis of	Treatment
12th Dec'89		To remove the bad effects of the prolonged use of Cortisone group of ointments.	Cortisone, 200C 1 globule Organon, F.N. §246 (5th ed); §275 (6th ed)]; globule size number X [Size of the poppy-seed i.e. the exactly classical way, F.N. §285 (5th ed)]; to be dispensed in 4 ounce bottle or in a glass with distilled water [vide §272 (6th ed), §288 (5th ed)]; to be taken in sips throughout the day (approximately in every hour), stir thoroughly before every sip [vide §246, §247 & §280 (6th ed) every dose should be deviated from the former].
27th Jan'90	No appreciable change; skin conditions same.	Wait and watch with patience for movement of symptoms.	Wait and watch.
28th Feb'90	No appreciable change. Absolute standstill but no deterioration of the status.	I had already waited for two and a half months and there was no appreciable change but no deterioration, even so I planned to repeat the same potency.	Cortisone 200C This time the same medicated water, being divided into two equal halves 2 doses made from that single poppy-seed sized globule; and the patient was asked to sip the 1st dose on the first day, throughout the day, stir and take in sips; whilst the 2nd dose to be taken after 48 hours of the completion of the 1st dose (viz. alternate day, if the 1st to be taken on Monday, the 2nd dose on Wednesday).
2nd Apr'90	There was absolutely no change.	As it was already four months since the first prescription was made and there had been no changes, I planned to change the remedy.	Sulphur 0/1 (LM1), 8 doses (One globule in water divided into 8 doses). Each to be taken alternate mornings.
4th May'90	No change in these four weeks, rather, the skin is getting more dry and itchy.	Changed the plan of scale.	Sulphur 1000 1 dose in water.

Date	Report After Last Medication	Prescription done on the Basis of	Treatment
9th Jun '90	Absolutely no change and patient is as a whole no better; discomfort, itchy, more stubborn and gloomy.	I was feeling with my experience that the medicine was not holding him. Anyway, I thought it is better to wait about four weeks more before making another final decision to change the plan of treatment (i.e. the remedy). I always try to be sure before making a change of the remedy.	Wait and watch.
6th Jul '90	No change.	So a change in the plan of treatment considering; i) Pustular eruptions on face. Dr. N.M. Chowdhury in his Materia Medica says Croton eruptions are also vesicular in type. ii) Itching(+++) → desire to scratch → but skin gets raw, sore, and hypersensitive and bleeds → so better by gentle rubbing. Itching aggravates at night as any symptoms of Croton also aggravate at night. iii) Burning and smarting pain. iv) Profuse watery, yellowish stool, urging aggravates after meals. v) Crampy pain in abdomen, before stool; and gets exhausted from passing of profuse quantity of stool. vi) Dr. Guernsey mentions about otorrhoea (as quoted by Dr. Clarke). vii) Warm milk aggravates the abdominal pain (Ref. Dr. Clarke). viii) Gloomy, morose, weakness of memory; these features of this patient are also covered by Croton. ix) The strong psoric background (with the features of itchy skin) on which tubercular components are superimposed.	Croton Tig. 30C 2 doses in distilled water.

Date	Report After Last Medication	Prescription done on the Basis of	Treatment
8th Aug'90	Face clearing up. Cervical glands are also better.	Wait and watch.	Wait and watch.
6th Sep'90	Improved but now standstill.	Repeat the same potency.	Croton Tig. 30C 2 doses in water.
16th Oct'90	Standstill.	Higher potency given.	Croton Tig. 200C 2 doses in water.
22nd Nov'90	Face almost cleared up. Glands diminished. Much better in all aspects, mentally and physically.	No treatment required at this stage.	Wait and watch.
5th Jan'91	All eruptions disappeared. Glands also completely diminished.	Satisfactory cure.	Wait and watch.

*Readers may view the pictures of the case (before and after treatment) in our website under Dermatological Diseases (**Case No. D003**- A case of Atopic Dermatitis in a young 5 years old boy, completely cured by Croton Tiglium)*

CASE-3

A DIAGNOSED CASE OF CYSTIC HYGROMA ON THE NECK

Name of the Patient Mast. S.M., 3 months old baby (as on 17th November, 1998)

PRESENTING COMPLAINTS

(1) A large lump on the right side of neck. At birth there was a nodule of the size of a small lime which rapidly grew and by the age of 2 months it was almost the size of a large grapefruit. The mass was not painful but soft, cystic in texture.
(2) The paediatric surgeon gave the diagnosis and advised surgery but also mentioned there were chances of recurrence afterwards. The parents have decided not to opt for surgery but elected Homoeopathy.
(3) The baby had had an acute cough, for the last 15 days which might be due to exposure to cold, also occasional vomiting with expectoration of white mucous.
(4) Stool - Offensive, dry, hard, occasionally contained mucous.
(5) Temperament- Mild, generally quiet and appeared to be in his own world, not very much communication. The mother of the baby said he was decidedly hot, tended to kick off coverings; if covered, became cranky.
(6) Cervical lymph gland on the other side (left) of the neck was swollen+++.
(7) Food desire - Sweet++, sour+, salt+, cold food+. (This was not revealed initially because he was a tiny baby and did not have any particular preference for flavours but this was established at the age of 16 months).
(8) Thirsty +.
(9) Sleep- Nothing to report.
(10) Sweat – Profuse on head. Occasionally smelled sour.

CASE ANALYSIS, MIASMATIC DIAGNOSIS AND FINAL PRESCRIPTION

This case is a wonderful example which illustrates the depth and beauty of Classical Homoeopathy which can handle such pathology. As the parents of the baby were not happy with the prognosis given by the surgeon, therefore Homoeopathy accepted the challenge.

PSORA	SYCOSIS	SYPHILIS	TUBERCULAR
• Acute cough from exposure to cold • Expectoration of white mucus • Stool, dry, hard • Mild, generally quiet and appears to be in his own world • Desires sweet • Sweat smells sour	• Large lump • Lump soft, cystic in texture • Sweats profusely on head		• Desires cold food • Cervical lymph gland on the other side (left) of the neck was swollen

Psora 6   Sycosis 3   Syphilis 0   Tubercular 2

Mixed miasmatic case with Psora-Sycotic preponderance

This is a good example of a case of large tumour with Psora-Syco-Tubercular preponderance. As the surface miasm is predominately Sycotic (manifestation is tumour) and the second layer is Psoric therefore we have to think of a medicine which is either mixed miasmatic (covers all the miasms) or has similar Syco-Psoric-Tubercular preponderance. The Calcarea group is tri-miasmatic with Syco-Tubercular preponderance whereas the Iodum group is preponderantly tubercular. Therefore Calcarea Iod will exactly cover the miasmatic dyscrasia of the case. Calcarea Iod also has the capability of taking care of such cystic swellings and covers the totality, and is therefore an appropriate medicine covering the surface miasm as well as the surface symptoms.

FINAL PRESCRIPTION MADE ON THE BASIS OF

(1) Large lump of the neck.
(2) Started as a nodule, grew larger and became a soft cystic mass.
(3) Stool dry, hard.
(4) Mental Symptoms - Mild, generally quiet and appears to be in his own world, not very much communication (I understood this to be withdrawn).
(5) Hot patient.
(6) Cervical lymph gland on the other side (left) of the neck swollen+++. Glandular involvement.
(7) Desire - sweet++, sour+, salt+, cold food+
(8) Thirsty+.
(9) Sweats profusely on head. Occasionally smells sour.
(10) Miasmatic coverage.

FINAL PRESCRIPTION

CALCAREA IODATUM, 200C 1 globule (No. 10 poppy seed size) in sugar of milk sachet, the powder was dissolved in 8 ounces of pure water (preferably in his feeding bottle) The bottle was shaken and sipped throughout the day, some water was saved at the bottom, topped up the next morning, and sipped throughout the next day. Generally I give instruction to my patients to dilute the medicated water as many times as s/he likes. The patient will continue like this for 7 days. Then 7 days of no medicine. Followed by another dose to be shaken and sipped for 7 days in the same way.

PRESCRIPTION CHART

Date	Prescription done on the basis of WATCH THIS CHART PRINTER	Treatment
17th Nov, 98	As discussed above.	Calc. Iod. 200C, 2 doses
25th Nov, 98	Patient's parent thinks the baby is little better.	Wait and watch
15th Feb, 99	Doing better. Mass is better; stool okay.	Wait and watch
12th Apr, 99	Mass is reducing.	Wait and watch
15th Jun, 99	Doing better. Mass is better. Some skin eruption appeared, could be surfacing of Psora. Wait and watch. Ask to apply some plain coconut oil and nothing else. Report to me if aggravation or if there is a spread.	Wait and watch
10th Aug, 99	Mass decreased. Skin disease better. Emotionally more communicative and becoming restless. Sleep okay, stool okay. As a whole, swelling 60% better.	Wait and watch
12th Oct, 99	Symptoms same as before. Wait and watch.	Wait and watch
4th Dec, 99	Appears to be standstill status.	Calc. Iod, 200C 2 doses
4th Feb, 00	No further appreciable change.	Calc. Iod, 1M, 1 dose
8th Apr, 00	Little better. As a whole swelling, 70% better.	Wait and watch
3rd Jun, 00	No further appreciable change.	Calc.Iod., 1M, 2 doses
15th Jul, 00	Little better. As a whole swelling 80% better. Mentally more alert and reactive.	Wait and watch
12th Sep, 00	No further appreciable change. Mass – Standstill.	Calc.Iod. 10M, 1 dose
27th Oct, 00	Mass is reducing in size. Wait and watch.	Wait and watch
22nd Dec, 00	Mass is better almost 95% gone but appears to be standstill since mid November 2000.	Calc.Iod. 50M 1 dose
28th Jan, 01	Mass completely disappeared.	

Remedy Reaction

I began with **CALCAREA IODATUM 200C** and gradually ascended up to **50M** in two years.. Within three months of starting homoeopathic treatment, the mass started reducing and within eight months, it came down to the size of a small lime. In two years, it had totally disappeared.

*Readers may view the pictures of the case (before and after treatment) in our website under Neoplastic Diseases (**Case No. NEO 002** - A case of Cystic Hygroma (massive swelling in the side of the neck) in a young 6 months old baby, completely cured by Calcarea Iodata).*

CASE-4

A CASE OF BALDNESS
MIASMATIC APPROACH OF PRESCRIBING

Name of the Patient Mr. G.M., 20 years.

PRESENTING COMPLAINTS
(1) Complete hair loss, almost shiny baldness.
(2) Hair started falling out about nine years ago, which patient thinks was after delayed convalescence of typhoid fever (enteric fever).
(3) For about the last fourteen months, there has been complete baldness.
(4) At the initial stage of hair falling, it used to aggravate (increased hair falling) after showering, and during rainy season.
(5) Gas and distension of abdomen, since typhoid fever, aggravates from rich and spicy food. Appetite has also become poor.
(6) Extreme weakness, easy fatigueability, from least exertion.
(7) Bouts of nausea come on during the day, more after heavy meals, since typhoid fever.
(8) Weakness aggravated by exertion and motion, better by complete rest.
(9) HEAD- Hot flushes from vertex with occasional burning when gets irritated, ends up with headache which is long lasting.
(10) EYES - Nothing particular.
(11) EARS- H/O (History of) glue ear (discharge from ear) during childhood. Now better.
(12) NOSE- Catches cold easily. It starts with a runny nose → sneezing.
(13) MOUTH- Apthous ulcer (recurrent). Foetor oris.
(14) TEETH - Occasional swelling of the gums from cold.
(15) TONGUE- Thick, moist, slight imprint of the teeth.
(16) THROAT - When catches cold, pain left side of the throat.
(17) LUNGS - Occasional dry cough.
(18) HEART- As a result of weakness, occasional palpitation, < while fast walking, < from exertion, < from emotional upsets.
(19) ABDOMEN- (i) Distension of abdomen, especially. upper and middle portion. (ii) Eructation ameliorates. (iii) Since typhoid fever, his digestive capacity has become extremely poor.
(20) STOMACH - Appetite poor.
(21) SWEAT- Average, no specific odour.
(22) URINE - Regular, no odour.
(23) STOOL - (i) Stool not clear. (ii) Mucus +. (iii) Offensive odour +(iv) Sensation as if not finished so has to wait a long time in the bathroom.
(24) UPPER EXTREMITIES - Nothing particular.
(25) PALMS- Occasional perspiration in palms when he feels extremely frustrated.
(26) LOWER EXTREMITIES - Nothing particular.
(27) MALE GENITAL ORGANS - Sexual desire strong. Prolonged History of masturbation, which he thinks has weakened him. Wet dreams - occasionally.
(28) ANUS - Nothing particular.
(29) SKIN (i) Delayed healing. (ii) Pityriasis- more in the trunk, for the last two years, aggravates during summer.
(30) TEMPERAMENT- Extremely irritable, objects to parental guidance in every way. Whimsical, suicidal. Likes to leave home (escape).
(31) TENDENCIES - Suicidal tendency.
(32) HABITS (i) Silent habits. (ii) Dirty habits.
(33) LIFE and HATRED- Desire for death, disgusted with life.
(34) MEMORY - Weak, gradual loss of memory.
(35) WEEPING - Weeping mood, involuntary sighing.

(36) SYMPATHY - Sympathetic - average.
(37) ACTIONS - Slow.
(38) PERCEPTIONS - Dull.
(39) FEARS - Fear of darkness, thunderstorms, incurable diseases, failure.
(40) Causative Factors/Aetiology - Bad effects of masturbation; he thinks weakness occurred since the loss of semen; profuse loss of vital-fluids; weakness. Bad effects of typhoid fever delayed convalescence. Hair falling started thereafter. N.B.W.S- excessive mental labour; mental worries, anxiety, memory weakness since. Has suffered from a skin condition, Pityriasis and has applied some lotions.
(41) Habits - Alcohol, smoking, taking opium. No such bad effects from them.
(42) Past Medical History - Typhoid, skin disease, measles.
(43) Vaccination History - Regular vaccinations. Has not suffered from chicken pox or any other infective / childhood disorders.
(44) What is the first cause of breakdown of health? Typhoid fever - N.B.W.S.

HOMOEOPATHIC GENERALITIES:

(1) Heat and cold relationship - Chilly ++. Hates rain. Catches cold easily.
(2) Desire and aversion for foodstuffs - Sweet ++, sour +, pungent and hot ++, salt +, salty ++, bitter +. Bread +, milk – aversion to, potato +, vegetables and spinach +, onion +, fruit +, fish ++, meat and chicken ++, egg (boiled and fried) +. Rich, spicy and fat food ++, warm food- no, cold food +++ Warm drinks - no, cold drinks +. Thirsty ++.
(3) Sleep - Disturbed sleep, wakes up 4 a.m. and cannot sleep again. Dreams of robbers, dead people.
(4) Discharges - Stool, urine, sweat, only stool has offensive odour. Sweat and urine are normal.
(5) Family history (i) Uncle - cancer of the stomach. (ii) Maternal aunt - diabetes.
(6) History of treatment - Has had lots of allopathic, Ayurvedic and homoeopathic medicines without any lasting improvement. Patient cannot name the medicines, oils, and lotions applied, but there were plenty.

CASE ANALYSIS, MIASMATIC DIAGNOSIS AND FINAL PRESCRIPTION

I started the case with Typhoidinum considering the bad effects being caused by the enteric (typhoid) fever and as the patient mentioned that he is N.B.W.S. (never been well since). According to Dr. D.M. Foubister's approach, Typhoidinum was given in order to clear up the bad effects caused by the disease and to restore the vitality. The patient had improved to a certain extent with Typhoidinum and I presume that the block had been removed. After a considerable period of waiting (W.W.W. = Wait, Watch with Wisdom) with the indicated remedy, there was no further movement of symptoms, so I decided to make a change in the plan of treatment and according to the totality, Thyroidinum was prescribed and the result was extremely satisfying.

MIASMATIC ANALYSIS

PSORA	SYCOSIS	SYPHILIS	TUBERCULAR
• Gas in the abdomen • Appetite poor • Caches cold easily • Dry cough • Silent habits, dirty habits • Fear of thunderstorms • Fear of darkness • Fear of incurable disease • Fear of failure • Desire for pungent and hot foods • Extreme weakness, easy fatigue, from least exertion (Tubercular miasm joins) • Weakness aggravates from exertion, motion, ameliorates from complete rest • Weak, gradual loss of memory • Weeping mood, involuntary sighing (Sycosis can join) • Actions slow • Food desires-sweet++, sour +, pungent and hot++	• Hot flushes from vertex • Thick tongue • Strong sexual desire • Dreams of robbers • Hair falling, used to (at the initial stage) increase during rainy season • Sexual desire strong	• Burning in head • Apthous ulcer, recurrent (Tubercular joins) • Foetor oris • Mucous in stool with offensive odour • Delayed healing of skin • Dull perception • Complete hair loss, almost shiny baldness • History of glue ear (discharge from ear) (Tubercular miasm joins) • Pityriasis more in the trunk, for last two years which aggravates during summer • Suicidal • Desire for death, disgusted with life • Dull	• Swelling of the gums from cold • Palpitation • Extremely irritable, objects to parental guidance (Syco-tubercular) • Whimsical • Likes to leave home • Weakness from loss of semen • Prolonged history of masturbation, which he thinks weakens him so much • Catches cold easily; starts with a runny nose, and sneezing • When catches cold, pain in left side of the throat (recurrent) • Chilly ++, Catches cold easily • Desires cold food +++

Psora 16   Sycosis 6   Syphilis 12   Tubercular 11

This is an interesting case of hair falling though considering the extreme bald appearance of the scalp it feels like the case has Syphilitic preponderance, but interestingly we can see other miasms are present as well. Thyroidinum is a deep acting mixed miasmatic medicine, it has wonderfully taken care of the maladjustment aspect of the case as well as the totality and covers the miasmatic status of the patient. We see wonderful improvement through the action of Thyroidinum in this case.

MIASMATIC SUM-UP (MIASMATIC TOTALITY)
So, it is a mixed miasmatic case with Syphilo-tubercular preponderance (or surface miasm). Therefore the selected medicine should cover the symptomatic totality as well as the miasmatic totality.

FINAL PRESCRIPTION

(1)   Thyrodinum was selected on the basis of maladjustment, hormonal and emotional, resulting in impaired coordination, metabolic, nervous and vascular, resulting altered growth and development, here hair falling.
(2)   Hair falling started about nine years ago, which patient thinks commenced after delayed convalescence from typhoid fever (enteric fever). I took this as a shock to the system resulting impaired growth and development of hair.
(3)   Extreme weakness, easy fatigue from least exertion.
(4)   NOSE - Catches cold easily and starts with a runny nose, and sneezing.
(5)   MOUTH - Apthous ulcer (recurrent). Foetor oris.

(6) TEETH - Occasional swelling of the gums from cold.
(7) THROAT - When catches cold, pain left side of the throat.
(8) MALE GENITAL ORGANS - Sexual desire strong.
(9) SKIN DISEASE - Delayed healing.
(10) TEMPERAMENT - Extremely irritable, objects to parental guidance in every way. Whimsical, suicidal. Likes to leave home.
(11) TENDENCIES - Suicidal tendency.
(12) LIFE and HATRED - Desire for death, disgusted with life.
(13) MEMORY - Weak, gradual loss of memory.
(14) WEEPING - Weeping mood, involuntary sighing.
(15) FEARS - Fear of darkness, thunderstorms, incurable diseases, failure.
(16) Excessive mental labour, mental worries, anxiety, memory weakness since.
(17) Chilly ++. Hates rainy season. Catches cold easily.
(18) Desires sweet ++.

THYROIDINUM Miasmatics - Psora++, Sycosis+++, Syphilitic++, Tubercular+++ Chilly.

(1) In this case, there are Psora + Syphilitic preponderances → so Psora + Syphilis = Tubercular miasm, according to John Henry Allen, (Ref. Psora-Pseudo Psora).
(2) Thyroidinum does cover Tubercular miasm.
(3) Basically I was looking for a deep acting mixed miasmatic medicine. Therefore, Thyroidinum came in my mind for its mixed miasmatic status as well as being deep in action and it covers the aforesaid symptoms of the case and also:
   (i) Emotional maladjustment → In-coordination → Temper tantrums.
   (ii) Altered development → maladjustment → In-coordination → Hair falling.
   (iii) Mental in-coordination e.g. manic depression.
   (iv) Vital in-coordination e.g. low energy.
   (v) Maladjustment acts as a trigger (aetiological factor) → results in-coordination → which can be hormonal.

I have started the case with Typhoidinum, 200C, went up to 1M and 10M consecutively with proper wait and watch. Then Thyroidinum was prescribed and the result was simply marvellous. The medicine was given in water to sip for 7 days as usual.

Date	Prescription done on the basis of	Treatment
7th Sep'90	Considering the bad effects of typhoid fever N.B.W.S. (His entire vitality deranged since). Gas and distension and lowered digestive function.	Typhoidinum 200C 2 doses. To sip (with water) the 1st dose for 7 days; 7 days off; then the 2nd dose to sip for 7 days.
5th Oct'90	No appreciable change. Standstill. Wait.	Wait and watch
12th Nov'90	No appreciable change. So went higher.	Typhodinum 1000 (1M), 2 doses (Same way as mentioned above)
17th Dec'90	Digestion better, gas and distension as little less, but no change in bald hair, weakness etc. Wait for further movement of symptoms.	Wait and watch
30th Jan'90	Digestive power has improved to a certain extent and then standstill. Absolutely no other changes. Wait for any further reaction.	Wait and watch
25th Feb'91	Standstill, went higher.	Typhoidinum 10,000, 2 doses
28th Mar'91	No further change. Wait and watch.	Wait and watch.

Date	Prescription done on the basis of	Treatment
6th May'91	Absolute standstill. Change in the plan of treatment. Considering conditions which point towards loss of balance in the human economy due to strain, during some particular period of development, due to climatic variations or due to some other mental or emotional factors, Thyroidinum to be thought of. Want of metabolic adjustment - Thyroidinum exercises a general regulating influence over the mechanism of the organs of nutrition, growth and development. Chilly, sensitive to cold, and catches cold easily. Deep syphilitic miasmatic preponderance (for generalised shining baldness). Mental irritability, whimsical moods. Temperamental disturbances of adolescence. Generalised and profound weakness, easy fatigue. Decided craving for sweets. Palpitation from emotion, exertion. Flatulence, distended abdomen. Long lasting headache from irritability. Suicidal tendencies.	Thyroidinum 1M 2 doses.
10th Jun'91	Started feeling better but no change in bald hair. Wait and watch.	Wait and watch
8th Jul'91	Weakness much better. Temperament better, calmer. Gas and distension much improved. Digestive process improved. Nausea better.	Wait and watch
10th Aug'91	Improved but standstill. Repeat.	Thyroidinum 1000 (1M) 2 doses (procedure as above).
26th Sep'91	Hair growth started. Doing better n every way. Temperament much better. Wait and watch.	Wait and watch
2nd Nov'91	Hair is growing. Temperament and suicidal thoughts much improved.	Wait and watch
22nd Dec'91	Hair growth steadily improving.	Wait and watch
3rd Jan'92	Hair growth improving.	Wait and watch
14th Feb'92	Sudden attack of depression and suicidal thoughts. Patient appears to be standstill, so went higher in potency.	Thyroidinum (10M), 2 doses (same way as mentioned above)
26th Mar'92	Again temperament, whimsical thoughts and depression is much improved. Hair growth steadily improving.	Wait and watch
20th Apr'92	Much better. Almost normal appearance of the hair.	Wait and watch
26th May'92	Cured.	Stopped treatment.

Remedy Reaction Thyroidinum 1M and then I went gradually up to 10M and cured the case in about twenty months.

*Readers may view the pictures of the case (before and after treatment) in our website under Dermatological Diseases (**Case No. D002** - A case of total Baldness in a 24 years aged person, completely cured by Thyroidinum).*

CASE-5

A CASE OF BRAIN TUMOUR COMPLETELY CURED BY HOMOEOPATHY

Mrs. P.R.J., 23 years, Hindu Female, brought to me first on 8th of August 1988 with the following complaints:

PRESENTING COMPLAINTS (Started in February 1988.)

(1) Recurrent vomiting followed by sweat. Sweat also on little exertion.
(2) Loss of sleep.
(3) Slurring of speech aggravated in the morning and night, ameliorated after warm drinks.
(3) Dimness of the vision, aggravated by excitement and better by rest.
(4) Vertigo with dizziness especially while walking.
(5) Loss of appetite.
(6) Dull, heavy headache.
(7) Aggravation in the morning and night (esp. vomiting and vertigo).
(8) Aggravation from motion, exertion, better by rest.
(9) Better in open air.
(10) Worse from warmth in general.
(11) Headache ameliorated by pressure.
(12) Better by sleep.
(13) Better by consolation.
(14) Dull and heavy ache, giddiness.
(15) Occasional apthous ulcers.
(16) Occasional dry cough with pain right side of the chest.
(17) Occasional palpitation especially after emotion.
(18) Gas and distension in the upper abdomen.
(19) Extremely poor appetite, though slight hunger felt between 9 a.m. to 10 a.m.
(20) Sweat ++, especially in the back parts. No odour. Sweat on exertion. Vomiting followed by sweat.
(21) Stool - White mucus. No ineffectual urging. Neither diarrhoeic nor constipated. Mucus present +.
(22) Coldness of the extremities especially after the vomiting.
(23) Sexual desire ++, history of masturbation during youth, before marriage.
(24) Menses - Started at 14 years of age, occasional pain, menstruation is scanty, occasional flow with scanty periods.
(25) White discharge after periods.
(26) Mind was at first clear – then there was gradual stupefaction.
(27) Gloomy ++; absent minded +; forgetful ++. Wants to be alone. Fear of death (occasional).
(28) Memory weak.
(29) Weepy +. Sympathetic +. Slow & dull.
(30) Fear of darkness, incurable disease.
(31) Past History- History Of- Recurrent vomiting at 7 years. of age; also H/O school going diarrhoea treated allopathically; H/O measles in childhood.
(32) What is the first cause of breakdown of health? Cannot co-relate.
(33) Chilly patient. Sensitive to cold and damp. Likes to take baths regularly. Does not catch cold easily.
(34) Desire and aversion for foods - Sweet +, sour +, pungent and hot +, salt +, salty +, bitter No. Bread +, milk No, potato +, vegetables and spinach +, onion No, fruit +, fish ++, meat and chicken +, egg (boiled/fried) +. Rich, spicy and fat food +, warm food No, cold food ++. Warm drinks No, cold drinks +. Ice cream +.
(35) Thirstless.

(36) Loss of sleep may be from worry.
(37) Married for four years.
(38) Family History- i) Mother – rheumatism ii) Father - asthma.
(39) Treated by one Calcutta's leading Homoeopath's with Causticum without effect.

INVESTIGATION DONE BEFORE DR. BANERJEA'S TREATMENT

(1) 20/7/88 - E.E.G. Mildly abnormal E.E.G. indicating interseizure pattern of left temporal region.
(2) 20/7/88- C.T. Scan of Brain C.T.study reveals an irregularly enhanced cystic midline S.O.L. (space occupying lesion) in the posterior fossa. Findings are suggestive of Haemangioblastoma. Cystic astrocytoma cannot be ruled out on these findings.
(3) 6/11/89- C.T.Scan of Brain - Normal Scan.
(4) Provisional diagnosis - Brain Tumour ? (Haemangioblastoma or Cystic Astrocytoma)
(5) Miasmatic diagnosis - Psora-Sycotic.
(6) Constitutional remedy - Gelsemium

PRESCRIPTION CHART

Date	Prescription done on the basis of	Treatment
8th Aug '88		Gelsemium 200C - 2 doses. To sip (with water) the 1st dose for 5 days; 2 days off; then the 2nd dose to sip for 5 days.
25th Aug '88	No change.	Wait and watch
24th Sept '88	No change, standstill but no further deterioration.	Gelsemium 200C – 2 doses
12th Oct '88	Standstill, no worsening.	Wait and watch.
16th Nov '88	Standstill, so go higher	Gelsemium 1000 (1M) – 2 doses
13th Dec '88	Improved. Vomiting is less. Vertigo and weakness are better.	Wait and watch
15th Feb '89	Better in every way. Patient has conceived. L.M.P. 18/12/88	Wait and watch
27th Mar '89	Better in every way. Pregnancy is progressing nicely and there are no complications.	Wait and watch
26th April '89	More or less cured, no major presenting complaints. Weakness occasionally, headaches etc. Patient is reluctant to continue any further treatment as she has to travel about 120 km to get to the city.	Wait and watch

MIASMATIC INTERPRETATION & DISCUSSION

General nature of the Sycotic miasm
Sycosis produces in-coordination everywhere; over-production, growth infiltration in forms of warts, condylomata, tumours & fibrous tissues etc.

Organs/tissues are affected by this stigmata (Sycosis)
Entodermal tissues, soft tissues etc. (-- whereas Psora affects ectodermal tissues, Syphilis affects mesodermal tissues).

Psychic manifestations of Sycotic stigmata in relation to the case in concern
Sycosis the in-coordinating miasm, manifests in-coordination in psychic sphere also. As if the association fibres of the cerebrum and the linking fibres of the autonomic nervous system with central nervous system have become out of gear. This in-coordination is manifested in the field of memory by forgetfulness of what she has just thought, said and done.

General manifestations of Sycotic Stigmata

All "hypers" are Sycotic or (-- whereas "hypos" are generally Psoric and "dyses" are generally Syphilitic). Hyperplasia of the tissues of the case in concern is Sycotic.

MIASMATIC INTERPRETATION

PSORA	SYCOSIS	SYPHILIS	TUBERCULAR
1) Dimness of vision better by rest 2) Loss of appetite 3) Vertigo aggravated by movement and ameliorated by rest 4) Headache better by sleep 5) Dry cough 6) Gas and distension in upper abdomen 7) Coldness of extremities 8) Scanty menstruation 9) Gradual stupefaction 10) Fear of death 11) History of school going diarrhoea (during childhood) 12) Loss of sleep from worry 13) Wants to lie down day and night which ameliorates her trouble 14) Weepy and depressed 15) Various fears, of darkness, of incurable disease 16) Anamnesis from P/H 17) Craves sweet + 18) Craves pungent & hot food 19) Aversion to milk 20) Paresis and functional paralysis (Sycosis joins)	1) Recurrent vomiting 2) Sweats on little exertion 3) Slurring of speech 4) Vertigo while walking 5) Headache ameliorated by pressure 6) Sweat ++ especially on the back 7) Sexual desire ++ 8) Leucorrhoea after menses 9) Absent-minded 10) Weepy + 11) Sensitive to damp 12) Rheumatism with mother (F/H) 13) Asthma with father (F/H) 14) Absentminded 15) Desires salt (can be tubercular as well) and salty food 16) Anamnesis from F/H (family history of Rheumatism with mother and Asthma with father).	1) Vertigo worse at night 2) Apthous ulcers 3) White mucous 4) Gloomy ++ 5) Forgetful 6) Slow and dull	1) Vertigo better in open air 2) Palpitation 3) Desires cold food

Psora 20   Sycosis 16   Syphilis 6   Tubercular 3

This is a case of brain tumour which was diagnosed by C.T. scan as a case of haemangioblastoma or astrocytoma. Haemangioblastoma is Syco-Tubercular and it is a tumour of vascular origin, whereas astrocytoma is Syphilo-Sycotic and it is a space occupying lesion in the brain with degenerative changes. The neurologist and neurosurgeon were of the opinion that as the patient had deteriorated so quickly and was almost bedridden within a few months, it was more likely to be an astrocytoma which is a malignant tumour of Syco-Syphilitic variety.

One can observe the Syco-Syphilitic preponderance of the case in a Psoric background, from the above miasmatic assessment therefore we have to think of a medicine which covers Syco-Syphilitic dyscrasia. Gelsemium covers the totality including the emotional state of the case as well as the miasmatic background. One can see the wonderful results of Gelsemium in this case and with the right selection of the medicine and the dose a patient of such advanced pathology has improved so dramatically which reflects the powerful penetrating dynamic capabilities of homoeopathy.

SYCOTIC TAINT OF GELSEMIUM   Dr.Clarke refers a case of Hydrosalpirgitis of gonorrhoeal origin cured by Gels 1M.

POINTS IN FAVOUR OF GELSEMIUM

(1) Slurring of speech which was > by warm drinks (patient as a whole was not fond of warm drinks, but she found sipping warm water relieved (particular modality of the complaint Dr.Clarke refers stimulants ameliorate).
(2) Dim vision < from excitement (In Gelsemium we have general < from emotion & excitement).
(3) Vertigo > in open air (Boericke).
(4) Dull headache > by pressure and compression.
(5) Complete relaxation and prostration of the whole muscular system lack of muscular coordination (Clarke).
(6) Coldness of extremities (Kent).
(7) Insomnia from worry (Clarke).
(8) Dr. Harvey Farrington refers weakness and languor are the earliest symptom to appear. Patient feels tired and weary and wants to lie down. Dr. Farrington clearly emphasized that the excessive weakness is the prodromal state of practically all the complaints where Gelsemium is indicated. Dr.Clarke refers that the lassitude is expressed by the patient (--not expressed, Mur.Acid.).
(9) Desire to be let alone.
(10) Thirstless.
(11) Mind was first clear - gradual or insidious stupefaction.
(12) Listless attitude. Wants to lie down and rest (Clarke).
(13) Apathy regarding illness.
(14) Anamnesis of the P/H of school-going diarrhoea.
(15) Dr. Clarke refers functional paralysis (paresis) of all descriptions.
(16) Appearance   Heavy, dull appearance of the face (expression) of the countenance (Clarke). Apathy regarding her illness; "discernings are lethargic" (Ref.Boericke).

NOTES ON GELSEMIUM -

1) When there is presence of many group of symptoms of various ailments and if according to the indications Gelsemium being prescribed at the outset, it can really abort the entire disease. (Ref. Ghatak).
2) Due to absence of deep-acting anti-Psoric base, Gelsemium cannot prevent the frequent relapse of the complaints due to Psoric stigmata. Dr. Nilmoni Ghatak refers that one might think that when Gelsemium has the capability to cure many deep-seated diseases, like paralysis, then how can it be possible that the medicine does not posses deep-seated anti-Psoric stigmata, but this may be noted that when the exciting cause excites the latent/dormant Psora to explore and thereby occurs manifestation of paralytic symptoms, Gelsemium having inability to prevent the said explosion of latent Psora and thereby annihilating the problem permanently like, Sulphur, Causticum, etc., does, which also corresponds miasmatically to the case. But Gelsemium has the capability of aborting the ailment when indicated by its totality, especially at the outset.

*Readers may view the pictures of the case (before and after treatment) in our website under Neoplastic Diseases (**Case No. NEO 001**- A case of Brain Tumour in a 23 years young married woman, completely cured by Gelsemium).*

CASE-6

A CASE OF INFERTILITY ASSOCIATED WITH PELVIC INFLAMMATORY DISEASE & BILATERAL LARGE OVARIAN CYSTS COMPLETELY CURED BY HOMOEOPATHY

PRESENTING COMPLAINTS:

Mrs. S. D. K., aged about 32 years first came to me on 9th October, 1995 with the following complaints -

(1) Irregular menstruation, delayed, profuse and clots.
(2) Trying to conceive for last three years, but not happening.
(3) Clinically diagnosed by Gynaecologist as a case of large right ovarian cyst and also left ovarian enlargement with cyst, associated with P.I.D. (Pelvic Inflammatory disease) Confirmed by Ultrasonographies.

HEAD TO FOOT SCANNING OF SYMPTOMS
(1) Head- No headaches. Sweat on back and front of head; sour smelling.
(2) Eyes- Nothing particular.
(3) Nose- Stoppage of nose < night. Catches cold easily and has a tendency of profuse and yellow discharge.
(4) Mouth- Foetor oris.
(5) Tongue- Blackish, prominent papillae.
(6) Throat- Prone to swelling of tonsils < cold (this symptom since childhood).
(7) Lungs- Nothing particular.
(8) Heart- Palpitation from least exertion.
(9) Chest- Whenever catches cold → cold extends downwards → tickling cough << warm room, << indoors.
(10) Abdomen- Can not bear tight clothing around abdomen.
(11) Appetite- Average.
(12) Sweat- Profuse perspiration, especially on head and back. Sour smelling.
(13) Urine- 8 - 10 times per 24 hours. Occasionally offensive or sourish smell.
(14) Stool- Constipated. Dry and occasionally with mucus. Sour smelling.
(15) Upper Extremities- Nothing particular.
(16) Lower Extremities- Backache < on sitting, < stooping.
(17) Female Genital Organs-
 (a) Sexual desire- Poor.
 (b) Menstruation - Puberty - 12 years of age. Onset - delayed. Duration - 4 - 5 days. Character - fishy, darkish. Quantity - profuse. Clots. Frequency - 40 days apart generally. Associated symptom during menses - i) Profound weakness, ii) Sharp cutting pain in the right ovarian region.
 (c) Leucorrhoea- Occasional yellowish discharge < before period.
(18) Rectum- Nothing particular.
(19) Skin Diseases- Occasional allergy from jewellery, contact allergy, small rash with itching.
(20) Mental Symptoms- (a) Mild, (b) Fault finding, (c) Absent minded, (d) Shy, (e) Wants to be alone, (f) Memory weak, absent minded, (g) Sympathetic, (h) Fears thunderstorms, accidents, failure.
(21) Exciting Causes/Causative Factors- No history of- (i) Injury, (ii) Mental grief or disappointments, (iii) Handling chemicals, (iv) Sexual excesses, (v) Excessive mental labours, (vi) History of S.T.D. etc.

(22) Past Medical History- Nothing particular.
(23) First Cause of Breakdown of Health- Cannot correlate.
(24) Homoeopathic Generalities-
    (a) Heat and Cold Relationship- Hot patient; but catches cold easily.
    (b) Desires and Aversions to Food Stuffs
        Desires: i) Sweet++, ii) Sour +, iii) Salt +, iv) Salty +, v) Fruits +,
        vi) Egg +++, vii) Cold food +, viii) Cold drinks +, ix) Ice-creams +,
        Aversions- i) Bitter, ii) Meat.
    (c) Thirst- Average.
    (d) Sleep- Okay. No particular dreams.
    (e) Discharges- Sweat, stool and urine all have a sourish smell.
(25) Marital Status-
Married for four years and trying to conceive for last three years, but cannot conceive.
(26) Family History-
    (i) Paternal side- Cancer
    (ii) Maternal side- Heart and rheumatic problems.
(27) Previous Medical Treatment-
    (i) Allopathic (conventional medicine) mainly hormonal drugs but reacted with feeling of discomfort and hot flushes → so stopped.
    (ii) Homoeopathic Pulsatilla, Graphites, Sepia etc. in various potencies from other homoeopaths.
(28) Medical Reports-
    (a) 17th April, 1995 - USG - Pelvis Good sized right ovarian cyst. 8.3 x 6.0 cm. Uterus normal. Left ovary enlarged and cystic.
    (b) 27th September, 1995 - H.S.G. (Hystero-Salpingography). Patent both fallopian tubes.
    USG Bilateral ovarian cyst.
    O/E cystic swelling in P.O.D.
    (c) 8th November, 1994 - Husband's Semen T.C. 92×10^6. Active motile 1st hr. - 70%, 2nd hr. - 55%, 3rd hr. - 30%.
    (d) 9th October, 1996 - USG pelvis Right ovarian Cyst. 5 cm x 2 cm & P.I.D. (Pelvic Inflammatory Disease).
    (e) 23rd January, 1998 USG Pelvis Right ovary 4.5 x 3.9 cm (Just bulky, no cysts). Left ovary 2.5 x 2.5 cm (Normal).

(29)   Miasmatic Diagnosis- Syco-Tubercular.

PSORA	SYCOSIS	SYPHILIS	TUBERCULAR
• Sour smelling sweat • Catches cold easily • Stool dry and constipated • Mild • Shy • Wants to be alone • Fear of thunderstorms, accidents, failure • Desires sweet • Sweat, stool, urine – sourish smell	• Sweat on back and front of head • Profuse and yellow discharge from nose • Blackish papillae on tongue, (hyper pigmentation) • Cannot bear tight clothing around abdomen (hypersensitivity) • Urine increased • Menstruation has fishy odour • Cutting pain in the right ovarian region during menstruation • Irregular menstruation (hormonal imbalance, in-coordination, sycosis) • Cystic mass and ovarian enlargement • Yellowish leucorrhoea • Absent minded • Married four years, trying to conceive for last three but cannot conceive (in-coordination also, fallopian tubes are patent, so no blockage; yet inability to conceive, therefore hormonal imbalance, sycotic) • From ultrasound (USG) report – ovarian cyst • Pelvic inflammatory disease (diagnosed by Gynaecologist)	• Stoppage of nose, < night • Foetor oris	• Recurrent swelling of tonsils < cold • Palpitation from least exertion • Menstrual blood – profuse and clots • Profound weakness during menstruation • Allergy from jewellery (nickel) • Fault finding • Desires cold food • Tendency to catch cold easily

Psora   9   Sycosis   14   Syphilis   2   Tubercular   8

This is a case where the patient primarily came because she couldn't conceive even after three years of trying. This could be due to hormonal imbalance or in-coordination which is Sycotic. From the Gynaecologist's point of view the patient has patent fallopian tubes (H.S.G. report) and also has bi-lateral ovarian cysts, this is Sycotic. So from the clinical and pathological point of view Sycotic miasm is coming as the surface miasm, from the miasmatic totality we can see it is a mixed miasmatic case with Sycotic preponderance. Accordingly we need a mixed miasmatic medicine with Sycotic preponderance and here Calcarea Iodata entirely fits such miasmatic dyscrasica as well as covering the totality.

After the action of Calcarea Iodata, in the follow up sonography report one can see that not only the cysts have improved but the patient also conceived which reflects the wonderful capability of homoeopathy in solving the problem.

(30) **Remedy Diagnosis-** Calcarea Iodata.

(31) **Remedy Discussion**

    (A)   Features of Calcarea Carbonica -

        (i)   Sweat on back of head, sour smelling.
        (ii)   Yellowish nasal discharge.
        (iii)   Tendency to catch cold easily.
        (iv)   Cannot bear tight clothing around abdomen.
        (v)   Profuse perspiration, head and back, sour smelling.
        (vi)   Constipated, sour smelling stool.
        (vii)   Profuse menses with clots.
        (viii)   Fearful temperament.
        (ix)   Desires sweet, sour, egg, cold food, ice-creams.
        (x)   Aversion to meat.

    (B)   Features of Iodum

        (i)   Offensive odour from month.
        (ii)   Catches cold easily → cold extends downwards → tickling cough → << warm room and indoor (Ref. Dr. Boericke).
        (iii)   Palpitation from least exertion.
        (iv)   Profound weakness during menses.
        (v)   Irregular period.
        (vi)   Sharp pain in right ovarian region.
        (vii)   Hot patient.

    (C).   Features of Calcarea Iodata

        i)   Nasal discharge has a tendency to be profuse and yellow.
        ii)   Takes cold easily.
        iii)   Prone to swelling of tonsils predisposition to glandular enlargements.
        iv)   Yellowish leucorrhoeal discharge.
        v)   Allergic skin rash with itching.
        vi)   Ovarian enlargement = interpreted as glandular swelling.

(32) **Prescription Chart**

Date	Prescription done on the basis of	Treatment
9th Oct'95	Features of Calcarea in hot constitution (other points in favour of prescription discussed earlier).	Calc. Iod., 200 C 2 doses. To sip (with water) the 1st dose for 7 days; 7 days off; then the 2nd dose to sip for 7 days.
17th Nov'95	Menses – 4 days, normal, regular, L.M.P. 28th Oct '95.	Wait and watch
20th Dec'95	L.M.P(Last Menstrual Period) - 18th Nov'95 L.M.P. - 17th Dec'95	Wait and watch
2nd Feb'96	L.M.P. 19th Jan'95 menses regular.	Wait and watch
1st Mar'96	Occasional pain in left side of abdomen. L.M.P. 17th Feb'96	Calc. Iod., 200 C 2 doses
12th Apr'96	As a whole doing better.	Wait and watch
3rd May'96	As a whole doing better.	Wait and watch

Date	Prescription done on the basis of	Treatment
17th Jun'96	L.M.P. - 16th Mar'96 L.M.P. - 16th Apr'96	Wait and watch
15th Jul'96	Delayed menses L.M.P. - 20th May'96 L.M.P. 27th Jun'96	Wait and watch
14th Aug'96	L.M.P. – 4th Aug'96	Calc. Iod, 200 C 2 doses
20th Sep'96	No problem externally. Regular menses L.M.P. – 4th Sep'96	Wait and watch.
9th Oct'96	Menstruation regular. L.M.P. - 4th Oct'96	Wait and watch.
29th Nov'96	L.M.P. - 27th Oct'96 L.M.P. - 20th Nov'96	Calc. Iod., 1 M 2 doses
13th Jan'97	L.M.P. - 20th Dec'96	Wait and watch.
7th Feb'97		Calc. Iod., 1 M 2 doses, 10 M 1 dose
28th Mar'97	Threaten abortion happened 19th Mar'97. L.M.P. 20th Dec'96. Now physically fit.	Wait and watch.
12th May'97		Wait and watch.
23rd Jun'97	Menstrual cycle regular	Wait and watch.
18th Aug'97	M.C. regular L.M.P. 27th Jul'97. Trying to conceive, but not happening, dropped.	Calc. Iod., 200 C / 2 doses
3rd Oct'97	Wait & watch.	Wait and watch.
21st Nov'97	Wait & watch.	Wait and watch.
22nd Dec'97	M.C. → regular. L.M.P. - 26th Nov'97	Wait and watch.
16th Feb'98	M.C. → 28th Jan'98 OVARIAN CYST CURED	Wait and watch.
6th Apr'98	Menstrual cycle →28th Jan'98, 3rd Mar'98, 2nd Apr'98	Wait and watch.
1st Jun'98	L.M.P. – 9th May'98	Calc. Iod., 50 M 2 doses
13th Jul'98	L.M.P. – 7th Jun'98 & 7th Jul'98	Wait and watch.
19th Aug'98	L.M.P. – 5th Aug'98	Wait and watch.
23rd Sep'98	No change of anything → standstill L.M.P. – 9th Sep'98	Calc. Iod., CM 2 doses
30th Oct'98	L.M.P. – 8th Oct'98	Wait and watch.
14th Dec'98	L.M.P. - 10th Nov'98, 10th Dec'98 Normal cycle. Stool - one daily – clear. Sleep – sound. Appetite - normal.	Wait and watch.
3rd Feb'99	L.M.P. – 8th Jan'99 Stool - clear. Appetite - normal. M.C. ON REGULAR TIME.	Wait and watch.

Patient got pregnant in March'99 and delivered a normal baby.

*Readers may view the pictures of the case (before and after treatment) in our website under Gynaecological Diseases (**Case No. GY 002**- A case of Ovarian Cyst in a 32 years old married woman, completely cured by Calcarea Iodata.).*

PART — IX
MIASMATIC PRESCRIBING :
LOOK AND DIAGNOSE THE MIASM

1) **PSORA:**

Hair: Dry, harsh, dandruff++

Face: Bluish appearance

Facial expression: Anxious, nervous, apprehensive, fearful

Lips: Dry, features of cyanosis

PSORA

Skin: Dry, harsh

Nails: Dry, harsh

Dress: Wears light colours

Personality: Affectionate, amiable, caring, cautious, collector, compassionate, conservative, considerate, dutiful (over the top Sycosis joins), easy-going, emotional, forsaken, kind, naïve, peace-maker, perceptive, private, reserved, sensitive, thoughtful, worrier.

Hobbies: Watching TV, video, films (cinema), reading, board games, playng cards

Occupation: Carer, clerical, nurse, nursery-nurse

2) **SYCOSIS:**

Hair: Fishy smell, alopecia in circular spots

Face: Yellowish colour, puffy, oedematous congenital/acquired overgrowth

Facial expression: Greedy, cunning, exploitative, jealous, suspicious, mischievous

Lips: Thickened

SYCOSIS

Skin: Thickened, fish-scale, vesicular

Nails: Thick, ridged, ribbed corrugated, convex

Dress: Wears yellow/bright colours (ostentatious and fatuous)

Personality: Aggressive, ambitious, arrogant, assertive, bossy, charismatic, enthusiastic, fanatic (if destructive Syphilis joins), faultfinding, friendly, gregarious, humorous, intense, list maker, manipulative, outgoing (if changeable Tubercular joins), perfectionist, planner, possessive, ritualistic serious, sincere, sociable (Tubercular joins)

Hobbies: Gambling, casinos, bingo, fast dancing (rock and roll), shopping (excess due to greed)

Occupation: Accountant, chief executive officer, dictator (successful), doctor (Psora also present), lawyer, pimp, policeman, politician, receptionist, stockbroker (Syphilis joins), under-cover agent

3) **SYPHILIS:**

Hair: Falling from all over the body

Face: Reddish appearance, cleft palate and allied congenital abnormalities

Facial expression: Cruel, brutal, vindictive, spiteful, dull, depressed

Lips: Cracked

Skin: Cracks and fissures, ulcerative

SYPHILIS

Nails: Thin, break easily, channelled, pitted, concave (spoon shaped)

Dress: Wears non-matching colours (lack of conception and realisation), dark colours, black

Personality: Abusive, closed, depressed, dogmatic, pessimistic, revengeful, rude

Hobbies: Hunting, wrestling, boxing, martial arts, archery, ten-pin bowling, speedway, coarse fishing (sea fishing)

Occupation: Butcher, manual labourer, publican

4) **TUBERCULAR:**

Hair: Breaks, splits and sticks together

Face: Purple colour, flushed cheeks

Facial expression: Indifferent, discontented, independent, stubborn, changeable

Lips: Bright red, flushing

TUBER-CULAR

Skin: Flushing, bleeding

Nails: Glossy, white spots, flush easily

Dress: Wears red, purple and pinkish colours

Personality: Adventurous, artistic, bubbly, changeable, creative, fearless, fun loving, independent, rebellious

Hobbies: Creative hobbies (cooking, knitting, drawing, acting), traveling, horse riding, motor racing, golf, skiing, music, gardening, lake fishing, swimming, shopping (likes changes)

Occupation: Actor, air hostess, artist, craftsman/artisan, detective, driver, gardener, kindergarten nurse (Psora joins), postman, salesman, teacher

INDEX

Abdominal symptoms
    comparison of 102-4
Accessory miasm 13
Action, pace of 54, 143
Acute miasm 13
Aggravation 138, 175
AIDS
    clinical tips on 183-6
Amelioration 138-9
Anamnesis 21
Ancestral tips, miasmatic 28, 173-188
Anti-miasmatic medicines 12
    leading 251-2
Anti-psoric medicines
    leading 251
Anti-sycotic medicines
    leading 251
Anti-syphilitic medicines
    leading 251
Anti-tubercular medicines
    leading 252
Anxiety 44
Appearance
    of extremities 134
    of face 83
    of skin 125-6
Appendicitis 175
Artificial chronic disease 9
Attitude 48
Aversions 101, 156
Awareness 43
Bacteria & miasm 31
Bacteriology, modern 20
Behaviour 49, 56, 144
Bronchospasm
    clinical tips on 178-9
Cancer
    clinical tips on 180
    prophylactic aspect of
      homoeopathic medicine in 180
Cardiac symptoms
    comparison of 92-95
Cause
    exciting 21-3
    fundamental 21
    initial 21
    remote 22-3
Characteristics
    comparison of 52-9
    synopsis 140-157
Characteristics & nature
    comparison of 52-9
Chronic disease
    order of progression in 19
Chronic miasm 11, 13, 16
Classical miasmatic prescribing 3
Classification of miasm 13
Clinical tips
    of natural characteristics 173-5
    on AIDS 183-6
    on bronchospasm 178-9
    on cancer 180
    on dementias 177

    on eczema 182
    on influenza 176
    on migraine 187-8
    on nutrition & foods 188
    on paediatric characteristics 176
    on pimples 176
    on rheumatism 181
Clinical utility of miasmatic theory 17
Clinicals
    abdominal 102, 164
    cardiac 92, 162-3
    dermatological 122, 167-8
    ear, of the 73, 161
    extremities, of the 130, 168-9
    eye, of the 70
    gastric 163-4
    mixed miasmatic, classification of 170-1
    nasal symptoms 76
    nose, of the 161
    ophthalmalogical 160
    oral 80, 161
    psora-sycotic 170
    psora-sycotic-syphilitic 170-1
    psora-syphilitic 170
    psychiatric 159-60
    rectal symptoms 105
    rectum, of the 165
    respiratory system, of the 86, 161-2
    sexual 144, 166-7
    stomach 96
    urinary 110, 165-6
Coition 121
Common mother 34
Comparison of
    abdominal symptoms 102-4
    cardiac symptoms 92-5
    characteristics & nature 52-9
    characteristics, a synopsis 140-57
    dermatological symptoms 122-8
    ear symptoms 73-5
    extremity symptoms 130-5
    eye symptoms 70-2
    facial symptoms 83-5
    head & scalp symptoms 62-9
    mental symptoms 41-51
    modality symptoms 138-9
    nail symptoms 129
    nasal symptoms 76-9
    oral symptoms 80-2
    rectal symptoms 105-9
    respiratory symptoms 86-91
    sexual symptoms 114-21
    sleep symptoms 136-7
    stomach symptoms 96-101
    urinary symptoms 110-3
    vertigo symptoms 60-1
Complex energy field (CEF) 15
Conception
    Hahnemannian 20
    Kentian 33
Concomitants
    cardiac 94
    dermatological 125
    ear 75
    headache 64

    heart 94
    migraine 65-6
    mouth 81
    rectal 107
    respiratory 88
    sexual 116-7
    skin 125
    sleep 137
    stomach 98-9
    urinary 111
    vertigo 61
Conjoint picture 1-2
Constitution 55, 143
Consumptive miasm 12
Contagium vivum 6
Contaminated picture 1
Cough 88-9
Cravings 99
Criminality 50
Criteria
    basic, of the four great miasms 7
    of psora 7
    of sycosis 7
    of syphilis 8
    tubercular 8
Criterias
    miasmatic infection and its 9
    three criterias of miasmatic disease 16
Cruelty 44
Death 145
Degenerating miasm 52-9
Dementia
    clinical tips on 177
    senile 177
    terminal 177
Deranged vital force (DVF) 15
Dermatological symptoms
    comparison of 122-8
Desire 156
    sexual 119
Desires 100
Diathesis 11, 42, 54
Differentiation of pseudo-psora & tubercular miasms 6
Discharges 118
Disease
    artificial chronic 9
    chronic, order of progression in 19
    miasmatic, three criterias of 16
    nature of 54, 142
    one-sided 1-2, 5
Disease force (DF) 15-6
Dreams
    character of 136
Drug miasm 9
Drugs, recreational 175
Dynamic pathology 39
    of Hahnemann 14
Dynamism
    Hahnemannian 20
Ear 149
    infections 174
    symptoms, comparison of 73-5

Eczema
    clinical tips on 182
Emotional suppressions 2
Energy field
    complex (CEF) 15
    vital (VEF) 15
Enuresis 113
Eruptions 127-8
Exciting cause 21-3
Expectoration 89
Expression of miasm 14
Extremity symptoms
    comparison of 130-5
Eye 149
    symptoms, comparison of 70-2
Face 83-5
Facial symptoms
    comparison of 83-5
Fears 45, 57, 146
Fertility 119
Fixed miasm 13
Flow (urinary) 112
Foundation of all sickness 34
Fundamental cause 21
Future 5
General manifestations 52-3
General miasmatic dyscrasia (GMD) 15
General nature of miasm 53
General traits 174
Grief 173
Haemorrhoids 109
Hahnemann
    dynamic pathology of 14
    the father of modern bacteriology 20
Hahnemann's self contradiction 35
Hahnemannian
    conception & modern bacteriology 20
    dynamism 20
Hair 67, 148
Half-acute miasm 13
Half-spiritual miasm 13
Hay fever 79
Head
    shape of 68
    symptoms, comparison of 62-9
Head & scalp symptoms
    comparison of 62-9
Headache 62-4
Hearing 75
Heart 92-5, 151
Hereditary transmission 38
Hering's law of cure 17
Hunger 96-8, 174
Iatrogenic suppression 2
Infection
    ear 174
    miasmatic, & its criterias 9
    miasmatic, source of 9
    with chronic miasm 16
Infection & implementation 9
Inflammation, lung 174
Influenza
    clinical tips on 176
Initial cause 21
Intellect 49
Kentian conception 33
Kidneys 112
Latent psora 18
Law of cure, Hering's 17
Layers
    miasmatic, unfolding of 23
    of miasmatic states 21
    of predisposing weakness 22
    of predisposition 21
Leading
    anti-miasmatic medicines 251-2
    anti-psoric medicines 251
    anti-sycotic medicines 251
    anti-syphilitic medicines 251
    anti-tubercular medicines 252
    tri-miasmatic medicines 252
Life in general 174
Lips 84
Lung inflammation 174
Lymph-adenopathy 183
Malignancy 155
Manias 51
Manifestations
    AIDS, of 183-6
    cardiac 95
    general 52-3
    mental 58-9, 146-8
    psychic 55-8, 143-6
    rheumatic 181
Marsh miasm 13
Medicines
    anti-miasmatic 12
    leading anti-miasmatic 251-2
    leading anti-psoric 251
    leading anti-sycotic 251
    leading anti-syphilitic 251
    leading anti-tubercular 252
    leading tri-miasmatics 252
    miasmatic weightage of 243-50
Memory 46, 56, 145
Menses 175
Menstruation 120-1
Mental 173
    manifestations 58-9, 146-8
    symptoms, comparison of 41-51
Miasm
    accessory, of cowpox vaccine 13
    acute 13
    chronic 11, 16
    chronic, infection with 16
    classification of 13
    clinical & practical utility of 17
    consumptive 12
    drug 13
    expression of 14
    fixed 13
    general nature of 53, 141
    half-acute 13
    half-spiritual 13
    infection with chronic 16
    marsh 13
    philosophy of 6
    psoric 13, 20
    rationality of 14
    sycotic 13
    syphilitic 13
    theory, the scientific basis of 16
    transmission of 16
    tubercular 6
    why should we know? 4
Miasm & bacteria 31
Miasmatic
    ancestral tips 28, 173
    characteristics 30
    disease, three criterias of 16
    state 11
Miasmatic infection
    and its criterias 9
    source of 9
Miasmatic infection & dyscrasia, transmission of 9
Miasmatic interpretation of
    migraine 187
    the various symptomatic manifestations of AIDS 183-6
Miasmatic layers, unfolding of 23
Miasmatic prescribing
    interpretation in chronic prescribing 10
    implementation of miasms in prescribing 10
Miasmatic repertory
    abdominal symptoms 217-9
    cardiac symptoms 210-2
    ear symptoms 199-200
    extremity symptoms 236-9
    eye symptoms 197-8
    facial symptoms 205-6
    head symptoms 194-6
    mental symptoms 189-92
    modality symptoms 241-2
    mouth symptoms 203-4
    nail symptoms 235
    nose symptoms 201-2
    rectal symptoms 227-9
    respiratory symptoms 207-9
    sexual symptoms 220-3
    skin symptoms 240
    sleep symptoms 240
    stomach symptoms 213-6
    urinary symptoms 224-6
    vertigo symptoms 193
Miasmatic states
    layers of 21
    mixed 29
Miasmatic totality 3
Miasmatic treatment
    plan of 24
    Dr. Banerjea's approach to a plan of 24
Miasmatic weightage of medicines 243-50
Miasmatics of rheumatic
    manifestations 181
    modalities 181

Migraine 64-6
   clinical tips on 187
   miasmatic interpretation of 187
Mind
   avaricious sycotic 41-51
   destructive syphilitic 41-51
   dissatisfied tubercular 41-51
   inconsistent psoric 41-51
Misconception 32, 34, 38-9
Mixed miasmatic states 29
Modalities 156-7
   abdominal 104
   cardiac 94
   dermatological 124-5
   ear 74
   extremity 132-3
   eye 71-2
   headache 63
   migraine 65
   mind 51
   nasal 77
   rectal 106-7
   respiratory 87
   sexual 116
   skin 124-5
   sleep 137
   stomach 98
   urinary 111
   vertigo 60-1
Modality symptoms
   comparison of 138-9
Modern bacteriology 20
Modus operandi 15
Mouth 80-2
Nails 154
   symptoms, comparison of 129
Nasal symptoms
   comparison of 76-9
Natural characteristics
   clinical tips of 173-5
Nature
   comparison of 52-9
Nature of diseases 54, 142
Nose 149, 174
Nutrition & foods
   clinical tips on 188
One-sided disease 1-2, 5
Oral symptoms
   comparison of 80-2
Pace of action 54, 143
Paediatrics
   clinical tips on 176
Pains 155, 175
Parasites 128
Past 5
Pathology, dynamic 39
Perspiration 69
Philosophy
   & misconceptions 32
   of miasm 6
Physical suppression 2
Picture
   conjoint 1-2
   contaminated 1

Pimples
   clinical tips on 176
Plan of miasmatic treatment 24
Practical utility of miasmatic theory 17
Predilections 26
Predisposing weakness 22
Predisposition
   layers of 21
Prescribing
   classical miasmatic 3
Present 5
Primary psora 18, 26
Prophylactic aspect of homoeopathic medicine in cancer 180
Prostate 113
Pseudo-psora 6, 12, 28
   & tubercular miasms,
   differentiation of 6
Psora
   and its states 18
   common mother, the 34
   criteria of 7
   cure of 26
   extirpation of 25
   foundation of all sickness, the 34-5
   latent 18
   not a predisposition but a disease 25, 36
   origin of 32
   primary 18, 26
   qualifying condition of 18
   secondary 18
   sensitising miasm 52-9
   spiritual sickness, the 33
   tertiary 18
Psoric miasm 13, 25
Psychic manifestations 55-8, 143-6
Pulse 95, 151
Rationality of miasm 14
Recreational drugs 175
Rectal symptoms
   comparison of 105-9
Rectum 105-9
Remote cause 22-3
Repertory
   see Miasmatic repertory
Respiration 90
Respiratory symptoms
   comparison of 86-91
Responsive, reactive miasm 52-9
Restlessness 47-8
Rheumatism
   clinical tips on 181
Running 173
Scalp 68
   symptoms, comparison of 62-9
Scarcity of symptoms 1-2
Secondary psora 18
Secretions 174
Senile dementia 177
Sensitising miasm 52-9
Septum 78

Sexual 175
   desire 119
   symptoms comparison of 114-21
Skin 122-8, 153, 175
   appearance of 125-6
   colour of 127
Sleep 175
   character of 136
   symptoms, comparison of 136-7
Smell 78
Social interaction 46
Source of miasmatic infection 9
Spiritual sickness 33
States
   mixed miasmatic 29
Stomach
   symptoms, comparison of 96-101
Stool 107-9, 152
Strep throat 174
Suppression
   emotional 2
   iatrogenic 2
   physical 2
   removal of 23
Susceptibility
   the precondition 37
Sweat 128
Syco-psora 12
Sycosis
   criteria of 7
   miasm of incoordination 52-9
Sycotic miasm 13
Symptoms
   explosion of 22-3
   scarcity of 1-2
   totality of 3
Synopsis
   comparison of characteristics 140-57
Syphilis
   criteria of 8
   degenerating miasm 52-9
Syphilitic miasm 13
Taste 80-1
Teeth 81-2, 174
Temperament 49-50
Terminal dementia 177
Terminologies 11
Tertiary psora 18
Thoughts & flow of words 42-3
Tongue 81
Totality
   miasmatic 3
   of symptoms 3
Transmission
   hereditary 38
   of miasm 16
   of miasmatic infection & dyscrasia 9
Tri-miasmatic medicines
   leading 252
Tubercular
   miasm, criteria of 8

    & pseudo-psora miasms,
      differentiation of 6
    responsive, reactive miasm 52-9

Urinary symptoms
    comparison of 110-3

Urine 113

Vaccinosis
    miasmatic dyscrasia of sycosis 9

Vertigo 148
    symptoms, comparison of 60-1

Vital energy field (VEF) 15

Vital force (VF) 15
    deranged (DVF) 15

Voice 88

Waiting room, in the 173

Warts 175

Weightage of medicines, miasmatic 243-50

Work 55, 144

Worms 109